T0259493

Update on Osteoarthritis

Editor

DAVID J. HUNTER

RHEUMATIC DISEASE CLINICS OF NORTH AMERICA

www.rheumatic.theclinics.com

Consulting Editor
MICHAEL H. WEISMAN

February 2013 • Volume 39 • Number 1

ELSEVIER

1600 John F. Kennedy Boulevard • Suite 1800 • Philadelphia, Pennsylvania, 19103-2899
http://www.theclinics.com

RHEUMATIC DISEASE CLINICS OF NORTH AMERICA Volume 39, Number 1
February 2013 ISSN 0889-857X, ISBN 13: 978-1-4557-7328-2

Editor: Pamela Hetherington

Rheumatic Disease Clinics of North America (ISSN 0889-857X) is published quarterly by Elsevier Inc., 360 Park Avenue South, New York, NY 10010-1710. Months of issue are February, May, August, and November. Business and editorial offices: 1600 John F. Kennedy Boulevard, Suite 1800, Philadelphia, PA 19103-2899. Periodicals postage paid at New York, NY and additional mailing offices. Subscription prices are USD 317.00 per year for US individuals, USD 555.00 per year for US institutions, USD 156.00 per year for US students and residents, USD 374.00 per year for Canadian individuals, USD 684.00 per year for Canadian institutions, USD 444.00 per year for international individuals, USD 684.00 per year for international institutions, and USD 218.00 per year for Canadian and foreign students/residents. To receive student/resident rate, orders must be accompanied by name of affiliated institution, date of term, and the *signature* of program/residency coordinator on institution letterhead. Orders will be billed at individual rate until proof of status received. Foreign air speed delivery is included in all *Clinics* subscription prices. All prices are subject to change without notice. **POSTMASTER:** Send address changes to *Rheumatic Disease Clinics of North America,* Elsevier Health Sciences Division, Subscription Customer Service, 3251 Riverport Lane, Maryland Heights, MO 63043. **Customer Service: 1-800-654-2452 (US and Canada). From outside of the US and Canada: 314-447-8871. Fax: 314-447-8029. For print support, e-mail: JournalsCustomerService-usa@elsevier.com. For online support, e-mail: JournalsOnline Support-usa@elsevier.com.**

Reprints. For copies of 100 or more of articles in this publication, please contact the Commercial Reprints Department, Elsevier Inc., 360 Park Avenue South, New York, New York, 10010-1710; Tel.: (+1) 212-633-3813, Fax: (+1) 212-462-1935, and E-mail: reprints@elsevier.com.

Rheumatic Disease Clinics of North America is covered in *MEDLINE/PubMed (Index Medicus), Current Contents/Clinical Medicine, Science Citation Index, ISI/BIOMED,* and *EMBASE/Excerpta Medica.*

Printed and bound by CPI Group (UK) Ltd, Croydon, CR0 4YY

Transferred to digital print 2012

Contributors

CONSULTING EDITOR

MICHAEL H. WEISMAN, MD
Director, Division of Rheumatology; Professor of Medicine, Cedars-Sinai Medical Center, Los Angeles, California

EDITOR

DAVID J. HUNTER, MBBS, MSc, PhD, FRACP
Department of Rheumatology, Royal North Shore Hospital, St Leonards, New South Wales; Professor of Medicine, Northern Clinical School, University of Sydney, Sydney, New South Wales, Australia

AUTHORS

A. ABHISHEK, MD, MRCP
Academic Rheumatology, University of Nottingham, Nottingham, United Kingdom

ILANA N. ACKERMAN, BPhysio(Hons), PhD
Research Fellow, Department of Medicine, Melbourne EpiCentre, Royal Melbourne Hospital, The University of Melbourne, Parkville, Victoria, Australia

KIM L. BENNELL, BAppSci(physio), PhD
Professor, Department of Physiotherapy, Centre for Health, Exercise and Sports Medicine, School of Health Sciences; Faculty of Medicine, Dentistry and Health Sciences, The University of Melbourne, Parkville, Victoria, Australia

MEGAN A. BOHENSKY, BA, MPH, PhD
Department of Medicine, Melbourne EpiCentre, Royal Melbourne Hospital, The University of Melbourne, Parkville, Victoria, Australia

CAROLINE A. BRAND, MBBS, BA, MPH, FRACP
Senior Medical Staff Clinical Epidemiologist, Melbourne EpiCentre, Royal Melbourne Hospital, Melbourne Health, University of Melbourne, Parkville, Victoria, Australia; Adjunct Associate Professor, Centre for Research Excellence in Patient Safety, Monash University, Australia

MICHAEL DOHERTY, MD, FRCP
Academic Rheumatology, University of Nottingham, Nottingham, United Kingdom

JEFF DURYEA, PhD
Associate Professor of Radiology, Harvard Medical School; Department of Radiology, Brigham and Women's Hospital, Boston, Massachusetts

FELIX ECKSTEIN, MD
Director, Institute of Anatomy and Musculoskeletal Research, Paracelsus Medical University, Salzburg, Austria

JILLIAN EYLES, BAppSc(Physiotherapy)
Department of Physiotherapy, Royal North Shore Hospital, St Leonards, New South Wales, Australia

RICHARD B. FROBELL, PhD
Assistant Professor, Department of Orthopedics, Clinical Sciences Lund, Lund University, Lund, Sweden

ALI GUERMAZI, MD, PhD
Professor, Department of Radiology, Boston University School of Medicine, Boston, Massachusetts

DAICHI HAYASHI, MD, PhD
Research Assistant Professor, Department of Radiology, Boston University School of Medicine, Boston, Massachusetts

RANA S. HINMAN, BPhysio, PhD
Department of Physiotherapy, Centre for Health, Exercise and Sports Medicine; Faculty of Medicine, Dentistry and Health Sciences, The University of Melbourne, Victoria, Australia

MICHAEL A. HUNT, PT, PhD
Department of Physical Therapy, University of British Columbia, Vancouver, Canada

DAVID J. HUNTER, MBBS, MSc, PhD, FRACP
Department of Rheumatology, Royal North Shore Hospital, St Leonards, New South Wales; Professor of Medicine, Northern Clinical School, University of Sydney, Sydney, New South Wales, Australia

JAMES D. JOHNSTON, PhD
Assistant Professor, Department of Mechanical Engineering, University of Saskatchewan, Saskatoon, Saskatchewan, Canada

YOUNG-JO KIM, MD, PhD
Associate Professor, Department of Orthopedic Surgery, Harvard Medical School, Children's Hospital Boston, Boston, Massachusetts

BOON-WHATT LIM, MSc, PhD
School of Sports, Health and Leisure, Republic Polytechnic, Singapore

BARBARA R. LUCAS, BAppSc(Physiotherapy), MEd, MPH, FACP
Department of Physiotherapy, Royal North Shore Hospital, St Leonards, New South Wales, Australia

GLORIA L. MATTHEWS, DVM, PhD, DACVS
Senior Director, Orthopaedic and Regenerative Medicine Research, Genzyme, A Sanofi Company, Framingham, Massachusetts

EMILY J. McWALTER, PhD
Postdoctoral Fellow, Department of Radiology, Stanford University, The Lucas Center for MR Spectroscopy and Imaging, Stanford, California

TUHINA NEOGI, MD, PhD, FRCPC
Associate Professor of Medicine and Epidemiology, Boston University Schools of Medicine and Public Health, Boston, Massachusetts

JOHN M. O'DONNELL, MBBS, FRACS
Associate Professor, University of Melbourne, Richmond, Melbourne, Victoria, Australia

STEPHANIE Y. PUN, MD
Fellow in Orthopaedic Surgery, Young Adult and Adolescent Hip Unit, Harvard Medical School, Children's Hospital Boston, Boston, Massachusetts

JOHN C. RICHMOND, MD
Department of Orthopedic Surgery, New England Baptist Hospital, Boston, Massachusetts

EDWARD A. RIORDAN, BSc
School of Medicine, University of Sydney, Sydney, New South Wales, Australia

FRANK W. ROEMER, MD
Assistant Professor, Department of Radiology, Klinikum Augsburg, Augsburg, Germany; Associate Professor, Department of Radiology, Boston University School of Medicine, Boston, Massachusetts

DAVID R. WILSON, DPhil
Associate Professor, Department of Orthopaedics, Centre for Hip Health and Mobility, Vancouver Coastal Health Research Institute, University of British Columbia, Vancouver, British Columbia, Canada

TIM V. WRIGLEY, BSc, MSc
Department of Physiotherapy, Centre for Health, Exercise and Sports Medicine; Faculty of Medicine, Dentistry and Health Sciences, The University of Melbourne, Victoria, Australia

YUQING ZHANG, DSc
Professor of Medicine and Epidemiology, Boston University Schools of Medicine and Public Health, Boston, Massachusetts

Contents

Osteoarthritis (OA) is the most common form of arthritis in the United States and is a leading cause of disability. It is typically defined in epidemiologic studies by radiographic findings and consideration of symptoms. Its incidence and prevalence are rising, likely related to the aging of the population and increasing obesity. Risk factors for OA include numerous person-level factors, such as age, sex, obesity, and genetics, as well as joint-specific factors that are likely reflective of abnormal loading of the joints. In studying OA, several methodologic challenges exist that can hamper our ability to identify pertinent relationships.

Mechanics play a role in the initiation and progression of osteoarthritis. However, our understanding of which mechanical parameters are most important, and what their impact is on the disease, is limited by the challenge of measuring the most important mechanical quantities in living subjects. Consequently, comprehensive statements cannot be made about how mechanics should be modified to prevent, slow or arrest osteoarthritis. Our current understanding is based largely on studies of deviations from normal mechanics caused by malalignment, injury, and deformity. Some treatments for osteoarthritis focus on correcting mechanics, but there appears to be scope for more mechanically based interventions.

Osteoarthritis (OA), the commonest arthropathy, targets the knees, hips, finger interphalangeal joints, thumb bases, first metatarsophalangeal joints, and spinal facet joints, and displays marked heterogeneity of clinical presentation. Signs of OA include coarse crepitus, bony enlargement, reduced range of movement, and joint-line tenderness. Muscle wasting and joint deformity occur with severe OA. Painful periarticular disorders often coexist with OA. Inflammation is absent or only modest, although mild-moderate effusions are common at the knee. The diagnosis of OA may be made without recourse to radiographic or laboratory investigations in the at-risk age group with typical symptoms and signs.

role of muscle in the development and progression of knee osteoarthritis. The review also focuses on whether muscle deficits can be modified in knee osteoarthritis and whether improvements in muscle function lead to improved symptoms and joint structure. The review concludes with a discussion of exercise prescription for muscle rehabilitation in knee osteoarthritis.

article summarizes the evidence available for patient characteristics that have been analyzed as potential predictors of response to nonsurgical interventions for patients with hip and knee osteoarthritis. The specific variables targeted for this review include body mass index, psychological factors, muscle strength, tibiofemoral alignment, radiographic changes, and signs of inflammation. Several studies provide moderate to good evidence of potential predictors of response to nonsurgical treatments, and areas for future research are illuminated.

RHEUMATIC DISEASE CLINICS OF NORTH AMERICA

RELATED INTEREST

Orthopedic Clinics, November 2012
http://www.orthopedic.theclinics.com/current
Arthroplasty in the Lower Extremity – An online-only bonus issue
Giles R. Scuderi, MD, *Editor*

NOW AVAILABLE FOR YOUR iPhone and iPad

Foreword

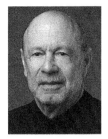

Michael H. Weisman, MD
Consulting Editor

David Hunter has provided us with an excellent example of a targeted approach to osteoarthritis with a focus on the knee and hip. He emphasizes the knee, for example, as a unit where contributions to the observed phenotype can come from a variety of sources, including cartilage, bone, periarticular soft tissues, as well as intra-articular soft tissues. The age-old question remains—is osteoarthritis a condition that begins in the cartilage or in the bone? That question is probably a bit outdated because many things can contribute the initiation and perpetuation of the process, including genes, weight, injury, crystal-induced, anatomic (congenital) abnormalities, and likely many others. The dimension of time is often neglected as the discussion on this volume focuses on the role of muscle activity and function and whether the process can be modified or even slowed down by muscle strengthening and conditioning. The volume herein addresses the patient with osteoarthritis and not just the disease itself—what are the goals of patient management and how much do they cost the patient, the family, and society? Finally, the discussion of management is not complete with addressing prevention—our ever-increasing problem of obesity, the metabolic syndrome, and repetitive sports injuries accompanying the fitness agenda should be a wakeup call to those policymakers who prioritize the health care dollar for us. This volume causes us to think broadly about osteoarthritis as a societal conundrum, and it is welcomed in 2013.

Michael H. Weisman, MD
Division of Rheumatology
Cedars-Sinai Medical Center
8700 Beverly Boulevard
Los Angeles, CA 90024, USA

E-mail address:
michael.weisman@cshs.org

Rheum Dis Clin N Am 39 (2013) xiii
http://dx.doi.org/10.1016/j.rdc.2012.12.001
0889-857X/13/$ – see front matter © 2013 Published by Elsevier Inc.
rheumatic.theclinics.com

Preface

Osteoarthritis

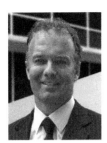

David J. Hunter, MBBS, MSc, PhD, FRACP
Editor

Osteoarthritis (OA) is the leading cause of disability among older adults. It is an incredibly prevalent condition affecting upward of 1 in 8 adults. Societal trends in aging, obesity, and increasing joint injury will lead to a doubling of the number of persons with OA in the next decade. In this context, this issue of *Rheumatic Disease Clinics of North America* is timely, as we envision this increasingly prevalent disabling condition in an era where health care expenditure is increasingly scrutinized.

Consideration of the impact of this condition in our society requires an understanding of the incidence and prevalence of this disease. Drs Neogi and Zhang provide a thoughtful appraisal of the epidemiology of OA illuminating us on how we define OA (both radiographic and symptomatic), the prevalence and incidence of OA, and risk factors for OA. As international leaders in these methods, they also highlight a number of methodologic challenges that exist in studying OA that can hamper our ability to identify pertinent relationships.

We now conceptualize OA as a disease of the whole joint organ. Critically the disease is no longer viewed as a passive, degenerative disorder but rather an active disease process with an imbalance between the repair and destruction of joint tissues driven primarily by mechanical factors. Mechanics plays a critical role in the initiation, progression, and successful treatment of OA. Dr Wilson, a true pioneer in this field, summarizes the methods for assessing joint mechanics, describes the current evidence for the role of mechanics in OA initiation and progression, and further describes some current treatment approaches that focus on modifying joint mechanics.

Drs Abhishek and Doherty provide a sagely review of the diagnosis and clinical presentation of OA with an emphasis on symptoms and signs at the key target sites. In patients with typical presentation at the target sites, clinical assessment alone is sufficient to allow a diagnosis of OA. Patients with OA should be assessed in a holistic manner, which should include a targeted examination for the associated comorbidities.

Dr Hunter is funded by an Australian Research Council Future Fellowship.

Rheum Dis Clin N Am 39 (2013) xv–xviii
http://dx.doi.org/10.1016/j.rdc.2012.11.005
0889-857X/13/$ – see front matter © 2013 Published by Elsevier Inc.

rheumatic.theclinics.com

Many define OA as a condition that primarily affects hyaline articular cartilage, including William Hunter, who in 1743 stated soberly, "From Hippocrates to the present age it is universally allowed that ulcerated cartilage is a troublesome thing and that once destroyed, is not repaired."[1] We now conceptualize OA as a disease of the whole joint organ. Conventional radiography has played an important role in confirming the diagnosis of OA, demonstrating late bony changes and joint space narrowing, and has been applied as an endpoint for disease progression in clinical trials. However, OA is a disease of the whole joint, including cartilage, bone, and intra-articular and periarticular soft tissues. Thus, the importance to image and assess all joint structures has been recognized in recent years largely using magnetic resonance imaging. Led by leaders in this field, Drs Guermazi, Hayshi, Eckstein, Hunter, Duryea, and Roemer review radiography and magnetic resonance imaging in OA but also give insight into other modalities such as ultrasound, scintigraphy, computed tomography, and computed tomographic arthrography and discuss their role in the diagnosis, follow-up, and research in OA.

There are a multitude of reasons a person can develop OA; hence, we term this multifactorial. This said, in today's society the 2 big risk factors for knee OA are obesity and joint injury. The risk for knee OA in our society attributed to these 2 risk factors accounts for approximately 80% of the reason for OA development. Both are eminently preventable; yet little is being done to reduce these risk factors.[2] Similarly, joint injuries, such as a tear of the cruciate ligament (ACL) or meniscus, increase the risk of knee OA by altering the contact mechanics of the joint environment (ie, the way weight-bearing load is distributed in the joint). ACL ruptures have been found to be linked to OA changes in 50% to 70% of the patients, 10 to 15 years following the injury.[3] Drs Riordan, Frobell, Roemer, and Hunter review the pattern of joint damage that accompanies an ACL rupture and the long-term structural changes that predispose the injured knee to the development of OA. The current evidence for the efficacy and cost-effectiveness of surgical and nonsurgical treatment strategies is also reviewed.

Sir William Osler, considered to be the Father of Modern Medicine, once said, "When an arthritis patient walks in the front door, I feel like leaving by the back door." For many clinicians this attitude still holds true; however, there is much the interested clinician can do rather than nihilistic waiting. In fact, there are a multitude of effective treatment options outlined in the many guidelines for management of OA and at times what is best for the individual patient can be unclear. In the face of so many choices, it would be helpful for clinicians to be able to base treatment decisions on the identification of specific clinical presentations that foretell a greater likelihood of success following a given treatment. Ms Eyles, Ms Lucas, and Dr Hunter review the evidence available for patient characteristics that have been analyzed as potential predictors of response to nonsurgical interventions for patients with hip and knee OA.

The challenge facing clinicians is dwarfed by the experience that persons with OA have to face. Any person with a chronic illness faces a personal daily battle with the condition itself; in the case of OA, the daily battle is further compounded by a nihilistic "broken" health care system. Drs Brand, Ackerman, Bohensky, and Bennell provide an insightful overview of the many issues currently facing patients, health care providers, funding providers, and policymakers, who are working to improve OA health outcomes. They suggest that a broad approach that considers individual and system quality-of-care outcomes is a useful way to identify future research and improvement opportunities.

No one denies that the management of OA is a challenge; however, modern clinicians are armed with a plethora of effective treatment options. Like other chronic diseases, there is no sole treatment or cure; instead, there are several strategies to use that can help manage the condition. Clinicians who manage patients with OA recognize that to maximize treatments it is best to use them as part of a package and incorporate many of the strategies together (eg, not just prescribing analgesics to manage symptoms, but also considering weight, fitness levels, and muscle strength, and evaluating daily patterns of activity). For the practicing clinician, arming themselves with knowledge of mechanisms and evidence for disease management is critical. It is important that symptomatic improvement serves the purpose of increasing tolerance for functional activity. Ultimately, an efficacious treatment for any progressive disorder should also control the factors and forces that drive disease progression.

Drs Bennell, Hunt, Wrigley, Lim, and Hinman provide a thorough review of the influence of muscle activity on knee joint loading, describe the deficits in muscle function observed in people with knee OA, and summarize available evidence pertaining to the role of muscle in the development and progression of knee OA. They focus on whether muscle deficits can be modified in knee OA and whether improvements in muscle function lead to improved symptoms and joint structure and conclude with a discussion of exercise prescription for muscle rehabilitation in knee OA.

The Holy Grail for many in this field is to the modification of the underlying structural changes to facilitate repair or reduce risk of further destruction. Dr Matthews reviews the evidence to suggest we can modify disease. This article also considers the methodologic approaches and other obstacles demonstrating efficacy of these agents in clinical trials. Unfortunately, many of the trials of disease-modifying agents to date have been in joints that have little if any tissue to preserve as the joint destruction of these trial participants has been quite severe. If we are to develop interventions for OA that target the joint before it is irreversibly damaged, we need to identify disease earlier and target the tissue that leads to the cascade of events we describe as joint failure.

Failing prior interventions, OA surgery may become necessary. Although the indications for arthroscopy have narrowed, joint replacement continues to play a pivotal role in disease management. Dr Richmond reviews the plethora of surgical options and the evidence to support their efficacy. Orthopedic surgeons continue to explore options less invasive than total knee replacement for isolated unicompartmental arthritis of the knee joint.

The prevalence of hip OA is about 9% in those aged over 65[4] and is also expected to increase as the population ages and the prevalence of obesity rises. Like the knee, recent evidence highlights the importance of local mechanical factors in leading to hip OA and 90% or more of hip OA cases can be attributed to anatomical abnormalities.[5] These anatomic/shape abnormalities are termed femoroacetabular impingement and this insight into the cause of hip OA is one of the most important and provocative new tenets in OA.[6] Drs Pun, O'Donnell, and Kim review this complex area and the nonarthoplasty surgical approaches to its management.

Looking forward, we are reminded by the late Sir Henry Tizard that "the secret of science is to ask the right question, and it is the choice of problem more than anything else that marks the man of genius in the scientific world." We have been afforded an opportunity to study a much maligned disease that is rapidly evolving. Let's learn from the insights our research is providing to focus even more on important modifiable risk factors, such as mechanics, injury, and obesity, as we develop the therapeutic armamentarium of the 21st century. Assuming we maintain a meaningful motivation with the patient at the forefront of our mind, we have an opportunity to make a difference in millions of peoples' lives. I look forward to the evolution ahead.

I would sincerely like to thank my friends and colleagues for their valuable contributions to this issue. They were a pleasure to work with and I am sure you will see from the contents that it reflects wonderful insight and appraisal of a complex and developing field.

David J. Hunter, MBBS, MSc, PhD, FRACP
Department of Rheumatology
Royal North Shore Hospital
Pacific Highway, St Leonards
NSW 2065 Australia

Department of Medicine
Northern Clinical School
University of Sydney, Sydney
NSW, Australia

E-mail address:
David.Hunter@sydney.edu.au

REFERENCES

1. Buchanan WW. William Hunter (1718-1783). Rheumatology 2003;42(10):1260–1.
2. Hunter DJ. Lower extremity osteoarthritis management needs a paradigm shift. Br J Sports Med 2011;45(4):283–8.
3. Lohmander LS, Ostenberg A, Englund M, et al. High prevalence of knee osteoarthritis, pain, and functional limitations in female soccer players twelve years after anterior cruciate ligament injury. Arthritis Rheum 2004;50(10):3145–52.
4. Lawrence RC, Helmick CG, Arnett FC, et al. Estimates of the prevalence of arthritis and selected musculoskeletal disorders in the United States [see comments]. Arthritis Rheum 1998;41(5):778–99.
5. Tanzer M, Noiseux N. Osseous abnormalities and early osteoarthritis: the role of hip impingement. Clin Orthopaed Relat Res 2004;429:170–7.
6. Ganz R, Parvizi J, Beck M, et al. Femoroacetabular impingement: a cause for osteoarthritis of the hip. Clin Orthopaed Relat Res 2003;417:112–20.

Epidemiology of Osteoarthritis

Tuhina Neogi, MD, PhD, FRCPC[a],*, Yuqing Zhang, DSc[b]

KEYWORDS

- Osteoarthritis • Epidemiology • Risk factors • Pain

KEY POINTS

- Osteoarthritis (OA) is the most common form of arthritis, with OA of the knee, hand, or hip having a similar prevalence of approximately 20% to 30% of adults in various populations.
- Person-level factors associated with OA include increasing age, female sex, overweight/obesity, and race/ethnicity, which may represent genetic or sociocultural influences.
- Joint-level factors associated with OA are reflective of mechanisms related to abnormal loading of the joints.
- Several methodologic challenges to the study of OA exist, which have affected our ability to identify important relationships.
- There is a need for ongoing epidemiologic and intervention studies regarding the prevention of incident and progressive OA and related pain.

INTRODUCTION

Osteoarthritis (OA) is the most common form of arthritis,[1] and one of the most common diagnoses in general practice.[2] Given its predilection for lower extremity joints such as the knee and hip, OA is the leading cause of lower extremity disability among older adults.[3]

DEFINING OSTEOARTHRITIS

OA is frequently defined by radiography, with the most commonly used radiographic grading system being the Kellgren and Lawrence (KL) grade, which scores OA severity on a scale of 0 to 4; definite radiographic OA is KL grade 2 or greater.[4] The KL grading system has been used for the hand, hip, and knee; however, at the knee it is only used to define tibiofemoral OA. Patellofemoral radiographic OA can also be assessed if appropriate radiographic views are obtained. The Osteoarthritis Research Society International Atlas provides a means to score individual radiographic features, such as osteophytes and joint-space narrowing, in a semi-quantitative manner,[5] and other

[a] Sections of Clinical Epidemiology Research, Training Unit and Rheumatology, 650 Albany Street, Suite X200, Boston University School of Medicine, Boston, MA, 02118, USA; [b] Sections of Clinical Epidemiology Research, Training Unit, 650 Albany Street, Suite X200, Boston University School of Medicine, Boston, MA, 02118, USA
* Corresponding author.
E-mail address: tneogi@bu.edu

Rheum Dis Clin N Am 39 (2013) 1–19
http://dx.doi.org/10.1016/j.rdc.2012.10.004
0889-857X/13/$ – see front matter © 2013 Elsevier Inc. All rights reserved.

methods are available to quantify joint-space width on radiographs.[6] Numerous joint structures that are not otherwise visualized on radiographs can be examined by magnetic resonance imaging (MRI). An MRI definition of OA has been proposed, but requires validation.[7] However, individual structural lesions on MRI are well described, including cartilage lesions, osteophytes, bone marrow lesions, synovitis, effusion, and subchondral bone attrition.[8,9] Of knees without radiographic evidence of tibiofemoral OA (KL 0) in adults 50 years or older, the enhanced sensitivity of MRI revealed that 89% had at least 1 such abnormality in the tibiofemoral joint, with similar prevalences in painful and painless knees.[10]

Symptomatic OA indicates the presence of radiographic OA in combination with knee symptoms attributable to OA. Not all individuals with radiographic OA have concomitant symptoms. OA may be described in a joint-specific manner (eg, knee OA, hip OA), or, when several joint areas are involved, it may be considered as being generalized (eg, involvement with OA of at least 1 of each joint area: knee, hip, and hand), although a standard definition for generalized OA does not yet exist.

INCIDENCE AND PREVALENCE OF OA

One estimate of the lifetime risk of developing symptomatic knee OA was approximately 40% in men and 47% in women, with higher risks among those who are obese.[11] Age- and sex-standardized incident rates for symptomatic hand, hip, and knee OA have been estimated to be 100, 88, and 240 cases per 100,000 person-years, respectively, with incidence rates rising sharply after age 50 and leveling off after age 70 years (**Fig. 1**).[12] However, the interpretation of the leveling off or decline in OA incidence at older ages should be made with caution, given the potential biases related to competing risks and depletion of susceptibles (see later discussion on methodologic

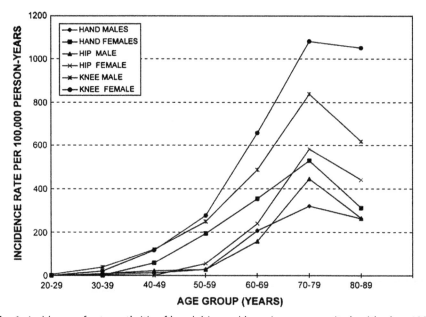

Fig. 1. Incidence of osteoarthritis of hand, hip, and knee in a community health plan, 1991 to 1992, by age and sex. (*Data from* Oliveria SA, Felson DT, Reed JI, et al. Incidence of symptomatic hand, hip, and knee osteoarthritis among patients in a health maintenance organization. Arthritis Rheum 1995;38:1134–41.)

challenges).[13] Recent estimates of incidence of hand OA derived from the Framingham Osteoarthritis Study were approximately 34% to 35% for OA incidence in any hand joint for both sexes, with incidence of symptomatic hand OA being 4% for men and 9.7% for women over a 9-year period.[14]

There has been an increase in OA prevalence, with an estimated 27 million United States adults in 2005 having clinical OA of their hand, knee, or hip joint, an increase from 21 million in 1995.[1] Such increases are likely due to aging of the population and the rising prevalence of obesity. In Framingham, the age-standardized prevalence of radiographic hand OA was 44.2% in women and 37.7% in men,[14] and 19% had knee OA among adults aged 45 years and older.[15] From the Johnston County Osteoarthritis Project, approximately 28% of African Americans and Caucasians aged 45 or older had knee OA and 28% had hip OA.[16,17] This latter estimate is higher than the 7% prevalence noted in the Study of Osteoporotic Fractures among Caucasian women older than 65 years.[18]

Symptomatic prevalence estimates for OA are lower because it requires the presence of radiographic OA with pain, aching, or stiffness in the joint. The age-standardized prevalence of symptomatic hand OA was 14.4% and 6.9% in women and men, respectively, in younger Framingham cohorts,[14] which increased to 26.2% and 13.4%, respectively, among those aged 71 and older in an older Framingham cohort.[19] The prevalence of symptomatic knee OA among adults 45 years and older was approximately 7% in Framingham,[15] whereas in the Johnston County OA Project it was approximately 17%.[16] Symptomatic hip OA was present in approximately 10% of the Johnston County cohort.[17] There has also been an increase in prevalence of symptomatic knee OA over the past 20 years by 4.1% and 6% among women and men, respectively, in the Framingham cohort.[20]

Racial/ethnic differences in the prevalence of OA and specific patterns of joint involvement have been noted. In the Johnston County OA Project, African American men had a higher prevalence of radiographic hip OA than Caucasian men (32.2% vs 23.8%), whereas there was no difference between African American and Caucasian women (40.3% vs 39.4%).[17] Individual radiographic features at the hip and knee were also noted to differ between the two groups.[21,22] In the Beijing Osteoarthritis Study, hand and hip OA were less prevalent among Chinese than Caucasians (age-standardized prevalences 44.5%–47% vs 75.2%–85% and 0.8% vs 3.8–4.5%, respectively), but knee OA was more prevalent among Chinese women than among Caucasian women (46.6% vs 34.8%).[23–25] A higher prevalence of lateral tibiofemoral knee OA was also noted in Beijing Chinese in comparison with Framingham Caucasian subjects.[26]

RISK FACTORS FOR RADIOGRAPHIC OA

OA can be thought of as the phenotypic manifestation of a series of different pathways leading to a common end-stage pathology (**Fig. 2**). As such, the disease has a multifactorial etiology, with different sets of risk factors (at a person and/or joint level) acting together to cause onset of OA in any given individual. Person-level factors are generally those that are thought to act at a systemic level on all relevant joints or are a characteristic of the individual, whereas joint-level factors generally refer to those that are joint specific and may be unique to a particular joint.

Person-Level Risk Factors

Age and sex

Age is one of the strongest risk factors for OA.[1] The exact mechanism is not known, but is likely related to a combination of changes in the capacity for joint tissues to

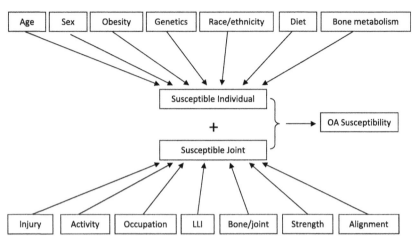

Fig. 2. Potential risk factors for susceptibility to incidence and progression of osteoarthritis (OA), each with varying degrees of evidence to support their association (see text for details). LLI, leg-length inequality.

adapt to biomechanical insults, and age being a proxy for the accumulation of a sufficient set of risk factors over the years.

Female sex is associated with higher prevalence and greater severity of OA.[27] The increase in prevalence and incidence of OA at the time of the menopause has led to hypotheses regarding the role of estrogen in OA, such as the loss of estrogen potentially unmasking the symptoms of OA by enhancing pain sensitivity. However, results from observational studies and clinical trials have been conflicting regarding estrogen effects on OA.[28–30] In the Heart and Estrogen/Progestin Replacement Study, there was no difference in knee pain in those randomized to receive estrogen replacement therapy compared with those receiving placebo.[29] On the other hand, in the Women's Health Initiative, unopposed estrogen therapy was associated with a borderline significant lower rate of joint arthroplasty, but no such association was noted for estrogen plus progestin in comparison with placebo.[30] A review of sex differences in MRI features of OA and biomarkers of joint metabolism noted variable findings.[31] Women may have thinner and more reduced volume of knee cartilage than men (even after taking into account differences in height, weight, and bone size); whether women have a more accelerated rate of loss of cartilage volume than men is not clear.

Obesity
Obesity has long been identified as a risk factor for knee OA.[32] In a meta-analysis, those who were obese or overweight had 2.96-times higher risk of incident knee OA compared with those of normal weight (95% confidence interval [CI] 2.56–3.43).[33] Assuming the prevalence of obesity in a hypothetical population to be 25%, the population-attributable risk percentage due to obesity would therefore be 29% (95% CI 24%–34%); this would be higher where obesity prevalence is higher.[34] Furthermore, those who were only overweight (not obese) had more than twice the chance of developing knee OA compared with their normal-weight counterparts.[33] Risk of incident knee OA increases with increasing body mass index (BMI; weight in kilograms divided by height in meters squared, ie, kg/m^2), regardless of knee alignment.[35] Decreasing BMI by 2 units or more over 10 years (~5 kg) was associated

with a 50% lower risk of developing symptomatic knee OA among women,[36] findings supported by a recent meta-analysis.[37] Duration of exposure to high BMI during adulthood confers risk of incident knee OA, suggesting the importance of weight control throughout life as a means of primary prevention of knee OA.[38] Obesity also contributes to symptoms in knee OA, with the Arthritis, Diet, and Activity Promotion Trial (ADAPT) and Intensive Diet and Exercise for Arthritis (IDEA) trial both demonstrating improvements in pain accompanying weight loss related to dietary and exercise interventions.[39,40]

In contrast to data supporting the role of obesity in the development of knee OA, high BMI was not associated with progressive radiographic knee OA in one study.[35] However, using the same data, Zhang and colleagues[41] demonstrated that high BMI increased the risk of both mild radiographic OA (KL = 2) and moderate to severe radiographic OA (KL = 3 or 4) among knees that were KL = 0 at baseline, respectively. Because knees that develop KL = 3 or 4 over time must have gone through the KL = 2 stage, this provides indirect evidence that obesity increases the risk of incident knee OA and also accelerates the progression of knee OA.

The effects of obesity on OA may be through both mechanical and systemic effects (eg, metabolic or inflammatory). There is no doubt about an effect of increased load related to overall body weight, but there may be differential systemic effects that depend on the degree of fat versus lean mass; unfortunately, BMI does not differentiate between the two. Recently, total body fat measured by dual-energy x-ray absorptiometry was associated with decreased cartilage thickness while lean mass was associated with increased cartilage thickness.[42] Adipose tissue is known to be metabolically active, secreting adipokines such as adiponectin, leptin, and resistin, but the role of these adipokines in OA is not yet clear.[43,44]

Obesity is also associated with both incident radiographic and symptomatic hand OA,[45,46] further supporting potential metabolic or inflammatory effects of obesity. By contrast, the association between obesity and hip OA has been variable and, where noted, less strong than for the knee or hand.[47-51]

Genetics

The heritable component of OA has been estimated to be 40% to 65%, and stronger for hand and hip OA than for knee OA.[52-54] To date 3 loci, *GDF5*, which encodes the growth differentiation factor 5 (a bone morphogenetic protein expressed in skeletal and articular structures), chromosome 7q22, and *MCF2L* have been associated with OA at genome-wide significance levels.[55-57] A recent large, well-powered study from the arcOGEN Consortium identified 5 new susceptibility loci for OA with genome-wide significance.[58] Two single-nucleotide polymorphisms (SNPs) were on chromosome 3, in linkage disequilibrium with each other within an exon of nucleostemin-encoding *GNL3*; one on chromosome 9 close to *ASTN2*; one on chromosome 6 between *FILIP1* and *SENP6*; one on chromosome 12 close to *KLHDC5* and *PTHLH*; and another on chromosome 12 close to *CHST11*.[58] Of note, the previously identified loci did not achieve genome-wide significance in this arcOGEN sample.

Pain severity related to OA may also have genetic contributions. A functional polymorphism (Val158Met) in the *COMT* gene, which has been associated with pain sensitivity in other clinical conditions, was associated with hip OA–related pain in one cohort study, but has not yet been replicated in other cohorts.[59] Other genes associated with pain sensitivity have also been studied in relation to OA pain. *TRPV1* and the PACE4 gene *Pcsk6* were associated with pain in knee OA in two separate meta-analyses,[60,61] while an association with a *SCN9* SNP could not be replicated.[62]

Bone mineral density

The material properties of bone may influence susceptibility to OA. Nevitt and colleagues[63] recently confirmed the previous observation that higher systemic bone mineral density (BMD) was associated with an increased risk of incident OA. Whether this finding is related to factors contributing to bone remodeling or peak bone mass that may be genetically determined,[64] or whether the higher systemic BMD represents higher BMI load over the years before onset of OA (itself a strong risk factor for OA), is not clear. Paradoxically, BMD was not associated with progressive OA in the same study.[63] Low BMD has been associated cross-sectionally with reduced joint-space width at the hip, which could be a reflection of effects of existing OA.[65] That is, once symptomatic OA has developed an individual may decrease his or her physical activity and therefore loading of the joint, which in turn can contribute to low BMD. Furthermore, there is evidence to suggest that although the apparent density of bone in OA may be increased, the bone itself is less mineralized, resulting in lower material density.[66]

Nutritional factors

The effects of readily modifiable dietary factors in humans have been inconclusive. Studies of the relationship between vitamin D and OA have been conflicting.[67–69] A recent randomized controlled trial of the effects of vitamin D on knee OA did not demonstrate a beneficial effect on cartilage loss on MRI.[70] One difficulty in the conduct of such a study is that it is unethical to conduct a fully placebo-controlled trial; whether the 400 IU/d given to the control arm was sufficient to account for the negative results is not clear. Antioxidant vitamins such as vitamins C and E have also been studied in relation to OA, with conflicting results.[71–76] Vitamin K, which has potential bone and cartilage effects, has been associated cross-sectionally with hand and knee OA, incident radiographic knee OA, and MRI-based cartilage lesions, and with potentially less hand OA progression among those who were deficient at baseline in a randomized trial, although the overall trial results were null.[77–80] Selenium and iodine deficiency has been associated with Kashin-Beck osteoarthropathy. In 2 observational cohort studies, both low and high levels of selenium have been associated with OA.[81,82]

Joint-Level Risk Factors

Occupation, physical activity, and injury

Repetitive joint use may predispose to OA. For example, squatting among Beijing Chinese,[83] and jobs requiring kneeling or squatting were associated with an increased risk of knee OA, particularly among those who were overweight or whose jobs required carrying or lifting, as well as worse cartilage morphology scores on MRI at the patellofemoral joint.[84–86] A recent meta-analysis noted a 1.6-fold increased risk of knee OA related to occupational activities, with most activities conferring increased risk other than standing.[87] Occupational lifting and prolonged standing have been associated with hip OA.[88–90] Occupations involving manual dexterity, particularly repeated pincer grip, have been associated with features of hand OA.[91,92] These data are also supported by an increase in OA found in the interphalangeal joint of the thumb and in the second and third proximal interphalangeal and metacarpophalangeal joints of the hand used to eat with chopsticks, compared with other joints of that same hand or any joint in the opposite hand among Beijing Chinese.[93]

Physical activity may have benefits for the joint by strengthening periarticular muscles to help stabilize the joint, but may potentially be detrimental if it places undue load on the joint, particularly one that is already vulnerable because of other risks.

General population studies have shown that habitual levels of activity are not associated with incident radiographic/symptomatic OA or new knee replacement, whereas more vigorous levels of activity appeared to increase the risk of OA.[94–96] A recent study reported that daily walking of more than 10,000 steps per day may be associated with worsening of certain MRI features; however, certain biases could not be ruled out.[97]

Although studies focused on former athletes have had conflicting results,[98–101] the mechanism by which vigorous or elite-level (or equivalent) physical activity/sports may be associated with increased risk of OA may be related to factors other than simple load bearing. In one study of athletes, the increased risk of OA appeared to be related to knee injury among soccer players, and increased BMI as well as squatting among weightlifters.[102] Several studies have demonstrated the importance of knee injury, such as injury related to meniscal tears requiring meniscectomy or anterior cruciate ligament injury, as a risk factor for onset of OA.[103,104] Two recent meta-analyses report knee injury to confer a 4-fold increased risk of developing knee OA.[33,105]

Beyond certain sports, some occupational activities may also increase the risk of meniscal tears, which are known to confer high risk of knee OA.[106] For example, floor layers, who spend much time kneeling, were more likely to have degenerative meniscal tears than were graphic designers with no knee demands.[107] Although the prevalence of meniscal abnormalities increases as the radiographic severity of knee OA increases,[108] surgical intervention has not been shown to reduce these risks.[109] These studies support the importance of maintaining an intact meniscus to protect against development of OA.

Muscle strength

The effect of knee injury on the risk of OA may be partially related to muscle strength. Muscle weakness and atrophy can occur as a consequence of OA related to disuse resulting from pain avoidance, but whether it is a risk factor for the development of OA is not clear. In some studies, quadriceps muscle weakness was associated with increased risk of structural knee OA.[110,111] In another study, discrepant findings were noted for low knee extensor strength being associated with incident symptomatic knee OA, but not with incident radiographic OA.[112] In this study, the patellofemoral joint was included in the evaluation of incident symptomatic whole knee OA, but was not included in the definition of incident radiographic tibiofemoral OA. On the other hand, greater quadriceps strength in the setting of malalignment and laxity was associated with increased risk of progression of tibiofemoral OA in one study,[113] but no association with tibiofemoral progression was noted in another study, where it was also associated with less cartilage loss in the lateral patellofemoral joint,[114] suggesting a more complex interrelationship.

Muscle strength could also potentially play a role in hand OA. For example, greater grip strength was associated with increased risk of developing radiographic hand OA.[115] However, potentially as a consequence of existing hand OA, a cross-sectional study found an inverse association between grip strength and prevalent OA of the first carpometacarpal joint, and between pinch strength and prevalent OA of the metacarpophalangeal joint.[116]

Alignment

Dynamic alignment (ie, the alterations in the knee that occur during gait) may be pertinent for understanding the specific load effects the joint is experiencing. In epidemiologic studies, however, static alignment from full-limb radiographs (mechanical axis) or from posteroanterior knee radiographs (ie, anatomic axis) is typically assessed according to feasibility. Prior studies have had conflicting findings regarding the effects of alignment on incident OA,[117,118] although more recent studies have reported that varus malalignment assessed by full-limb radiographs increased the incidence of both radiographic knee OA and cartilage damage.[119,120] Nevertheless, a best-evidence synthesis concluded there was a lack of sufficient evidence to draw a conclusion.[121]

Knee malalignment is one of the strongest predictors of progressive knee OA.[120] These findings may imply that the association between alignment and development of OA is a vicious cycle: joint-space narrowing (eg, due to cartilage and meniscal abnormalities) and alterations of bony contour occurring in OA may themselves lead to joint malalignment, and malalignment itself can further alter joint loading and accelerate disease progression. However, no study to date has documented slowing of disease progression if alignment is corrected. Of interest, in post hoc analysis of data from a randomized placebo-controlled trial of doxycycline in obese middle-aged women with unilateral knee OA, varus malalignment was found to negate the potential chondroprotective effects of doxycycline.[122] Using a computational modeling approach with finite or discrete element analysis, knees that developed incident symptomatic OA demonstrated higher maximal contact stress and larger area of engagement with higher contact stresses at baseline than control knees that did not develop symptomatic OA, suggesting a local biomechanical role in the development of symptomatic knee OA.[123]

Leg-length inequality
Leg-length inequality (LLI) is an easily modifiable abnormality. Persons with LLI of at least 2 cm in the Johnston County OA Project were almost twice as likely to have prevalent radiographic knee OA, but no association was noted for incident knee OA.[124,125] Similar findings were noted using data from The MOST Study, in which persons with LLI of 1 cm or more were almost twice as likely to have prevalent radiographic knee OA in the shorter limb.[126] An association with incident radiographic knee OA was not found in that study, although LLI was associated with incident symptomatic knee OA. This discordance, as discussed earlier, may be related to the inclusion of the patellofemoral joint in the definition of symptomatic whole knee OA, whereas it is excluded from incident radiographic tibiofemoral OA.

Bone and joint morphology
The anatomy or the shape of a joint may contribute to the risk of OA, given that biomechanical load distribution through the joint is partially dependent on the geometric shape over which that load is distributed in addition to the material properties of the joint tissues receiving that load. This aspect has perhaps been best studied and described in the hip in relation to OA where, using active shape modeling, the 2-dimensional shape of the hip has been associated with OA.[127,128] Even mild acetabular dysplasia has been associated with a risk of incident hip OA.[129] Pistol-grip deformity, or cam-type femoral acetabular impingement (FAI) syndrome, as well as the pincer-type FAI, have been associated with hip OA and hip pain.[130,131] More recently, using MRI data, 3-dimensional bone shape has been shown to predict the onset of knee OA.[132,133]

RECENT INSIGHTS INTO RISK FACTORS FOR KNEE PAIN

Clinical symptoms related to knee OA are known to be activity related in the early stages, progressing to more persistent symptoms in late stages of disease that are punctuated with intermittent increased pain.[134] In The MOST Study, approximately 40% of persons with or at high risk of knee OA had fluctuating knee pain; these individuals had less severe KL grades on radiography, fewer depressive symptoms, and less widespread pain.[135] In the Longitudinal Examination of Arthritis Pain, an observational cohort study of 287 adults with hip or knee OA in which pain assessments were conducted weekly over 12 weeks, psychological factors fluctuated with pain severity,[136] supporting an important link between the pain experience and psychological state. Indeed, because numerous factors (many of which may not be assessed in a particular study) can contribute to the pain experience, such as genetics, sociocultural environment, and medications, among others, in addition to psychological factors, a so-called structure-symptom discordance is often described in OA.

However, when such between-person variability and confounding factors are accounted for by using a within-person knee-matched study design (in which one knee has pain while the other does not), a strong association between radiographic severity and knee pain can be discerned, even at the earliest stages of radiographic knee OA (**Fig. 3**).[137] Such findings indicate that certain structural lesions within the knee may be a cause of knee pain. Furthermore, specific MRI features of OA that can change over time, including bone marrow lesions, synovitis, and effusions, have been associated with fluctuation of knee pain.[138] As structural lesions worsened, the likelihood that the knee would be painful increased. Similarly, a decrease in the structural abnormalities of a knee was associated with the pain in that knee having

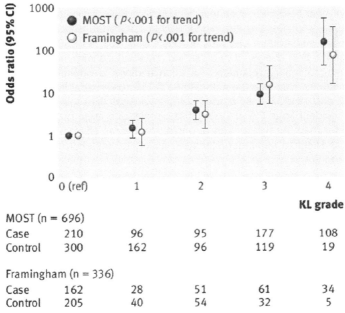

MOST (n = 696)					
Case	210	96	95	177	108
Control	300	162	96	119	19
Framingham (n = 336)					
Case	162	28	51	61	34
Control	205	40	54	32	5

Fig. 3. Associations of frequent knee pain with Kellgren and Lawrence (KL) grade among people with two knees discordant for frequent knee pain status. Number of case knees (ie, with knee pain) and control knees (ie, without knee pain) are shown beneath the graph for each KL grade. Note that the y-axis is logarithmically scaled. CI, confidence interval. (*Data from* Neogi T, Felson D, Niu J, et al. Association between radiographic features of knee osteoarthritis and pain: results from two cohort studies. BMJ 2009;339:b2844. http://dx.doi.org/10.1136/bmj.b2844.)

subsided. A recent systematic review supports an association of MRI-detected bone marrow lesions and synovitis with the pain experience of OA.[139]

METHODOLOGIC CHALLENGES IN THE STUDY OF INCIDENT AND PROGRESSIVE RADIOGRAPHIC KNEE OA

There are several methodologic challenges to the conduct, analysis, and interpretation of results from studies of OA, as discussed elsewhere[13,41] and reviewed briefly here.

Depletion of Susceptibles

Most risk factors for OA, such as obesity or BMD, are chronic in nature. These chronic factors are likely to be present long before subjects are enrolled in a study. If those chronic risk factors have already caused a substantial proportion of subjects to develop knee OA, it is quite possible that participants who are still exposed to such a risk factor without yet having developed OA are less susceptible to knee OA than are individuals who have never been exposed to such a risk factor. For example, long-standing exposures such as obesity may have caused OA at an earlier age than in those being studied, but such a true effect cannot be discerned because those individuals who already have knee OA are excluded from studies of incident disease. Individuals who have been obese for a long time and who are free of OA at study onset may in fact be less susceptible to developing OA. Thus observational studies evaluating the association between a chronic exposure and incident knee OA may not be able to detect the true magnitude of effect. Such a phenomenon has been observed in other fields. For example, studies that have assessed BMI in midlife (in one's 40s, 50s, and 60s) find that higher BMI is associated with an increased risk of death over the subsequent decades (in one's 60s, 70s, and 80s). However, many investigations of BMI at age 70 or older find associations with mortality that are less clear.[140] One potential explanation for such findings is depletion of susceptibles among the elderly. Because the risk of knee OA increases rapidly around the middle 50s to 60s, one would ideally study subjects younger than this age to identify risk factors for incident knee OA. If OA studies consist of a large proportion of subjects who are older than the typical age of onset, the overall effect of a specific chronic risk factor is likely to be underestimated, owing to depletion of those who were susceptible to OA.

Loss to Follow-up and Competing Risks

The risk of developing new-onset OA is difficult to determine because of several challenges. OA is a chronic disease whose onset is typically unknown. In most OA cohort studies, repeated study visits with imaging may occur with a substantial interval between each study visit. As a result, there is a potential for loss to follow-up. For example, in 2 large cohort studies where knee radiographs were repeated after 4 and 9 years, respectively, both studies reported that approximately 40% did not undergo radiography at the follow-up visit.[141,142] Given that OA is a disease with onset in middle or older ages, death attributable to other causes than OA (competing risks) makes risk estimation difficult and prone to bias. In most cases, estimates of the risk of OA can only be obtained among subjects who provide both baseline and follow-up data. If loss to follow-up is associated with the occurrence of OA (as might be expected when older adults or obese participants are lost to follow-up, for example), the estimate of risk of OA based on those who are followed with complete data could be an underestimate.

Potential Discordant Findings for Risk Factors for Incident and Progressive Knee OA

Some risk factors associated with incident disease are not associated with or are even paradoxically protective against progressive OA. In observational studies of progression of OA, eligible knees consist of those that already have knee OA, that is, KL = 2 or KL = 3, representing a mixture of differing degrees of severity that may vary among exposed and nonexposed groups. The outcome is also heterogeneous: knees that progress from KL = 3 to KL = 4 are considered the same as those that progress from KL = 2 to KL = 3 or to KL = 4 over the same period of time. Finally, studies of OA progression are, in essence, conducted to assess an association between a risk factor that causes initiation of OA to progress to more severe OA. This approach results in conditioning on an intermediate stage of OA when assembling the study sample, that is, by limiting the study sample to those who already had mild to moderate knee OA at baseline. This limitation blocks the potential effect of a risk factor on the risk of OA progression if the risk factor of interest was present before any OA abnormality occurred.[41] Conditioning on an intermediate stage of OA can also result in collider bias. For example, in a hypothetical study of obesity as a risk factor for progressive radiographic OA, the assembled knees with KL = 2 or KL = 3 would be divided into those knees that belong to obese persons and those that belong to nonobese persons. Those knees with OA among the nonobese participants must have developed OA that was due to some other risk factors. Without accounting for those risk factors that led to the development of OA in those knees, the results of the study will be confounded, and will tend to be negatively biased (toward the null).

Discerning Independent Effects

Over the past several years, MRI has enabled identification of various pathologic changes in the joint. However, little is known about the true natural history of the occurrence of these structural lesions detected on MRI, particularly in relation to one another. There is often an attempt to include all structural lesions in a statistical regression model to compare the effect of each structural lesion on the outcome of interest. Without knowing the causal pathway and chronology of occurrence of these lesions, standard approaches of automatically mutually adjusting for all factors can lead to biased effect estimates and, moreover, the effect estimates for each structural lesion are not directly comparable with one another, resulting in incorrect interpretations of study findings.[143]

SUMMARY

OA poses a substantial public health burden, given its prevalence that continues to increase. Several risk factors have been recognized, including some modifiable ones such as obesity and avoiding joint injury. There are numerous methodologic challenges to studying risk factors for OA, therefore prevention of OA and its progression also remain challenging. There is a need for ongoing epidemiologic and intervention studies on the prevention of incident and progressive OA, as well as pain related to OA, with adoption of novel approaches to avoid some of the methodologic challenges identified.

REFERENCES

1. Lawrence RC, Felson DT, Helmick CG, et al. Estimates of the prevalence of arthritis and other rheumatic conditions in the United States. Part II. Arthritis Rheum 2008;58:26–35.

2. Hsiao CJ, Cherry DK, Beatty PC, et al. National ambulatory medical care survey: 2007 summary. Natl Health Stat Report 2010;27:1–32.
3. Guccione AA, Felson DT, Anderson JJ, et al. The effects of specific medical conditions on the functional limitations of elders in the Framingham Study. Am J Public Health 1994;84:351–8.
4. Kellgren JH, Lawrence JS. Atlas of standard radiographs. Oxford (United Kingdom): Oxford University Press; 1963.
5. Altman RD, Hochberg M, Murphy WA Jr, et al. Atlas of individual radiographic features in osteoarthritis. Osteoarthritis Cartilage 1995;3(Suppl A):3–70.
6. Buckland-Wright JC, Macfarlane DG, Lynch JA, et al. Joint space width measures cartilage thickness in osteoarthritis of the knee: high resolution plain film and double contrast macroradiographic investigation. Ann Rheum Dis 1995;54:263–8.
7. Hunter DJ, Arden N, Conaghan PG, et al. Definition of osteoarthritis on MRI: results of a Delphi exercise. Osteoarthritis Cartilage 2011;19:963–9.
8. Hunter DJ, Guermazi A, Lo GH, et al. Evolution of semi-quantitative whole joint assessment of knee OA: MOAKS (MRI Osteoarthritis Knee Score). Osteoarthritis Cartilage 2011;19:990–1002.
9. Peterfy CG, Guermazi A, Zaim S, et al. Whole-Organ Magnetic Resonance Imaging Score (WORMS) of the knee in osteoarthritis. Osteoarthritis Cartilage 2004;12:177–90.
10. Guermazi A, Niu J, Hayashi D, et al. Prevalence of abnormalities in knees detected by MRI in adults without knee osteoarthritis: population based observational study (Framingham Osteoarthritis Study). BMJ 2012;345:e5339.
11. Murphy L, Schwartz TA, Helmick CG, et al. Lifetime risk of symptomatic knee osteoarthritis. Arthritis Rheum 2008;59:1207–13.
12. Oliveria SA, Felson DT, Reed JI, et al. Incidence of symptomatic hand, hip, and knee osteoarthritis among patients in a health maintenance organization. Arthritis Rheum 1995;38:1134–41.
13. Neogi T, Zhang Y. Osteoarthritis prevention. Curr Opin Rheumatol 2011;23: 185–91.
14. Haugen IK, Englund M, Aliabadi P, et al. Prevalence, incidence and progression of hand osteoarthritis in the general population: the Framingham Osteoarthritis Study. Ann Rheum Dis 2011;70:1581–6.
15. Felson DT, Naimark A, Anderson J, et al. The prevalence of knee osteoarthritis in the elderly. The Framingham Osteoarthritis Study. Arthritis Rheum 1987;30: 914–8.
16. Jordan JM, Helmick CG, Renner JB, et al. Prevalence of knee symptoms and radiographic and symptomatic knee osteoarthritis in African Americans and Caucasians: the Johnston County Osteoarthritis Project. J Rheumatol 2007;34: 172–80.
17. Jordan JM, Helmick CG, Renner JB, et al. Prevalence of hip symptoms and radiographic and symptomatic hip osteoarthritis in African Americans and Caucasians: the Johnston County Osteoarthritis Project. J Rheumatol 2009;36: 809–15.
18. Nevitt MC, Lane NE, Scott JC, et al. Radiographic osteoarthritis of the hip and bone mineral density. The Study of Osteoporotic Fractures Research Group. Arthritis Rheum 1995;38:907–16.
19. Zhang Y, Niu J, Kelly-Hayes M, et al. Prevalence of symptomatic hand osteoarthritis and its impact on functional status among the elderly: the Framingham Study. Am J Epidemiol 2002;156:1021–7.

20. Nguyen US, Zhang Y, Zhu Y, et al. Increasing prevalence of knee pain and symptomatic knee osteoarthritis: survey and cohort data. Ann Intern Med 2011;155:725–32.
21. Braga L, Renner JB, Schwartz TA, et al. Differences in radiographic features of knee osteoarthritis in African-Americans and Caucasians: the Johnston county osteoarthritis project. Osteoarthritis Cartilage 2009;17:1554–61.
22. Nelson AE, Braga L, Renner JB, et al. Characterization of individual radiographic features of hip osteoarthritis in African American and White women and men: the Johnston County Osteoarthritis Project. Arthritis Care Res (Hoboken) 2010;62:190–7.
23. Nevitt MC, Xu L, Zhang Y, et al. Very low prevalence of hip osteoarthritis among Chinese elderly in Beijing, China, compared with whites in the United States: the Beijing osteoarthritis study. Arthritis Rheum 2002;46:1773–9.
24. Zhang Y, Xu L, Nevitt MC, et al. Comparison of the prevalence of knee osteoarthritis between the elderly Chinese population in Beijing and whites in the United States: the Beijing Osteoarthritis Study. Arthritis Rheum 2001;44:2065–71.
25. Zhang Y, Xu L, Nevitt MC, et al. Lower prevalence of hand osteoarthritis among Chinese subjects in Beijing compared with white subjects in the United States: the Beijing Osteoarthritis Study. Arthritis Rheum 2003;48:1034–40.
26. Felson DT, Nevitt MC, Zhang Y, et al. High prevalence of lateral knee osteoarthritis in Beijing Chinese compared with Framingham Caucasian subjects. Arthritis Rheum 2002;46:1217–22.
27. Srikanth VK, Fryer JL, Zhai G, et al. A meta-analysis of sex differences prevalence, incidence and severity of osteoarthritis. Osteoarthritis Cartilage 2005;13:769–81.
28. Hanna FS, Wluka AE, Bell RJ, et al. Osteoarthritis and the postmenopausal woman: epidemiological, magnetic resonance imaging, and radiological findings. Semin Arthritis Rheum 2004;34:631–6.
29. Nevitt MC, Felson DT, Williams EN, et al. The effect of estrogen plus progestin on knee symptoms and related disability in postmenopausal women: the Heart and Estrogen/Progestin Replacement Study, a randomized, double-blind, placebo-controlled trial. Arthritis Rheum 2001;44:811–8.
30. Cirillo DJ, Wallace RB, Wu L, et al. Effect of hormone therapy on risk of hip and knee joint replacement in the Women's Health Initiative. Arthritis Rheum 2006;54:3194–204.
31. Maleki-Fischbach M, Jordan JM. New developments in osteoarthritis. Sex differences in magnetic resonance imaging-based biomarkers and in those of joint metabolism. Arthritis Res Ther 2010;12:212.
32. Felson DT, Anderson JJ, Naimark A, et al. Obesity and knee osteoarthritis. The Framingham Study. Ann Intern Med 1988;109:18–24.
33. Blagojevic M, Jinks C, Jeffery A, et al. Risk factors for onset of osteoarthritis of the knee in older adults: a systematic review and meta-analysis. Osteoarthritis Cartilage 2010;18:24–33.
34. Zhang W. Risk factors of knee osteoarthritis—excellent evidence but little has been done. Osteoarthritis Cartilage 2010;18:1–2.
35. Niu J, Zhang YQ, Torner J, et al. Is obesity a risk factor for progressive radiographic knee osteoarthritis? Arthritis Rheum 2009;61:329–35.
36. Felson DT, Zhang Y, Anthony JM, et al. Weight loss reduces the risk for symptomatic knee osteoarthritis in women. The Framingham Study. Ann Intern Med 1992;116:535–9.

37. Christensen R, Bartels EM, Astrup A, et al. Effect of weight reduction in obese patients diagnosed with knee osteoarthritis: a systematic review and meta-analysis. Ann Rheum Dis 2007;66:433–9.
38. Wills AK, Black S, Cooper R, et al. Life course body mass index and risk of knee osteoarthritis at the age of 53 years: evidence from the 1946 British birth cohort study. Ann Rheum Dis 2012;71:655–60.
39. Messier SP, Loeser RF, Miller GD, et al. Exercise and dietary weight loss in overweight and obese older adults with knee osteoarthritis: the Arthritis, Diet, and Activity Promotion Trial. Arthritis Rheum 2004;50:1501–10.
40. Messier SP, Nicklas BJ, Legault C, et al. The Intensive Diet and Exercise for Arthritis Trial: 18-month clinical outcomes. Arthritis Rheum 2011;63:S281.
41. Zhang Y, Niu J, Felson DT, et al. Methodologic challenges in studying risk factors for progression of knee osteoarthritis. Arthritis Care Res (Hoboken) 2010;62:1527–32.
42. Ding C, Stannus O, Cicuttini F, et al. Body fat is associated with increased and lean mass with decreased knee cartilage loss in older adults: a prospective cohort study. Int J Obes (Lond) 2012. [Epub ahead of print].
43. Sandell LJ. Obesity and osteoarthritis: is leptin the link? Arthritis Rheum 2009; 60:2858–60.
44. Sowers MR, Karvonen-Gutierrez CA. The evolving role of obesity in knee osteoarthritis. Curr Opin Rheumatol 2010;22:533–7.
45. Carman WJ, Sowers M, Hawthorne VM, et al. Obesity as a risk factor for osteoarthritis of the hand and wrist: a prospective study. Am J Epidemiol 1994;139: 119–29.
46. Oliveria SA, Felson DT, Cirillo PA, et al. Body weight, body mass index, and incident symptomatic osteoarthritis of the hand, hip, and knee. Epidemiology 1999;10:161–6.
47. Grotle M, Hagen KB, Natvig B, et al. Obesity and osteoarthritis in knee, hip and/or hand: an epidemiological study in the general population with 10 years follow-up. BMC Musculoskelet Disord 2008;9:132.
48. Heliovaara M, Makela M, Impivaara O, et al. Association of overweight, trauma and workload with coxarthrosis. A health survey of 7,217 persons. Acta Orthop Scand 1993;64:513–8.
49. Karlson EW, Mandl LA, Aweh GN, et al. Total hip replacement due to osteoarthritis: the importance of age, obesity, and other modifiable risk factors. Am J Med 2003;114:93–8.
50. Tepper S, Hochberg MC. Factors associated with hip osteoarthritis: data from the First National Health and Nutrition Examination Survey (NHANES-I). Am J Epidemiol 1993;137:1081–8.
51. van Saase JL, Vandenbroucke JP, van Romunde LK, et al. Osteoarthritis and obesity in the general population. A relationship calling for an explanation. J Rheumatol 1988;15:1152–8.
52. Felson DT, Couropmitree NN, Chaisson CE, et al. Evidence for a Mendelian gene in a segregation analysis of generalized radiographic osteoarthritis: the Framingham Study. Arthritis Rheum 1998;41:1064–71.
53. Palotie A, Vaisanen P, Ott J, et al. Predisposition to familial osteoarthrosis linked to type II collagen gene. Lancet 1989;1:924–7.
54. Spector TD, Cicuttini F, Baker J, et al. Genetic influences on osteoarthritis in women: a twin study. BMJ 1996;312:940–3.
55. Evangelou E, Valdes AM, Kerkhof HJ, et al. Meta-analysis of genome-wide association studies confirms a susceptibility locus for knee osteoarthritis on chromosome 7q22. Ann Rheum Dis 2011;70:349–55.

56. Valdes AM, Evangelou E, Kerkhof HJ, et al. The GDF5 rs143383 polymorphism is associated with osteoarthritis of the knee with genome-wide statistical significance. Ann Rheum Dis 2011;70:873–5.

57. Day-Williams AG, Southam L, Panoutsopoulou K, et al. A variant in MCF2L is associated with osteoarthritis. Am J Hum Genet 2011;89:446–50.

58. arcOGEN Consortium, arcOGEN Collaborators. Identification of new susceptibility loci for osteoarthritis (arcOGEN): a genome-wide association study. Lancet 2012;380:815–23.

59. van Meurs JB, Uitterlinden AG, Stolk L, et al. A functional polymorphism in the catechol-O-methyltransferase gene is associated with osteoarthritis-related pain. Arthritis Rheum 2009;60:628–9.

60. Valdes AM, De Wilde G, Doherty SA, et al. The Ile585Val TRPV1 variant is involved in risk of painful knee osteoarthritis. Ann Rheum Dis 2011;70: 1556–61.

61. Malfait AM, Seymour AB, Gao F, et al. A role for PACE4 in osteoarthritis pain: evidence from human genetic association and null mutant phenotype. Ann Rheum Dis 2012;71:1042–8.

62. Valdes AM, Arden NK, Vaughn FL, et al. Role of the Nav1.7 R1150W amino acid change in susceptibility to symptomatic knee osteoarthritis and multiple regional pain. Arthritis Care Res (Hoboken) 2011;63:440–4.

63. Nevitt MC, Zhang Y, Javaid MK, et al. High systemic bone mineral density increases the risk of incident knee OA and joint space narrowing, but not radiographic progression of existing knee OA: the MOST study. Ann Rheum Dis 2010; 69:163–8.

64. Naganathan V, Zochling J, March L, et al. Peak bone mass is increased in the hip in daughters of women with osteoarthritis. Bone 2002;30:287–92.

65. Jacobsen S, Jensen TW, Bach-Mortensen P, et al. Low bone mineral density is associated with reduced hip joint space width in women: results from the Copenhagen Osteoarthritis Study. Menopause 2007;14:1025–30.

66. Li B, Aspden RM. Composition and mechanical properties of cancellous bone from the femoral head of patients with osteoporosis or osteoarthritis. J Bone Miner Res 1997;12:641–51.

67. Felson DT, Niu J, Clancy M, et al. Low levels of vitamin D and worsening of knee osteoarthritis: results of two longitudinal studies. Arthritis Rheum 2007;56:129–36.

68. Chaganti RK, Parimi N, Cawthon P, et al. Association of 25-hydroxyvitamin D with prevalent osteoarthritis of the hip in elderly men: the osteoporotic fractures in men study. Arthritis Rheum 2010;62:511–4.

69. McAlindon T, Felson DT. Nutrition: risk factors for osteoarthritis. Ann Rheum Dis 1997;56:397–400.

70. McAlindon T, LaValley M, Schneider E, et al. Effect of vitamin D supplementation on progression of knee pain and cartilage volume loss in patients with symptomatic osteoarthritis: a randomized controlled trial. JAMA 2013;309(2):155.

71. McAlindon TE, Jacques P, Zhang Y, et al. Do antioxidant micronutrients protect against the development and progression of knee osteoarthritis? Arthritis Rheum 1996;39:648–56.

72. Chaganti R, Tolstykh I, Javaid K, et al. Association of baseline vitamin C with incident and progressive radiographic knee OA: the MOST Study. Arthritis Rheum 2008;58:S897.

73. Peregoy J, Wilder FV. The effects of vitamin C supplementation on incident and progressive knee osteoarthritis: a longitudinal study. Public Health Nutr 2011;14: 709–15.

74. De Roos AJ, Arab L, Renner JB, et al. Serum carotenoids and radiographic knee osteoarthritis: the Johnston County Osteoarthritis Project. Public Health Nutr 2001;4:935–42.

75. Jordan JM, De Roos AJ, Renner JB, et al. A case-control study of serum tocopherol levels and the alpha- to gamma-tocopherol ratio in radiographic knee osteoarthritis: the Johnston County Osteoarthritis Project. Am J Epidemiol 2004;159: 968–77.

76. Wluka AE, Stuckey S, Brand C, et al. Supplementary vitamin E does not affect the loss of cartilage volume in knee osteoarthritis: a 2 year double blind randomized placebo controlled study. J Rheumatol 2002;29:2585–91.

77. Neogi T, Booth SL, Zhang YQ, et al. Low vitamin K status is associated with osteoarthritis in the hand and knee. Arthritis Rheum 2006;54:1255–61.

78. Neogi T, Felson DT, Sarno R, et al. Vitamin K in hand osteoarthritis: results from a randomised clinical trial. Ann Rheum Dis 2008;67:1570–3.

79. Misra D, Booth SL, Tolstykh I, et al. Vitamin K deficiency is associated with incident knee osteoarthritis. Am J Med, in press.

80. Oka H, Akune T, Muraki S, et al. Association of low dietary vitamin K intake with radiographic knee osteoarthritis in the Japanese elderly population: dietary survey in a population-based cohort of the ROAD study. J Orthop Sci 2009; 14:687–92.

81. Engstrom G, Gerhardsson de Verdier M, Nilsson PM, et al. Incidence of severe knee and hip osteoarthritis in relation to dietary intake of antioxidants beta-carotene, vitamin C, vitamin E and Selenium: a population-based prospective cohort study. Arthritis Rheum 2009;60:S235–6.

82. Jordan JM, Fang F, Arab L, et al. Low selenium levels are associated with increased risk for osteoarthritis of the knee. Arthritis Rheum 2005;52:S455.

83. Zhang Y, Hunter DJ, Nevitt MC, et al. Association of squatting with increased prevalence of radiographic tibiofemoral knee osteoarthritis: the Beijing Osteoarthritis Study. Arthritis Rheum 2004;50:1187–92.

84. Amin S, Goggins J, Niu J, et al. Occupation-related squatting, kneeling, and heavy lifting and the knee joint: a magnetic resonance imaging-based study in men. J Rheumatol 2008;35:1645–9.

85. Coggon D, Croft P, Kellingray S, et al. Occupational physical activities and osteoarthritis of the knee. Arthritis Rheum 2000;43:1443–9.

86. Felson DT, Hannan MT, Naimark A, et al. Occupational physical demands, knee bending, and knee osteoarthritis: results from the Framingham Study. J Rheumatol 1991;18:1587–92.

87. McWilliams DF, Leeb BF, Muthuri SG, et al. Occupational risk factors for osteoarthritis of the knee: a meta-analysis. Osteoarthritis Cartilage 2011;19:829–39.

88. Croft P, Coggon D, Cruddas M, et al. Osteoarthritis of the hip: an occupational disease in farmers. BMJ 1992;304:1269–72.

89. Croft P, Cooper C, Wickham C, et al. Osteoarthritis of the hip and occupational activity. Scand J Work Environ Health 1992;18:59–63.

90. Yoshimura N, Sasaki S, Iwasaki K, et al. Occupational lifting is associated with hip osteoarthritis: a Japanese case-control study. J Rheumatol 2000;27: 434–40.

91. Hadler NM, Gillings DB, Imbus HR, et al. Hand structure and function in an industrial setting. Arthritis Rheum 1978;21:210–20.

92. Lawrence JS. Rheumatism in cotton operatives. Br J Ind Med 1961;18:270–6.

93. Hunter DJ, Zhang Y, Nevitt MC, et al. Chopstick arthropathy: the Beijing Osteoarthritis Study. Arthritis Rheum 2004;50:1495–500.

94. Hannan MT, Felson DT, Anderson JJ, et al. Habitual physical activity is not associated with knee osteoarthritis: the Framingham Study. J Rheumatol 1993;20: 704–9.
95. McAlindon TE, Wilson PW, Aliabadi P, et al. Level of physical activity and the risk of radiographic and symptomatic knee osteoarthritis in the elderly: the Framingham study. Am J Med 1999;106:151–7.
96. Wang Y, Simpson JA, Wluka AE, et al. Is physical activity a risk factor for primary knee or hip replacement due to osteoarthritis? A prospective cohort study. J Rheumatol 2011;38:350–7.
97. Dore DA, Winzenberg TM, Ding C, et al. The association between objectively measured physical activity and knee structural change using MRI. Ann Rheum Dis 2012. [Epub ahead of print].
98. Lane NE, Oehlert JW, Bloch DA, et al. The relationship of running to osteoarthritis of the knee and hip and bone mineral density of the lumbar spine: a 9 year longitudinal study. J Rheumatol 1998;25:334–41.
99. Panush RS, Schmidt C, Caldwell JR, et al. Is running associated with degenerative joint disease? JAMA 1986;255:1152–4.
100. Marti B, Knobloch M, Tschopp A, et al. Is excessive running predictive of degenerative hip disease? Controlled study of former elite athletes. BMJ 1989;299:91–3.
101. Spector TD, Harris PA, Hart DJ, et al. Risk of osteoarthritis associated with long-term weight-bearing sports: a radiologic survey of the hips and knees in female ex-athletes and population controls. Arthritis Rheum 1996;39:988–95.
102. Kujala UM, Kettunen J, Paananen H, et al. Knee osteoarthritis in former runners, soccer players, weight lifters, and shooters. Arthritis Rheum 1995;38:539–46.
103. Lohmander LS, Ostenberg A, Englund M, et al. High prevalence of knee osteoarthritis, pain, and functional limitations in female soccer players twelve years after anterior cruciate ligament injury. Arthritis Rheum 2004;50:3145–52.
104. Roos EM, Ostenberg A, Roos H, et al. Long-term outcome of meniscectomy: symptoms, function, and performance tests in patients with or without radiographic osteoarthritis compared to matched controls. Osteoarthritis Cartilage 2001;9:316–24.
105. Muthuri SG, McWilliams DF, Doherty M, et al. History of knee injuries and knee osteoarthritis: a meta-analysis of observational studies. Osteoarthritis Cartilage 2011;19:1286–93.
106. Englund M, Guermazi A, Roemer FW, et al. Meniscal tear in knees without surgery and the development of radiographic osteoarthritis among middle-aged and elderly persons: The Multicenter Osteoarthritis Study. Arthritis Rheum 2009;60:831–9.
107. Rytter S, Egund N, Jensen LK, et al. Occupational kneeling and radiographic tibiofemoral and patellofemoral osteoarthritis. J Occup Med Toxicol 2009;4:19.
108. Englund M, Guermazi A, Gale D, et al. Incidental meniscal findings on knee MRI in middle-aged and elderly persons. N Engl J Med 2008;359:1108–15.
109. Lohmander LS, Englund PM, Dahl LL, et al. The long-term consequence of anterior cruciate ligament and meniscus injuries: osteoarthritis. Am J Sports Med 2007;35:1756–69.
110. Brandt KD, Heilman DK, Slemenda C, et al. Quadriceps strength in women with radiographically progressive osteoarthritis of the knee and those with stable radiographic changes. J Rheumatol 1999;26:2431–7.
111. Slemenda C, Heilman DK, Brandt KD, et al. Reduced quadriceps strength relative to body weight: a risk factor for knee osteoarthritis in women? Arthritis Rheum 1998;41:1951–9.

112. Segal NA, Torner JC, Felson D, et al. Effect of thigh strength on incident radiographic and symptomatic knee osteoarthritis in a longitudinal cohort. Arthritis Rheum 2009;61:1210–7.

113. Sharma L, Dunlop DD, Cahue S, et al. Quadriceps strength and osteoarthritis progression in malaligned and lax knees. Ann Intern Med 2003;138:613–9.

114. Amin S, Baker K, Niu J, et al. Quadriceps strength and the risk of cartilage loss and symptom progression in knee osteoarthritis. Arthritis Rheum 2009;60: 189–98.

115. Chaisson CE, Zhang Y, Sharma L, et al. Higher grip strength increases the risk of incident radiographic osteoarthritis in proximal hand joints. Osteoarthritis Cartilage 2000;8(Suppl A):S29–32.

116. Dominick KL, Jordan JM, Renner JB, et al. Relationship of radiographic and clinical variables to pinch and grip strength among individuals with osteoarthritis. Arthritis Rheum 2005;52:1424–30.

117. Brouwer GM, van Tol AW, Bergink AP, et al. Association between valgus and varus alignment and the development and progression of radiographic osteoarthritis of the knee. Arthritis Rheum 2007;56:1204–11.

118. Hunter DJ, Niu J, Felson DT, et al. Knee alignment does not predict incident osteoarthritis: the Framingham osteoarthritis study. Arthritis Rheum 2007;56:1212–8.

119. Sharma L, Chmiel JS, Almagor O, et al. The role of varus and valgus alignment in the initial development of knee cartilage damage by MRI: the MOST study. Ann Rheum Dis 2012. [Epub ahead of print].

120. Sharma L, Song J, Dunlop D, et al. Varus and valgus alignment and incident and progressive knee osteoarthritis. Ann Rheum Dis 2010;69:1940–5.

121. Tanamas S, Hanna FS, Cicuttini FM, et al. Does knee malalignment increase the risk of development and progression of knee osteoarthritis? A systematic review. Arthritis Rheum 2009;61:459–67.

122. Mazzuca SA, Brandt KD, Chakr R, et al. Varus malalignment negates the structure-modifying benefits of doxycycline in obese women with knee osteoarthritis. Osteoarthritis Cartilage 2010;18:1008–11.

123. Segal NA, Anderson DD, Iyer KS, et al. Baseline articular contact stress levels predict incident symptomatic knee osteoarthritis development in the MOST cohort. J Orthop Res 2009;27:1562–8.

124. Golightly YM, Allen KD, Helmick CG, et al. Hazard of incident and progressive knee and hip radiographic osteoarthritis and chronic joint symptoms in individuals with and without limb length inequality. J Rheumatol 2010;37:2133–40.

125. Golightly YM, Allen KD, Renner JB, et al. Relationship of limb length inequality with radiographic knee and hip osteoarthritis. Osteoarthritis Cartilage 2007;15: 824–9.

126. Harvey WF, Yang M, Cooke TD, et al. Association of leg-length inequality with knee osteoarthritis: a cohort study. Ann Intern Med 2010;152:287–95.

127. Gregory JS, Waarsing JH, Day J, et al. Early identification of radiographic osteoarthritis of the hip using an active shape model to quantify changes in bone morphometric features: can hip shape tell us anything about the progression of osteoarthritis? Arthritis Rheum 2007;56:3634–43.

128. Lynch JA, Parimi N, Chaganti RK, et al. The association of proximal femoral shape and incident radiographic hip OA in elderly women. Osteoarthritis Cartilage 2009;17:1313–8.

129. Lane NE, Lin P, Christiansen L, et al. Association of mild acetabular dysplasia with an increased risk of incident hip osteoarthritis in elderly white women: the study of osteoporotic fractures. Arthritis Rheum 2000;43:400–4.

130. Doherty M, Courtney P, Doherty S, et al. Nonspherical femoral head shape (pistol grip deformity), neck shaft angle, and risk of hip osteoarthritis: a case-control study. Arthritis Rheum 2008;58:3172–82.

131. Reid GD, Reid CG, Widmer N, et al. Femoroacetabular impingement syndrome: an underrecognized cause of hip pain and premature osteoarthritis? J Rheumatol 2010;37:1395–404.

132. Bredbenner TL, Eliason TD, Potter RS, et al. Statistical shape modeling describes variation in tibia and femur surface geometry between Control and Incidence groups from the osteoarthritis initiative database. J Biomech 2010; 43:1780–6.

133. Neogi T, Bowes M, Niu J, et al. MRI-based 3D bone shape predicts incident knee OA 12 months prior to its onset. Osteoarthritis Cartilage 2011;19(Suppl 1):S51–2.

134. Hawker GA, Stewart L, French MR, et al. Understanding the pain experience in hip and knee osteoarthritis—an OARSI/OMERACT initiative. Osteoarthritis Cartilage 2008;16:415–22.

135. Neogi T, Nevitt MC, Yang M, et al. Consistency of knee pain: correlates and association with function. Osteoarthritis Cartilage 2010;18:1250–5.

136. Wise BL, Niu J, Zhang Y, et al. Psychological factors and their relation to osteoarthritis pain. Osteoarthritis Cartilage 2010;18:883–7.

137. Neogi T, Felson D, Niu J, et al. Association between radiographic features of knee osteoarthritis and pain: results from two cohort studies. BMJ 2009;339: b2844.

138. Zhang Y, Nevitt M, Niu J, et al. Fluctuation of knee pain and changes in bone marrow lesions, effusions and synovitis on MRI: the Most Study. Arthritis Rheum 2011;63:691–9.

139. Yusuf E, Kortekaas MC, Watt I, et al. Do knee abnormalities visualised on MRI explain knee pain in knee osteoarthritis? A systematic review. Ann Rheum Dis 2011;70(1):60–7. http://dx.doi.org/10.1136/ard.2010.131904.

140. Manson JE, Bassuk SS, Hu FB, et al. Estimating the number of deaths due to obesity: can the divergent findings be reconciled? J Womens Health (Larchmt) 2007;16:168–76.

141. Cooper C, Snow S, McAlindon TE, et al. Risk factors for the incidence and progression of radiographic knee osteoarthritis. Arthritis Rheum 2000;43: 995–1000.

142. Felson DT, Zhang Y, Hannan MT, et al. Risk factors for incident radiographic knee osteoarthritis in the elderly: the Framingham Study. Arthritis Rheum 1997;40:728–33.

143. Robins JM, Greenland S. Identifiability and exchangeability for direct and indirect effects. Epidemiology 1992;3:143–55.

The Measurement of Joint Mechanics and Their Role in Osteoarthritis Genesis and Progression

David R. Wilson, DPhil[a],*, Emily J. McWalter, PhD[b],
James D. Johnston, PhD[c]

KEYWORDS

- Osteoarthritis • Biomechanics • Knee • Hip • Kinematics

KEY POINTS

- Mechanics play a role in the initiation, progression and successful treatment of osteoarthritis. Many of the hypotheses proposed to explain why osteoarthritis begins and progresses center on mechanics.
- Not enough is known about which specific mechanical parameters are most important, and what their impact is on the disease process, so comprehensive statements cannot be made about how mechanics should be modified to prevent, slow or arrest osteoarthritis.
- Our understanding of the role of mechanics in osteoarthritis is limited by the challenge of measuring the most important mechanical quantities in living subjects.
- Our current understanding of the role of mechanics in osteoarthritis is based largely on studies of deviations from normal mechanics caused by malalignment, injury, and deformity.
- Some treatments for osteoarthritis focus on correcting mechanics, but there appears to be scope for more mechanically based interventions for osteoarthritis.

INTRODUCTION

Mechanics play a role in the initiation, progression, and successful treatment of osteoarthritis (OA). However, not enough is known about which specific mechanical parameters are most important and what their impact is on the disease process, so

This work was supported by grants from the Canadian Institutes of Health Research, the Canadian Arthritis Network (Networks of Centres of Excellence of Canada), and the Natural Sciences and Engineering Research Council of Canada.
[a] Department of Orthopaedics, Centre for Hip Health and Mobility, Vancouver Coastal Health Research Institute, University of British Columbia, Room 3114, 910 West 10th Avenue, Vancouver, British Columbia V5Z 4E3, Canada; [b] Department of Radiology, Stanford University, The Lucas Center for MR Spectroscopy and Imaging, Mail Code 5488, Route 8, Stanford, CA 94305-5488, USA; [c] Department of Mechanical Engineering, University of Saskatchewan, 57 Campus Drive, Saskatoon, Saskatchewan S7N 5A9, Canada
* Corresponding author.
E-mail address: david.wilson@ubc.ca

Rheum Dis Clin N Am 39 (2013) 21–44
http://dx.doi.org/10.1016/j.rdc.2012.11.002
0889-857X/13/$ – see front matter © 2013 Elsevier Inc. All rights reserved.

rheumatic.theclinics.com

comprehensive statements cannot be made about how mechanics should be modified to prevent, slow, or arrest the disease process. The idea of a mechanical role in OA is often made clear to the patient: OA is wear-and-tear arthritis, and joint surfaces need to be replaced because of wear in advanced stages of the disease, much like bearing surfaces in an engine that have worn down after too many revolutions. The parallels with machines are sometimes (at least superficially) obvious: obese people load their joints more and have a higher prevalence of OA, which is analogous to higher loads on a bearing increasing the rate of wear on its surfaces, a well-known mechanical phenomenon. Sufficiently high loads can destroy any tissue, so there is a level of joint loading that can injure cartilage irreversibly, leading to erosion from the joint surface. However, the usefulness of drawing parallels with machines is limited. Cartilage is avascular and aneural, but it is a living tissue with the capacity to adapt to its mechanical environment; it endures apparently unscathed through the most active decades of life in most people. Many surgical procedures and other treatment and prevention approaches are currently based implicitly or explicitly on the assumption that they improve or correct joint mechanics, and that this improvement or correction is required to protect the joint from OA. Justifying and improving mechanically based treatment and prevention approaches requires a critical understanding of the methods used to study joint mechanics and the current evidence for the role of mechanics in OA. This article summarizes methods for assessing joint mechanics and their relative merits and limitations, describes current evidence for the role of mechanics in OA initiation and progression, and describes some current treatment approaches that focus on modifying joint mechanics.

MECHANICAL HYPOTHESES ABOUT OA

Many of the hypotheses proposed to explain why OA begins and progresses center on mechanics. A widely accepted hypothesis regarding OA pathogenesis is that acute trauma destroys chondrocytes and disrupts the extracellular matrix, resulting in proteoglycan depletion, cartilage breakdown, and subsequent OA.[1,2] Surface damage, proteoglycan loss,[3] and chondrocyte death[1] are seen commonly in OA, and similar observations have been made with in vitro impact studies on human and animal specimens.[4–6] Recent research suggests that even moderate loading can induce biologic damage at levels less than those required to produce detectable macroscopic damage, and could be an early event in OA pathogenesis.[7] Prolonged exposure to overloading caused by obesity[8] and/or altered joint mechanics[9,10] are also hypothesized to be detrimental to long-term joint health.

Altered kinematics and associated increased shear stress, in particular are thought to be key initiating factors explaining idiopathic forms of OA.[10] In the articulating joint, cartilage is exposed to compressive loading (tending to compress the cartilage) and simultaneous shear loading (tending to change the shape of the cartilage) (**Fig. 1**) as the 2 cartilage surfaces slide relative to one another. Abnormal motion (perhaps caused by an anterior cruciate ligament [ACL] injury, joint laxity, or aging) results in a shift in the region of loading to a cartilage zone not conditioned to frequent load bearing.[10] This shift results in cartilage fibrillation at the cartilage surface, which is commonly seen in early stages of OA.[11,12] Following fibrillation there is an increase in friction that increases the tangential shear load at the cartilage surface, resulting in increased shear stress in the collagen network and further fibrillation. Cartilage metabolic activity depends on the type of loading (eg, hydrostatic compression, shear) and exhibits a particularly negative response to excessive shear stress.[13,14] Because of fibrillation, friction, and increased shear stresses, there is a metabolic upregulation

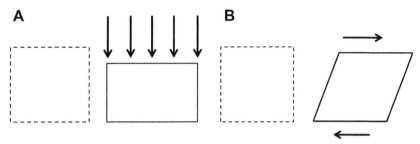

Fig. 1. The compressive component of stress (*A*) compresses the material from its initial state, shown with dashed lines. The shear component of stress (*B*) changes the shape of the material from its initial state, shown with dashed lines.

of catabolic factors detrimental to cartilage health (eg, matrix metalloproteinase and interleukins),[13,14] resulting in further cartilage degeneration.[10]

Another group of hypotheses suggest that OA progresses because of mechanical changes in subchondral bone.[15] An early view was that, because of impulse loading (loading that changes rapidly over time) and cumulative trauma, microfractures are created in the trabeculae that are repaired by fracture callus. As the trabeculae become thicker and new trabeculae are added, the repair process stiffens the subchondral bone, in effect acting as a support for the end plate, which causes the subchondral region to become less compliant, resulting in increased cartilage stresses and eventual degradation.[16,17] Variable subchondral bone stiffening across the joint surface also results in stiffness gradients and subsequent increased cartilage shear stresses.[15] A more recent, and generally accepted, hypothesis speculates that microfractures within the subchondral cortical end plate (as opposed to adjacent trabeculae), result in subchondral thickening. These microfractures, attributed to impulse loading and repetitive stress, are hypothesized to increase biological activity at the site of injury and result in increased bone turnover and reactivation of the secondary center of ossification, resulting in subchondral thickening, cartilage thinning, and increased cartilage stresses.[18]

Although evidence is emerging from animal studies in support of some of these hypotheses, little work has been done in humans. Studies are emerging that examine the role of bone in OA using traditional bone mineral density (BMD) measures. For example, cartilage thinning correlates with bone structure losses in the contralateral compartment in subjects with tibiofemoral OA.[19] Ratios of medial to lateral compartment BMD have also been associated with compartmental tibiofemoral OA.[20] In particular, higher BMD in the medial compartment was associated with medial joint space narrowing, and medial sclerosis and higher BMD in the lateral compartment was associated with lateral joint space narrowing and lateral sclerosis.[20] However, it is important to note that these findings were made using two-dimensional measurements of bone density, and similar findings were not found when using tomographic methods.[21] Improved tools for measuring bone, cartilage, and joint mechanics may ultimately allow the testing of these and other hypotheses in vivo in humans.

METHODS FOR ASSESSING JOINT MECHANICS
The Challenges of Study Design

It is difficult to test hypotheses about the role of mechanics in OA initiation and progression and the effects of changes in mechanics on OA because appropriate in vivo human studies present major challenges. First, studies require a well-characterized population that has, or is at risk for, OA, and such populations can be difficult to identify. Large populations are generally needed for studies to have appropriate statistical power, which adds to the cost and difficulty of managing the study. Second, studies require a means of assessing OA incidence or progression. Radiographic measurements of OA (eg, Kellgren-Lawrence[22] grade) are often insensitive to early OA and to small increments of progression. Advanced magnetic resonance imaging (MRI) techniques have shown potential for more sensitive, quantitative measurement of OA progression,[23] but these measures are more time-consuming and expensive than radiographic approaches. Most critically, such studies require in vivo assessments of joint mechanics. Standard clinical measurements used as surrogates for mechanics have been employed in several studies, but they have many limitations. More direct measurements of mechanics (with fewer limitations than the clinical surrogate measures) have been developed, but studies have generally only been done in small populations because the measurements are expensive and time consuming.

What Do We Need to Measure and What are the Obstacles?

The hypotheses about the links between mechanics and OA, and these hypotheses define the mechanical quantities of primary interest to researchers. However, the most interesting quantities are among the most difficult to measure. Compressive and tangential shear forces on the joint surfaces are key quantities in many hypotheses, but they can only be measured directly by implanting a measurement device into the joint, which is too interventional (in the case of the natural joint) for most in vivo studies of humans. Force distribution on the cartilage surface is also widely thought to be important: a moderate force transmitted through a small contact area may produce local stresses that cause cartilage damage, whereas the same force transmitted through a large contact area would produce no cartilage injury. Although there are sensors available to measure force distribution,[24] they must also be implanted, which carries the same limitations in vivo as direct measurements of force. Loading rate has been postulated to play a role in OA.[25] Assessing loading rate requires rapid measurements of force (typically hundreds per second), which is more challenging than static force measurements. There is also interest in how force is transmitted through joint structures such as cartilage and bone (stress). Measuring stress in simple machines and structures is a challenge, and stress has not been measured in joints in vivo. Some approaches are emerging for measuring strain, or deformation of the joint tissues in response to stress,[26–29] but the relationship between stress and strain is more complex in joint tissues than in, for example, steel or glass, which makes it difficult to use strain measurements to predict stress. Kinematics (joint movement) are easier to measure and several methods for accurately quantifying joint kinematics in vivo have been developed. Kinematics describe how the bones that make up the joint move relative to each other, which can reflect where load is transmitted through the surfaces and the lines of action of structures that transmit forces.

Ex Vivo Studies and Joint Models

Current understanding of joint mechanics is founded on ex vivo studies, which are inappropriate for linking mechanics with clinical symptoms. In ex vivo studies, kinematics and contact mechanics have been measured in cadaver specimens loaded in mechanical rigs.[30–37] Although studies of this type have improved understand of the biomechanics of healthy joints, their central limitation for studying OA is that morphologic adaptations caused by the disease process or the healing process and mechanical links to clinical symptoms such as pain and ongoing processes such as cartilage degeneration cannot be studied in cadavers. An alternative that avoids some of the limitations of mechanical measurements that can be made in vivo is to predict joint mechanics using mathematical models. Models are limited primarily by the assumptions that must be made to formulate them. Models incorporating sophisticated descriptions of joint structures have been developed, validated,[38–43] and used to answer specific clinically motivated questions.[44–48] Two primary limitations of mathematical models are that (1) many simplifying assumptions must be made about the properties of the joint, which limits their validity and applicability; and (2) like ex vivo studies, they are inappropriate for studying links with ongoing processes and symptoms in vivo, unless these changes are measured and incorporated into the model.

Subject-specific finite element (FE) modeling is an emerging technique in musculoskeletal research that has potential for providing information on the role of mechanics in OA initiation and progression.[49] FE modeling is a computational engineering technique used to evaluate how a structure with complex geometry and composed of a range of materials behaves when subjected to loading. Its basic premise is to divide a complicated object into a finite number of small, manageable pieces (elements). The behavior of each element can be described mathematically and evaluated computationally.[50] Using clinical computed tomography (CT) or MRI, a joint's bone, cartilage, and soft tissue geometry can be acquired. Tissue material properties (eg, elastic modulus, stiffness) can also be estimated using CT or MRI.[51,52] Image-derived geometry and material properties can then be used to create a subject-specific FE model that can be analyzed under varying loading scenarios (eg, repetitive walking, impact-intensive running) to simulate bone and cartilage responses to loading. Unique information that is impossible to measure experimentally (eg, internal stress and strain distributions in both bone and cartilage) can be acquired using FE modeling and linked with in vivo symptoms and OA processes. The FE method can also be applied longitudinally to evaluate bone and cartilage structural behavior following OA-related morphologic and mechanical alterations to these tissues. However, application of subject-specific FE modeling to address OA-related questions is in its infancy. To date, research using subject-specific FE modeling has been primarily restricted to addressing osteoporosis-related research questions (eg, fracture strength) of bony structures not necessarily affected by OA (eg, radius, femoral neck).[53,54] This lack of OA-related FE research is likely due to difficulties associated with validating FE models comprising numerous complex joint tissues. Validating models requires direct measurements of mechanical quantities such as stress and strain, which, as we have described earlier, are difficult to measure directly. However, new methods have recently been developed[27,55] that have potential to validate internal strain distributions in bone and cartilage acquired using FE modeling, and that can be applied using intact joints. These developments, combined with improvements in CT and MRI technologies and computing power, have made subject-specific FE modeling a candidate technique for addressing specific questions regarding the role of mechanics in OA initiation and progression. However, application of the approach to large populations is limited by long data analysis (segmentation) and processing times and the challenge of model validation.

Radiographic Measures of Alignment

Most of the measures used clinically to quantify joint mechanics assess joint alignment. For example, tibiofemoral alignment is often quantified with the femorotibial angle, or hip-knee-ankle angle.[56] A range of measures has emerged for quantifying patellofemoral alignment, with particular emphasis on medial-lateral position and patellar tilt. A central limitation of this approach is that the measures describe the joint (whose primary function is to move) at only 1 static position. In addition, although it is intuitive that these alignment measures are related to how load is transmitted in the joint, for most measures it is unclear by how much any given change in alignment measure would change force distribution in the joint. A further limitation is that the accuracy and repeatability of these measures are affected by their two-dimensional nature. Two-dimensional radiographic measurements are prone to errors caused by magnification and subject positioning. MRI and CT collect three-dimensional information about joint anatomy, which has been used in such applications as quantifying femoral neck deformities thought to be associated with hip OA.[57] However, in many cases the three-dimensional data are still reduced to a two-dimensional measurement, which does not adequately describe three-dimensional deformities.

Gait Analysis

Gait analysis (often more generally referred to as motion analysis) is an important modality for estimating joint mechanics in activity. In motion analysis, movement of the joint segments is tracked (most often with an optoelectronic system), and loads applied to the body (eg, ground reaction forces) are measured. Mechanical analysis can then be used to assess the resultant forces and moments at the joints for each position for which a complete set of measurements is available. The resultant forces and moments at the joints, which are output by most commercial motion analysis systems, are different from the contact forces (also known as the bone-on-bone forces) in the joint. Determining contact forces requires further analysis using joint models[58] and the measured joint segment positions and loads applied to the body. One advantage of gait analysis is that movement is unconstrained by the measurement system, and therefore a large range of activities can be studied. One key limitation of gait analysis is that joint segments are typically tracked with markers fixed to the skin that move substantially relative to the bones. However, it is often difficult to identify the joint center (or axis of rotation), particularly at the hip, and it is difficult to assess how well the measured marker positions correspond with motion at the joint (differences have been found to be on the order of 10° for knee flexion[59]). The use of large groups of skin-mounted markers has reduced the error caused by skin movement, although error will still be influenced by body habitus.[60] A second key limitation is that the models and analysis needed to determine joint contact forces require many simplifications and assumptions, limiting the accuracy with which these loads can be measured.[61] Models have often been based on the anatomy of a single specimen or participant, as opposed to using subject-specific anatomic measurements, which limits the usefulness of these models,[62] particularly when pathologic joints are involved.

Roentgen Stereophotogrammetric Analysis and In Vivo Radiography

Some of the limitations of motion analysis have been addressed with radiography-based methods for measuring motion, including roentgen stereophotogrammetric analysis (RSA; also known as radiostereometric analysis) and fluoroscopy. Three-dimensional knee kinematics have been measured during activity in vivo using single-plane fluoroscopy and subsequent image processing. This measurement has been done in joints after arthroplasty[63] and in natural joints.[64] A limitation of the single-plane approach is that measurement errors out of the imaging plane are large. More accurate three-dimensional measurements of kinematics can be made with biplanar fluoroscopy[65] and biplanar radiography, which have been used to study kinematics in the knees,[66,67] hip,[68] shoulder,[69] and other joints. Although many biplanar radiography studies have been done using a series of static positions, high-speed biplanar radiography has made possible accurate measurements of kinematics during dynamic activity.[70,71] Because these measurements are so accurate, combining kinematics with known joint geometry yields predictions of joint contact interactions.[68,72] In some approaches, markers (typically small tantalum spheres) have been implanted into the bones, which is an invasive procedure and therefore a limitation. However, recent work using model-based approaches suggests that measurements can be made accurately and precisely enough to be clinically useful without using implanted markers.[68,73,74] A key limitation of all these approaches is that they expose patients to ionizing radiation. Radiation doses vary with the joint of interest and the size of the subject. Such exposure always carries some risk and limits the number of repeat assessments that can be made, although, in general, imaging of the extremities is less of a concern than whole-body imaging because the body core can be shielded from radiation.

MRI Measurements of Kinematics

MRI has been used to assess joint kinematics and has the advantages that soft tissues are easily visualized and that no ionizing radiation is required, making it ideal for use in longitudinal studies. The different MRI-based approaches for assessing kinematics are distinguished from one another other by whether they describe two-dimensional or three-dimensional movement, whether they are assessed while the joint is actively loaded, and whether the movement is measured continuously. Many MRI studies of kinematics have focused on the patellofemoral joint, largely because patellar tracking is difficult to measure with other techniques such as gait analysis because of difficulties tracking skin-mounted markers on this small bone. Two-dimensional techniques have been used to assess kinematics at sequential static angles of knee flexion, dynamically over a range of knee flexion, and unloaded and loaded in a supine, lateral, or standing position.[75-80] Loading in the supine or lateral position is performed by applying, respectively, an axial force to the foot or a torsional load to the shank using custom-designed rigs. The primary limitation of two-dimensional studies is that they neglect at least half of the movement, because describing any joint's movement completely requires 6 quantities of movement (typically 3 rotations and 3 translations).[79,81] Planar studies can measure a maximum of 3 quantities.

Three-dimensional MRI-based kinematic methods, which measure the 6 quantities of movement, have also been developed and can be categorized in the same way as the two-dimensional techniques (sequential static vs dynamic, unloaded vs loaded).[82-92] The static three-dimensional methods have used standard MRI sequences, whereas the dynamic methods have used ultrafast gradient echo,[86] cine-MRI,[87-90,93,94] phase-contrast MRI,[91] and spoiled gradient echoes with radial acquisitions.[85] Although promising, these techniques have some limitations, most notably that static postures in a supine position do not necessarily represent normal activities of daily living, and dynamic methods either require subjects to extend their knees very slowly, which is not necessarily representative of normal motion, or to flex and extend their knees through many cycles that are averaged, which can cause errors if the motion is not repeated perfectly between cycles. Accuracy of these techniques ranges from approximately 1 mm and 1°[82,83] to approximately 2 mm and 3°.[95] Clinically important differences are likely in this range. Not all techniques have been rigorously validated and, therefore, care should be taken when interpreting data.

There are inherent trade-offs between static and dynamic methods and loaded and unloaded methods, as well as noteworthy limitations to these techniques. Substantial differences in two-dimensional patellar kinematic measures have been observed between unloaded, sequential static assessments and unloaded, dynamic assessments.[75] Substantial differences were similarly observed between static, loaded assessments and dynamic, loaded assessments in a three-dimensional analysis.[86]

These results suggest that differences exist between static and dynamic cases, regardless of applied load. To further support this, 2 other studies have shown differences in two-dimensional patellar kinematics assessed dynamically between a supine low-load scenario and an upright 45% body weight scenario[96] and in three-dimensional patellar kinematics assessed statically in the supine position at 0%, 15%, and 30% body weight scenario.[97] Most methods apply low loads to the limb (0%–50% body weight load, open chain and closed chain), because of the limitations of loading the leg in the closed-bore MRI scanner. Open configuration MRI allows greater loads to be applied because the subject can stand upright (at least 45% body weight in weightbearing). However, these scanners have lower field strengths, limiting image quality and increasing scan times, and are not widely available. The range of flexion angles that can be studied is also limited by the MRI scanner configuration. Depending on knee size, flexion angles of up to approximately 50° can be assessed in closed-bore systems. With open configuration scanners, angles of 60° and greater can be assessed. In addition to these differences, the definition of the kinematic quantities differs between studies, which makes comparing results between studies challenging. An additional limitation is that most of this work has focused on the knee; few data are available for kinematics of the hip, shoulder, elbow, or hand.

MRI Measurements of Contact Area

Joint contact areas are fundamental to the understanding of load transmission through the joint and its relationship to local damage in OA. Contact areas, contact loads, contact stresses, and tissue stresses would ideally be measured. However, currently the only measure possible in vivo is contact area. Contact area measurements are useful because they provide information about where loads are transmitted on the cartilage surface and they can be used to find average contact stress (if joint loads can be estimated). Several groups have developed methods of assessing contact area in vivo from MRI.[76,80,84,98–115] All of these methods have used gradient echo techniques with fat suppression, which is optimized to view cartilage. These scans have been acquired using traditional scanners (1.5 and 3.0 T) and open-configuration scanners (0.5 T) using the loading methods similar to those used for kinematic assessments. Contact area is generally assessed at sequential static, loaded angles of knee flexion, although it was measured during continuous flexion in a recent study.[110] Axial and sagittal scans have been used. The chosen plane should be the one that provides the most information about the contact periphery. Once the MRI scans are acquired, they must be processed to calculate contact areas, which can be done by delineating the contact region in a slice-by-slice manner and multiplying the length of each contact line by slice thickness[76,98–100,104–106] or interpolating between slices and summing the areas of discrete patches.[84,103,108] Alternatively, adjacent cartilage plates can be segmented separately and contact can then be calculated by either expanding 1 surface by a pixel and defining overlap as contact[80,101,102] or by performing a proximity analysis.[107] The coordinates of the contact centroid have also been reported on occasion.[84,108,116] These may provide valuable information about changes in contact location and are most useful when reported in a relevant coordinate system, such as that used for kinematic assessment. Validation of MRI-based techniques has been limited. Only 3 studies have examined agreement with a reference standard, 2 using cadaver specimens,[100,117] and 1 using a phantom.[99] Errors, expressed as coefficient of variation, were found to range from 3% to 11%. Intraobserver, interobserver, and intrasubject repeatability have also been assessed in vivo and have ranged from 3% to 10%.[80,99,104,117] Many of the factors that affect measures of patellar kinematics, such as loading, range of motion, and tibiofemoral angle, are equally applicable to measures of contact area. Most studies have focused on the patellofemoral joint,[76,80,84,98–106,108,109,112,113,116] whereas others have examined contact areas in the elbow[109,118,119] and tibiofemoral joint.[111,114,115] Little or no work has addressed the hip, shoulder, wrist, or hands.

The Future

Technologic advances hold promise for more and better in vivo mechanical measurements. Many of the methods described in this article are now beginning to be used to study patient populations. One area with promise is MRI mapping of cartilage strain, which had been done ex vivo in the knee[26,120,121] and the hip.[122] This work is challenging because achieving the resolution required to detect small changes in cartilage thickness in a short imaging time requires scanners with very high field strengths. As these scanners become more widely available for clinical use, there will be the potential to begin assessments of strain in vivo. Groups are also beginning to integrate mechanical measures with other OA disease indicators. For example, a recent study combined measures of contact area with measures of T1rho and T2 relaxometry; individuals with OA had longer T1rho and T2 relaxation times and greater contact areas.[112] Integration of mechanical measurements with MR techniques designed to detect early degenerative changes may be useful for improving understanding of the causes of OA. CT technology is also improving, with scans becoming faster and requiring lower doses of ionizing radiation. This progress raises the possibility of wider use of CT to assess joint kinematics and other mechanical quantities as well as integrating these measures with radiographic and MRI-based measures of tissue degeneration and OA. In addition, developments in nanotechnology suggest the feasibility of developing implantable transducers that transmit measurements through telemetry. This has been done on a limited scale[123] but, as technology improves, it may become more widespread.

CURRENT EVIDENCE FOR THE ROLE OF MECHANICS IN OA INITIATION AND PROGRESSION
Distinction Between Normal Aging and OA

OA is often thought of as a disease of aging that is mechanical in origin.[124] However, it is likely that there are some changes in mechanics over time that are a result of normal aging and not necessarily the OA disease process. For example, 1 study found, in participants without radiographic signs of OA, a significant increase in valgus alignment with age at a rate of 0.03° and 0.04° per year in men and women, respectively.[125] In the same study, participants with OA tended to show increasing varus angulation. Another study showed, through principal component analysis, that patterns of gait differed between young (23.9 ± 2.6 years) and older (65.5 ± 5.2 years) participants when climbing stairs.[126] These findings suggest that patterns of changes in joint mechanics may differ not only with OA but also with normal aging, which highlights the need for establishing age-dependent population norms for studying OA.

Alignment

Joint malalignment or incongruence leads to altered loading patterns at the cartilage surface, and joint alignment is therefore associated with OA. Tibiofemoral alignment has been studied extensively in individuals who have tibiofemoral and/or patellofemoral OA.[127–132] However, this relationship is not necessarily straightforward, with 1 study reporting that tibiofemoral alignment did not predict incident tibiofemoral OA, suggesting that instead tibiofemoral alignment may be a marker of disease or progression.[133] Another paradigm is that increased body mass index is a risk factor for incident OA but in one study it only affected OA progression in knees with moderate malalignment (odds ratio [OR] 1.23), not neutral knees.[134] A subsequent study showed that a high body mass index increased risk of OA progression only in neutral and valgus knees (OR 1.4 and 1.8, respectively).[135] These results are conflicting, indicating that further examination is necessary. Regardless, tibiofemoral alignment has also been shown to be protective against cartilage loss in the less loaded compartment, as assessed by MRI (OR 3.7 and 6.0 for the protected lateral and medial compartments, respectively).[136] Tibiofemoral alignment has also been shown to be associated with patellofemoral OA.[127,128,131,137] Varus tibiofemoral malalignment increases the odds of medial compartment radiographic patellofemoral OA progression (OR 1.85) and valgus tibiofemoral malalignment increases the odds of lateral compartment patellofemoral OA progression (OR 1.64).[127] More recently, the relationship between alignment and cartilage tissue properties, as assessed noninvasively by MRI, has also been studied. For example, in a study using delayed gadolinium-enhanced magnetic resonance imaging of cartilage as a measure of cartilage health, knees in valgus tended to have lower dGEMRIC values (less proteoglycan) in the lateral compartment, and knees in varus tended to have lower dGEMRIC values in the medial compartment.[138] T2 relaxation times have also been shown to be increased in the medial compartment of individuals with varus malalignment.[139] Together, these data suggest that tibiofemoral alignment plays an important role in OA but, in some instances, this role is part of a complex interaction with other mechanical risk factors.

Patellar alignment, along with tibiofemoral alignment, plays an important role in patellofemoral OA. Lateral patellar alignment has been associated with lateral joint space narrowing (OR 8.26),[140] lateral osteophytes (OR 3.07),[140] lateral cartilage loss (OR 3.4),[141] and lateral bone marrow lesions (OR 3.2).[142] Medial patellar alignment has been associated with medial joint space narrowing (OR 2.85).[140] In a study of OA progression, medial displacement of the patella increased the risk of medial patellofemoral joint space narrowing progression (OR 2.2), whereas it was protective of lateral patellofemoral joint space narrowing progression (OR 0.4), and increasing lateral tilt was protective of medial patellofemoral joint space narrowing progression (OR 0.2).[143] It has also been shown that patella alta (a high-riding patella) is associated with lateral joint space narrowing (OR 2.77),[140] lateral osteophytes (OR 1.67),[140] medial and lateral cartilage loss (OR 2.0–2.4 and 1.5–2.0, respectively),[141,144] and medial and lateral bone marrow lesions (OR 2.5–2.9)[141,144] and medial and lateral subchondral bone attrition (OR 2.2 and 3.5, respectively).[144] There is a high prevalence of medial patellofemoral OA that is independent of alignment.[145] This highlights that alignment alone does not explain all patellofemoral OA and perhaps more complex techniques, such as assessments of three-dimensional kinematics and contact area, may be required to understand the relationship between mechanics and patellofemoral OA.

Other Surrogates for High Joint Forces

Several studies have found associations between surrogate measures of high joint forces and OA. As discussed previously, joint forces cannot be measured directly, but estimates based on anthropometry, joint congruency or alignment, gait analysis, and activities of daily living can be used to study the effect of higher joint forces. Several mechanical factors have been associated with radiographic and/or MRI-based definitions of OA such as obesity,[135,146–148] patellar alignment,[140–142] knee height,[149] squatting,[150] and meniscectomy.[132,151] Although these are not direct measures of mechanics, these associations suggest that mechanics play a role in OA. For example, knee height, which contributes to increased moments about the knee and associated higher theoretic contact forces in the joints, was associated with an increasing prevalence of symptomatic and radiographic knee OA.[152] More specifically, increased knee height, measured from the ground to the femoral condyles when sitting, was associated with radiographic patellofemoral OA in men (OR 1.7) and was associated with symptomatic patellofemoral OA in women (OR 2.2).[152] Prolonged squatting (which theoretically produces high forces in the knee) in elderly Chinese men was also associated with higher risk for knee OA.[150] Obesity has been identified as a risk factor of both patellofemoral OA and tibiofemoral OA.[146,147] Obesity puts individuals at greater risk of radiographic patellofemoral OA than radiographic tibiofemoral OA (OR 3.5, 7, and 1.9 for isolated patellofemoral, combined, and tibiofemoral OA, respectively).[146] Gait analysis is probably the most widely used tool to estimate joint loads in OA. One of the strongest relationships established using gait analysis is that knee adduction moment is associated with OA.[153–155] A more recent study showed that cumulative knee adductor load was better than the peak knee adduction moment at discriminating between healthy and OA groups.[156] Gait analysis has also revealed that mechanics at other joints such as the hip and ankle can affect OA at the knee. For example, medial tibiofemoral compartment OA is associated with hip adduction moments and higher axial loading rates at the hip, knee, and ankle.[157] Gait parameters at the hip, knee, and ankle also vary, depending on the severity of OA.[158] It has been suggested that the changes in gait mechanics may be a compensatory mechanism to reduce pain by reducing loads at the affected joint.[159–161] Asymmetric gait patterns have also been shown in subjects who have advanced hip OA[162] and in subjects with unilateral knee OA.[163] In the latter study, individuals with bilateral OA did not display the same asymmetry in gait patterns. Ankle mechanics have been studied to a lesser extent than knee and hip mechanics, but it has been shown that a greater toe-out angle[164] and load[157] is associated with the progression of medial tibiofemoral OA. All these surrogate measures of joint loading provide information about the relative magnitudes of force being transmitted through the joint, but they do not indicate where on the joint surface these loads are transmitted. Advances in weight-bearing imaging may provide this information in the future.

Injury

Joint fractures and acute injury to the menisci and ACL are all associated with the development of OA, but the specifics of how injury affects mechanics, and how mechanical changes lead to OA, are not clear. Fractures of the joint surface at the hip, knee, and ankle are associated with high rates of OA, and the development of OA is related to increased contact stress caused by the fracture.[165] Meniscal and ACL injuries are well-known factors in the development of early knee OA.[166] Forty-three percent of subjects who had undergone meniscectomy because of meniscal tears had radiographic evidence of OA after 16 years,[167] meniscectomy increases risk of developing OA (OR 2.6),[151,168–171] 51% of female soccer players with ACL injury had radiographic evidence of OA after 12 years,[172] and 41% of male soccer players with ACL injury had radiographic evidence of OA after 14 years.[173] A study of ACL injury in a population of individuals with symptomatic knee OA found that a complete ACL tear increased the risk for medial tibiofemoral cartilage thinning compared with those with intact ACL or partial ACL tears (OR 1.8, adjusted for age, body mass index, and gender).[174] However, once an adjustment for medial meniscal tears was included in the regression model, a complete ACL tear was not an independent risk factor of cartilage thinning (OR 1.1).[174] Bone marrow lesions were associated with ACL tears in the same cohort.[175] Although these acute injuries are associated with OA, and change in joint mechanics produced by the injuries plays a role in the causes of OA, many other factors related to the patient, injury, and treatment affect whether OA develops after injury, and at what rate.[166] Researchers have proposed hypotheses detailing the cascade of events involving the effect of ACL injury on knee mechanics, the resulting change in loading patterns, and the cartilage response.[176]

Deformity

In contrast with knee OA, hip OA is generally associated with either instability or deformity, with primary hip OA considered rare. Although the association between severe hip deformity and OA has been understood for decades, interest has more recently focused on the role of more subtle deformities. It is well accepted that many cases of idiopathic hip OA can be attributed to bony deformity.[177] The hypothesis that femoroacetabular impingement (FAI - contact between the femur and acetabulum due to deformity and/or extreme movement) is a major causal factor leading to hip OA has growing support in the orthopedic literature.[28,29,178] Two mechanisms by which the cartilage and labrum are affected by FAI have been described.[179] Cam impingement is a result of a nonspherical femoral head abutting against the acetabular rim in flexion and internal rotation (**Fig. 2**). The abutment causes damage to the anterosuperior acetabular cartilage. Pincer impingement occurs as a result of linear contact between the femoral head-neck junction and the acetabular rim. In support of the FAI hypothesis, many studies have shown associations between features of impingement and cartilage damage. For example, in a study of 149 hips with mild or no radiographic OA, patients with radiological features of cam impingement (26 hips) had damage to the anterosuperior acetabular cartilage, whereas patients with radiological features of pincer impingement (16 hips) had a narrow strip of circumferential cartilage damage.[180] Specific radiological features characteristic of FAI predicted progression to hip OA (over at least 10 years) in patients with a pistol-grip deformity.[181] Early cartilage changes were present in hip cartilage in participants with cam deformities who had not complained of osteoarthritic symptoms.[182] FAI is of particular concern given its high prevalence. The prevalence of cam deformities in young men was reported to be 24%,[183] and the prevalence of specific cam and pincer deformity signs was higher in men than in women.[184] Although hip deformity seems to be related to OA, it is not clear what dictates whether or not FAI deformities will lead to OA, how many patients with the symptoms of FAI have cartilage changes, at what stage osteoarthritic changes begin in FAI, how they progress, and whether they can be prevented or reversed.

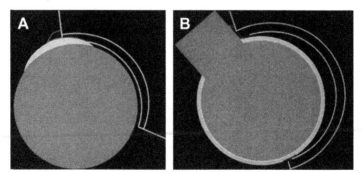

Fig. 2. Schematic illustrations of cam impingement (*A*) and pincer impingement (*B*). (*From* Ganz R, Parvizi J, Beck M, et al. Femoroacetabular impingement: a cause for osteoarthritis of the hip. Clin Orthop 2003;112–20; with permission.)

THE ROLE OF MECHANICS IN OA TREATMENT

Because of the clear role of mechanical factors in OA incidence and progression, some treatment approaches focus on modifying joint mechanics. Approaches include surgery, bracing, wedging, gait modification, walking aids, and muscle stretching and strengthening exercises. ACL repair is the treatment of choice for ligament rupture, with a leading justification for the procedure being protection of the joint from OA. Joint reconstruction including repair of the posterior cruciate ligament, medial collateral ligament, menisci, acetabular labrum, and many smaller structures is now widespread, and cartilage repair using grafts or engineered tissue is used to treat small lesions in young patients with traumatic damage to the cartilage. High tibial osteotomy is a surgical procedure used to treat tibiofemoral OA associated with abnormal tibiofemoral malalignment. In high tibial osteotomy, a wedge of bone from the proximal tibia is resected (closing wedge) or added (opening wedge) to realign the lower limb, placing more force on the lateral compartment of the knee (generally) in an effort to reduce pain and delay cartilage degeneration in the medial compartment.[185] Several groups have reported that high tibial osteotomy either arrests cartilage degeneration[186] or leads to cartilage regeneration[56,187] in the diseased compartment. Surgical correction of hip deformity associated with femoroacetabular impingement syndrome improves symptoms in most patients without advanced OA or chondral damage in the short term.[188] However, the longer term success of these procedures is not clear.[189] Conservative approaches to modifying mechanics include gait retraining, bracing, muscle stretching and training, modifying footwear with the objective of redistributing forces in the compartments of the knee, and using walking aids such as poles and canes to reduce or redistribute load in the knee.[190]

There is no simple explanation for why more mechanically based interventions are not being pursued. Weight loss is difficult, and exercise regimens require dedication. Insoles and braces can be uncomfortable and cumbersome. Joint reconstruction surgery is designed to protect the joint from OA in many instances, but its success is generally judged more on return to joint function in the short term rather than long-term incidence of OA. High tibial osteotomy is technically demanding, requires a long recovery, has yielded only mixed clinical success,[191,192] and has unicompartmental arthroplasty as an appealing alternative. Hip deformity correction is rapidly gaining interest, but is technically demanding. More generally, many surgeons are reluctant to operate on asymptomatic or mildly symptomatic joints, but intervening to restore joint integrity or correct a joint deformity may restore mechanics to normal and prove effective at averting the OA disease process.

SUMMARY

A lot has been learned about the links between mechanics and osteoarthritis (OA) in recent years. The findings are not always straightforward because OA and joint biomechanics are complex, and more knowledge is needed in this area. New and better methods for measuring joint mechanics promise to accelerate the pace of discovery. There is substantial scope for improving understanding of mechanically based treatments for OA and for developing new treatments that better address this prevalent and disabling condition.

ACKNOWLEDGMENTS

The authors are grateful to Dr Michael Hunt (Department of Physical Therapy, University of British Columbia) and Dr Angela Kedgley (Department of Bioengineering, Imperial College London, UK) for their valuable contributions to this article.

REFERENCES

1. Blanco FJ, Guitian R, Vazquez-Martul E, et al. Osteoarthritis chondrocytes die by apoptosis. A possible pathway for osteoarthritis pathology. Arthritis Rheum 1998;41(2):284–9.
2. Aigner T, McKenna L. Molecular pathology and pathobiology of osteoarthritic cartilage. Cell Mol Life Sci 2002;59(1):5–18.
3. Mankin HJ, Dorfman H, Lippiello L, et al. Biochemical and metabolic abnormalities in articular cartilage from osteo-arthritic human hips. II. Correlation of morphology with biochemical and metabolic data. J Bone Joint Surg Am 1971; 53(3):523–37.
4. Green DM, Noble PC, Ahuero JS, et al. Cellular events leading to chondrocyte death after cartilage impact injury. Arthritis Rheum 2006;54(5):1509–17.
5. Huser CA, Davies ME. Validation of an in vitro single-impact load model of the initiation of osteoarthritis-like changes in articular cartilage. J Orthop Res 2006;24(4):725–32.
6. Whiteside RA, Jakob RP, Wyss UP, et al. Impact loading of articular cartilage during transplantation of osteochondral autograft. J Bone Joint Surg Br 2005; 87(9):1285–91.
7. Nishimuta JF, Levenston ME. Response of cartilage and meniscus tissue explants to in vitro compressive overload. Osteoarthritis Cartilage 2012;20(5): 422–9.
8. Anderson JJ, Felson DT. Factors associated with osteoarthritis of the knee in the first national Health and Nutrition Examination Survey (HANES I). Evidence for an association with overweight, race, and physical demands of work. Am J Epidemiol 1988;128(1):179–89.
9. Setton LA, Elliott DM, Mow VC. Altered mechanics of cartilage with osteoarthritis: human osteoarthritis and an experimental model of joint degeneration. Osteoarthritis Cartilage 1999;7(1):2–14.
10. Andriacchi TP, Mundermann A, Smith RL, et al. A framework for the in vivo pathomechanics of osteoarthritis at the knee. Ann Biomed Eng 2004;32(3):447–57.
11. Guilak F, Ratcliffe A, Lane N, et al. Mechanical and biochemical changes in the superficial zone of articular cartilage in canine experimental osteoarthritis. J Orthop Res 1994;12(4):474–84.
12. Maniwa S, Nishikori T, Furukawa S, et al. Alteration of collagen network and negative charge of articular cartilage surface in the early stage of experimental osteoarthritis. Arch Orthop Trauma Surg 2001;121(4):181–5.
13. Lane Smith R, Trindade MC, Ikenoue T, et al. Effects of shear stress on articular chondrocyte metabolism. Biorheology 2000;37(1–2):95–107.
14. Smith RL, Carter DR, Schurman DJ. Pressure and shear differentially alter human articular chondrocyte metabolism: a review. Clin Orthop Relat Res 2004;(Suppl 427):S89–95.
15. Radin EL, Rose RM. Role of subchondral bone in the initiation and progression of cartilage damage. Clin Orthop Relat Res 1986;(213):34–40.
16. Radin EL, Paul IL, Rose RM. Role of mechanical factors in pathogenesis of primary osteoarthritis. Lancet 1972;1(7749):519–22.
17. Radin EL, Parker HG, Pugh JW, et al. Response of joints to impact loading. 3. Relationship between trabecular microfractures and cartilage degeneration. J Biomech 1973;6(1):51–7.
18. Burr DB, Radin EL. Microfractures and microcracks in subchondral bone: are they relevant to osteoarthrosis? Rheum Dis Clin North Am 2003;29(4):675–85.

19. Lindsey CT, Narasimhan A, Adolfo JM, et al. Magnetic resonance evaluation of the interrelationship between articular cartilage and trabecular bone of the osteoarthritic knee. Osteoarthritis Cartilage 2004;12(2):86–96.
20. Lo GH, Zhang Y, McLennan C, et al. The ratio of medial to lateral tibial plateau bone mineral density and compartment-specific tibiofemoral osteoarthritis. Osteoarthritis Cartilage 2006;14(10):984–90.
21. Bennell KL, Creaby MW, Wrigley TV, et al. Tibial subchondral trabecular volumetric bone density in medial knee joint osteoarthritis using peripheral quantitative computed tomography technology. Arthritis Rheum 2008;58(9):2776–85.
22. Kellgren JH, Lawrence JS. Radiological assessment of osteo-arthrosis. Ann Rheum Dis 1957;16(4):494–502.
23. Burstein D, Gray ML. Is MRI fulfilling its promise for molecular imaging of cartilage in arthritis? Osteoarthritis Cartilage 2006;14:1087–90.
24. Wilson DR, Apreleva MV, Eichler MJ, et al. Accuracy and repeatability of a pressure measurement system in the patellofemoral joint. J Biomech 2003;36(12):1909–15.
25. Radin EL, Ehrlich MG, Chernack R, et al. Effect of repetitive impulsive loading on the knee joints of rabbits. Clin Orthop Relat Res 1978;(131):288–93.
26. Song Y, Greve JM, Carter DR, et al. Articular cartilage MR imaging and thickness mapping of a loaded knee joint before and after meniscectomy. Osteoarthritis Cartilage 2006;14(8):728–37.
27. Pan B, Wu DF, Wang ZY. Internal displacement and strain measurement using digital volume correlation: a least-squares framework. Meas Sci Technol 2012;23(4).
28. Banerjee P, McLean CR. Femoroacetabular impingement: a review of diagnosis and management. Curr Rev Musculoskelet Med 2011;4(1):23–32.
29. Leunig M, Beaule PE, Ganz R. The concept of femoroacetabular impingement: current status and future perspectives. Clin Orthop Relat Res 2009;467(3):616–22.
30. Ahmed AM, Burke DL, Yu A. In-vitro measurement of static pressure distribution in synovial joints–Part II: retropatellar surface. J Biomech Eng 1983;105(3):226–36.
31. Ahmed AM, Duncan NA. Correlation of patellar tracking pattern with trochlear and retropatellar surface topographies. J Biomech Eng 2000;122(6):652–60.
32. Ahmed AM, Duncan NA, Tanzer M. In vitro measurement of the tracking pattern of the human patella. J Biomech Eng 1999;121(2):222–8.
33. Huberti HH, Hayes WC. Contact pressures in chondromalacia patellae and the effects of capsular reconstructive procedures. J Orthop Res 1988;6(4):499–508.
34. Huberti HH, Hayes WC. Patellofemoral contact pressures. The influence of q-angle and tendofemoral contact. J Bone Joint Surg Am 1984;66(5):715–24.
35. Ateshian GA, Kwak SD, Soslowsky LJ, et al. A stereophotogrammetric method for determining in situ contact areas in diarthrodial joints, and a comparison with other methods. J Biomech 1994;27(1):111–24.
36. Brown TD, Shaw DT. In vitro contact stress distributions in the natural human hip. J Biomech 1983;16(6):373–84.
37. Apreleva M, Hasselman CT, Debski RE, et al. A dynamic analysis of glenohumeral motion after simulated capsulolabral injury. A cadaver model. J Bone Joint Surg Am 1998;80(4):474–80.
38. Blankevoort L, Huiskes R. Validation of a three-dimensional model of the knee. J Biomech 1996;29(7):955–61.

39. Elias JJ, Wilson DR, Adamson R, et al. Evaluation of a computational model used to predict the patellofemoral contact pressure distribution. J Biomech 2004;37(3):295–302.
40. Wismans J, Veldpaus F, Janssen J, et al. A three-dimensional mathematical model of the knee-joint. J Biomech 1980;13(8):677–85.
41. Blankevoort L, Kuiper JH, Huiskes R, et al. Articular contact in a three-dimensional model of the knee. J Biomech 1991;24(11):1019–31.
42. van der Helm FC. A finite element musculoskeletal model of the shoulder mechanism. J Biomech 1994;27(5):551–69.
43. Brown TD, DiGioia AM 3rd. A contact-coupled finite element analysis of the natural adult hip. J Biomech 1984;17(6):437–48.
44. Ahmad CS, Kwak SD, Ateshian GA, et al. Effects of patellar tendon adhesion to the anterior tibia on knee mechanics. Am J Sports Med 1998;26(5):715–24.
45. Kwak SD, Ahmad CS, Gardner TR, et al. Hamstrings and iliotibial band forces affect knee kinematics and contact pattern. J Orthop Res 2000;18(1):101–8.
46. Cohen ZA, Henry JH, McCarthy DM, et al. Computer simulations of patellofemoral joint surgery. Patient-specific models for tuberosity transfer. Am J Sports Med 2003;31(1):87–98.
47. Cohen ZA, Roglic H, Grelsamer RP, et al. Patellofemoral stresses during open and closed kinetic chain exercises. An analysis using computer simulation. Am J Sports Med 2001;29(4):480–7.
48. Hadley NA, Brown TD, Weinstein SL. The effects of contact pressure elevations and aseptic necrosis on the long-term outcome of congenital hip dislocation. J Orthop Res 1990;8(4):504–13.
49. McErlain DD, Milner JS, Ivanov TG, et al. Subchondral cysts create increased intra-osseous stress in early knee OA: a finite element analysis using simulated lesions. Bone 2011;48(3):639–46.
50. van Lenthe GH, Muller R. Prediction of failure load using micro-finite element analysis models: towards in vivo strength assessment. Drug Discov Today Tech 2006;3(2):221–9.
51. Helgason B, Perilli E, Schileo E, et al. Mathematical relationships between bone density and mechanical properties: a literature review. Clin Biomech (Bristol, Avon) 2008;23(2):135–46.
52. Samosky JT, Burstein D, Eric Grimson W, et al. Spatially-localized correlation of dGEMRIC-measured GAG distribution and mechanical stiffness in the human tibial plateau. J Orthop Res 2005;23(1):93–101.
53. MacNeil JA, Boyd SK. Bone strength at the distal radius can be estimated from high-resolution peripheral quantitative computed tomography and the finite element method. Bone 2008;42(6):1203–13.
54. Keyak JH, Rossi SA. Prediction of femoral fracture load using finite element models: an examination of stress- and strain-based failure theories. J Biomech 2000;33(2):209–14.
55. Bay BK. Methods and applications of digital volume correlation. J Strain Anal Eng 2008;43(8):745–60.
56. Kanamiya T, Naito M, Hara M, et al. The influences of biomechanical factors on cartilage regeneration after high tibial osteotomy for knees with medial compartment osteoarthritis: clinical and arthroscopic observations. Arthroscopy 2002;18(7):725–9.
57. Ito K, Minka MA, Leunig M, et al. Femoroacetabular impingement and the cam-effect. A MRI-based quantitative anatomical study of the femoral head-neck offset. J Bone Joint Surg Br 2001;83(2):171–6.

58. Morrison JB. The mechanics of the knee joint in relation to normal walking. J Biomech 1970;3(1):51–61.
59. Li K, Zheng L, Tashman S, et al. The inaccuracy of surface-measured model-derived tibiofemoral kinematics. J Biomech 2012;45(15):2719–23.
60. Andriacchi TP, Alexander EJ, Toney MK, et al. A point cluster method for in vivo motion analysis: applied to a study of knee kinematics. J Biomech Eng 1998; 120(6):743–9.
61. D'Lima DD, Fregly BJ, Patil S, et al. Knee joint forces: prediction, measurement, and significance. Proc Inst Mech Eng H 2012;226(2):95–102.
62. Cleather DJ, Bull AM. The development of lower limb musculoskeletal models with clinical relevance is dependent upon the fidelity of the mathematical description of the lower limb. Part 2: patient-specific geometry. Proc Inst Mech Eng H 2012;226(2):133–45.
63. Delport HP, Banks SA, De Schepper J, et al. A kinematic comparison of fixed- and mobile-bearing knee replacements. J Bone Joint Surg Br 2006;88(8): 1016–21.
64. Kanisawa I, Banks AZ, Banks SA, et al. Weight-bearing knee kinematics in subjects with two types of anterior cruciate ligament reconstructions. Knee Surg Sports Traumatol Arthrosc 2003;11(1):16–22.
65. Amiri S, Anglin C, Agbanlog K, et al. A model-free feature-based bi-planar RSA method for kinematic analysis of total knee arthroplasty. J Biomech Eng 2012; 134(3):031009.
66. Karrholm J, Brandsson S, Freeman MA. Tibiofemoral movement 4: changes of axial tibial rotation caused by forced rotation at the weight-bearing knee studied by RSA. J Bone Joint Surg Br 2000;82(8):1201–3.
67. Fleming BC, Peura GD, Abate JA, et al. Accuracy and repeatability of Roentgen stereophotogrammetric analysis (RSA) for measuring knee laxity in longitudinal studies. J Biomech 2001;34(10):1355–9.
68. Martin DE, Greco NJ, Klatt BA, et al. Model-based tracking of the hip: implications for novel analyses of hip pathology. J Arthroplasty 2011;26(1):88–97.
69. Fox AM, Kedgley AE, Lalone EA, et al. The effect of decreasing computed tomography dosage on radiostereometric analysis (RSA) accuracy at the gleno-humeral joint. J Biomech 2011;44(16):2847–50.
70. You BM, Siy P, Anderst W, et al. In vivo measurement of 3-D skeletal kinematics from sequences of biplane radiographs: application to knee kinematics. IEEE Trans Med Imaging 2001;20(6):514–25.
71. Goyal K, Tashman S, Wang JH, et al. In vivo analysis of the isolated posterior cruciate ligament-deficient knee during functional activities. Am J Sports Med 2012;40(4):777–85.
72. Anderst WJ, Tashman S. A method to estimate in vivo dynamic articular surface interaction. J Biomech 2003;36(9):1291–9.
73. Anderst W, Zauel R, Bishop J, et al. Validation of three-dimensional model-based tibio-femoral tracking during running. Med Eng Phys 2009;31(1):10–6.
74. Bey MJ, Zauel R, Brock SK, et al. Validation of a new model-based tracking technique for measuring three-dimensional, in vivo glenohumeral joint kinematics. J Biomech Eng 2006;128(4):604–9.
75. Brossmann J, Muhle C, Schroder C, et al. Patellar tracking patterns during active and passive knee extension: evaluation with motion-triggered cine MR imaging. Radiology 1993;187(1):205–12.
76. Salsich GB, Ward SR, Terk MR, et al. In vivo assessment of patellofemoral joint contact area in individuals who are pain free. Clin Orthop 2003;(417):277–84.

77. Draper CE, Besier TF, Fredericson M, et al. Differences in patellofemoral kinematics between weight-bearing and non-weight-bearing conditions in patients with patellofemoral pain. J Orthop Res 2010;29(3):312–7.

78. Draper CE, Santos JM, Kourtis LC, et al. Feasibility of using real-time MRI to measure joint kinematics in 1.5T and open-bore 0.5T systems. J Magn Reson Imaging 2008;28(1):158–66.

79. Powers CM, Ward SR, Fredericson M, et al. Patellofemoral kinematics during weight-bearing and non-weight-bearing knee extension in persons with lateral subluxation of the patella: a preliminary study. J Orthop Sports Phys Ther 2003;33(11):677–85.

80. von Eisenhart-Rothe R, Siebert M, Bringmann C, et al. A new in vivo technique for determination of 3D kinematics and contact areas of the patello-femoral and tibio-femoral joint. J Biomech 2004;37(6):927–34.

81. Muhle C, Brossmann J, Heller M. Kinematic CT and MR imaging of the patello-femoral joint. Eur Radiol 1999;9(3):508–18.

82. Fellows RA, Hill NA, Gill HS, et al. Magnetic resonance imaging for in vivo assessment of three-dimensional patellar tracking. J Biomech 2005;38(8):1643–52.

83. Fellows RA, Hill NA, Macintyre NJ, et al. Repeatability of a novel technique for in vivo measurement of three-dimensional patellar tracking using magnetic resonance imaging. J Magn Reson Imaging 2005;22(1):145–53.

84. Patel VV, Hall K, Ries M, et al. Magnetic resonance imaging of patellofemoral kinematics with weight-bearing. J Bone Joint Surg Am 2003;85(12):2419–24.

85. Kaiser J, Bradford R, Johnson K, et al. Measurement of tibiofemoral kinematics using highly accelerated 3D radial sampling. Magn Reson Med 2012. [Epub ahead of print].

86. d'Entremont AG, Nordmeyer-Massner JA, Bos C, et al. Do dynamic-based MR knee kinematics methods produce the same results as static methods? Magn Reson Med 2012. [Epub ahead of print].

87. Sheehan FT, Drace JE. Quantitative MR measures of three-dimensional patellar kinematics as a research and diagnostic tool. Med Sci Sports Exerc 1999; 31(10):1399–405.

88. Sheehan FT, Zajac FE, Drace JE. Using cine phase contrast magnetic resonance imaging to non-invasively study in vivo knee dynamics. J Biomech 1998;31(1): 21–6.

89. Sheehan FT, Zajac FE, Drace JE. In vivo tracking of the human patella using cine phase contrast magnetic resonance imaging. J Biomech Eng 1999;121(6):650–6.

90. Barrance PJ, Williams GN, Novotny JE, et al. A method for measurement of joint kinematics in vivo by registration of 3-D geometric models with cine phase contrast magnetic resonance imaging data. J Biomech Eng 2005;127(5):829–37.

91. Rebmann AJ, Sheehan FT. Precise 3D skeletal kinematics using fast phase contrast magnetic resonance imaging. J Magn Reson Imaging 2003;17(2): 206–13.

92. Lerner AL, Tamez-Pena JG, Houck JR, et al. The use of sequential MR image sets for determining tibiofemoral motion: reliability of coordinate systems and accuracy of motion tracking algorithm. J Biomech Eng 2003;125(2):246–53.

93. Barrance PJ, Williams GN, Snyder-Mackler L, et al. Do ACL-injured copers exhibit differences in knee kinematics?: An MRI study. Clin Orthop Relat Res 2007;454:74–80.

94. Barrance PJ, Williams GN, Snyder-Mackler L, et al. Altered knee kinematics in ACL-deficient non-copers: a comparison using dynamic MRI. J Orthop Res 2006;24(2):132–40.

95. Patel VV, Hall K, Ries M, et al. A three-dimensional MRI analysis of knee kinematics. J Orthop Res 2004;22(2):283–92.
96. Draper CE, Besier TF, Santos JM, et al. Patellofemoral kinematic differences exist between high-load and low-load conditions in patients with patellofemoral pain. Paper presented at: American Society of Biomechanics Annual Meeting. State College. Philadelphia, August 26-29, 2009.
97. McWalter EJ, Hunter DJ, Wilson DR. The effect of load magnitude on three-dimensional patellar kinematics in vivo. J Biomech 2010;43(10):1890–7.
98. Besier TF, Draper CE, Gold GE, et al. Patellofemoral joint contact area increases with knee flexion and weight-bearing. J Orthop Res 2005;23(2):345–50.
99. Gold GE, Besier TF, Draper CE, et al. Weight-bearing MRI of patellofemoral joint cartilage contact area. J Magn Reson Imaging 2004;20(3):526–30.
100. Heino Brechter J, Powers CM, Terk MR, et al. Quantification of patellofemoral joint contact area using magnetic resonance imaging. Magn Reson Imaging 2003;21(9):955–9.
101. Hinterwimmer S, Gotthardt M, von Eisenhart-Rothe R, et al. In vivo contact areas of the knee in patients with patellar subluxation. J Biomech 2005;38(10):2095–101.
102. Hinterwimmer S, von Eisenhart-Rothe R, Siebert M, et al. Patella kinematics and patello-femoral contact areas in patients with genu varum and mild osteoarthritis. Clin Biomech (Bristol, Avon) 2004;19(7):704–10.
103. Nakagawa S, Kadoya Y, Kobayashi A, et al. Kinematics of the patella in deep flexion. Analysis with magnetic resonance imaging. J Bone Joint Surg Am 2003;85(7):1238–42.
104. Powers CM, Ward SR, Chan LD, et al. The effect of bracing on patella alignment and patellofemoral joint contact area. Med Sci Sports Exerc 2004;36(7):1226–32.
105. Ward SR, Powers CM. The influence of patella alta on patellofemoral joint stress during normal and fast walking. Clin Biomech (Bristol, Avon) 2004;19(10):1040–7.
106. Ward SR, Terk MR, Powers CM. Patella alta: association with patellofemoral alignment and changes in contact area during weight-bearing. J Bone Joint Surg Am 2007;89(8):1749–55.
107. Connolly KD, Ronsky JL, Westover LM, et al. Differences in patellofemoral contact mechanics associated with patellofemoral pain syndrome. J Biomech 2009;42(16):2802–7.
108. Shin CS, Carpenter RD, Majumdar S, et al. Three-dimensional in vivo patellofemoral kinematics and contact area of anterior cruciate ligament-deficient and -reconstructed subjects using magnetic resonance imaging. Arthroscopy 2009;25(11):1214–23.
109. Lalone EA, McDonald CP, Ferreira LM, et al. Development of an image-based technique to examine joint congruency at the elbow. Comput Methods Biomech Biomed Engin 2012. [Epub ahead of print].
110. Borotikar BS, Sipprell WH 3rd, Wible EE, et al. A methodology to accurately quantify patellofemoral cartilage contact kinematics by combining 3D image shape registration and cine-PC MRI velocity data. J Biomech 2012;45(6):1117–22.
111. Hosseini A, Van de Velde S, Gill TJ, et al. Tibiofemoral cartilage contact biomechanics in patients after reconstruction of a ruptured anterior cruciate ligament. J Orthop Res 2012;30(11):1781–8.
112. Subburaj K, Souza RB, Stehling C, et al. Association of MR relaxation and cartilage deformation in knee osteoarthritis. J Orthop Res 2012;30(6):919–26.
113. Shin CS, Souza RB, Kumar D, et al. In vivo tibiofemoral cartilage-to-cartilage contact area of females with medial osteoarthritis under acute loading using MRI. J Magn Reson Imaging 2011;34(6):1405–13.

114. Yao J, Lancianese SL, Hovinga KR, et al. Magnetic resonance image analysis of meniscal translation and tibio-menisco-femoral contact in deep knee flexion. J Orthop Res 2008;26(5):673–84.
115. Yao J, Salo AD, Lee J, et al. Sensitivity of tibio-menisco-femoral joint contact behavior to variations in knee kinematics. J Biomech 2008;41(2):390–8.
116. Connolly KD, Ronsky JL, Westover LM, et al. Analysis techniques for congruence of the patellofemoral joint. J Biomech Eng 2009;131(12):124503.
117. McWalter EJ, O'Kane CO, FitzPatrick DP, et al. Validation of an MRI-based method to assess patellofemoral joint contact areas in loaded knee flexion in vivo. J Magn Reson Imaging, in press.
118. Goto A, Moritomo H, Murase T, et al. In vivo elbow biomechanical analysis during flexion: three-dimensional motion analysis using magnetic resonance imaging. J Shoulder Elbow Surg 2004;13(4):441–7.
119. Lalone EA, Peters TM, King GW, et al. Accuracy assessment of an imaging technique to examine ulnohumeral joint congruency during elbow flexion. Comput Aided Surg 2012;17(3):142–52.
120. Chan DD, Neu CP, Hull ML. Articular cartilage deformation determined in an intact tibiofemoral joint by displacement-encoded imaging. Magn Reson Med 2009;61(4):989–93.
121. Chan DD, Neu CP, Hull ML. In situ deformation of cartilage in cyclically loaded tibiofemoral joints by displacement-encoded MRI. Osteoarthritis Cartilage 2009; 17(11):1461–8.
122. Greaves LL, Gilbart MK, Yung A, et al. Deformation and recovery of cartilage in the intact hip under physiological loads using 7T MRI. J Biomech 2009;42(3): 349–54.
123. Halder A, Kutzner I, Graichen F, et al. Influence of limb alignment on mediolateral loading in total knee replacement: in vivo measurements in five patients. J Bone Joint Surg Am 2012;94(11):1023–9.
124. Felson DT. Osteoarthritis as a disease of mechanics. Osteoarthritis Cartilage 2012. [Epub ahead of print].
125. Laxafoss E, Jacobsen S, Gosvig KK, et al. The alignment of the knee joint in relationship to age and osteoarthritis: the Copenhagen Osteoarthritis Study. Skeletal Radiol 2012. [Epub ahead of print].
126. Reid SM, Graham RB, Costigan PA. Differentiation of young and older adult stair climbing gait using principal component analysis. Gait Posture 2010;31(2): 197–203.
127. Cahue S, Dunlop D, Hayes K, et al. Varus-valgus alignment in the progression of patellofemoral osteoarthritis. Arthritis Rheum 2004;50(7):2184–90.
128. Elahi S, Cahue S, Felson DT, et al. The association between varus-valgus alignment and patellofemoral osteoarthritis. Arthritis Rheum 2000;43(8):1874–80.
129. Harrison MM, Cooke TD, Fisher SB, et al. Patterns of knee arthrosis and patellar subluxation. Clin Orthop Relat Res 1994;(309):56–63.
130. Sharma L. The role of proprioceptive deficits, ligamentous laxity, and malalignment in development and progression of knee osteoarthritis. J Rheumatol Suppl 2004;70:87–92.
131. Sharma L, Song J, Felson DT, et al. The role of knee alignment in disease progression and functional decline in knee osteoarthritis. JAMA 2001;286(2): 188–95.
132. Sharma L, Eckstein F, Song J, et al. Relationship of meniscal damage, meniscal extrusion, malalignment, and joint laxity to subsequent cartilage loss in osteoarthritic knees. Arthritis Rheum 2008;58(6):1716–26.

133. Hunter DJ, Niu J, Felson DT, et al. Knee alignment does not predict incident osteoarthritis: the Framingham Osteoarthritis Study. Arthritis Rheum 2007; 56(4):1212–8.
134. Felson DT, Goggins J, Niu J, et al. The effect of body weight on progression of knee osteoarthritis is dependent on alignment. Arthritis Rheum 2004;50(12):3904–9.
135. Niu J, Zhang YQ, Torner J, et al. Is obesity a risk factor for progressive radiographic knee osteoarthritis? Arthritis Rheum 2009;61(3):329–35.
136. Moisio K, Chang A, Eckstein F, et al. Varus-valgus alignment: reduced risk of subsequent cartilage loss in the less loaded compartment. Arthritis Rheum 2011;63(4):1002–9.
137. Cerejo R, Dunlop DD, Cahue S, et al. The influence of alignment on risk of knee osteoarthritis progression according to baseline stage of disease. Arthritis Rheum 2002;46(10):2632–6.
138. Williams A, Sharma L, McKenzie CA, et al. Delayed gadolinium-enhanced magnetic resonance imaging of cartilage in knee osteoarthritis: findings at different radiographic stages of disease and relationship to malalignment. Arthritis Rheum 2005;52(11):3528–35.
139. Friedrich KM, Shepard T, Chang G, et al. Does joint alignment affect the T2 values of cartilage in patients with knee osteoarthritis? Eur Radiol 2010;20(6): 1532–8.
140. Kalichman L, Zhang Y, Niu J, et al. The association between patellar alignment on magnetic resonance imaging and radiographic manifestations of knee osteoarthritis. Arthritis Res Ther 2007;9(2):R26.
141. Kalichman L, Zhang Y, Niu J, et al. The association between patellar alignment and patellofemoral joint osteoarthritis features–an MRI study. Rheumatology (Oxford) 2007;46(8):1303–8.
142. Kalichman L, Zhu Y, Zhang Y, et al. The association between patella alignment and knee pain and function: an MRI study in persons with symptomatic knee osteoarthritis. Osteoarthritis Cartilage 2007;15(11):1235–40.
143. Hunter DJ, Zhang YQ, Niu JB, et al. Patella malalignment, pain and patellofemoral progression: the Health ABC Study. Osteoarthritis Cartilage 2007;15(10):1120–7.
144. Stefanik JJ, Zhu Y, Zumwalt AC, et al. Association between patella alta and the prevalence and worsening of structural features of patellofemoral joint osteoarthritis: the Multicenter Osteoarthritis Study. Arthritis Care Res (Hoboken) 2010; 62(9):1258–65.
145. Gross KD, Niu J, Stefanik JJ, et al. Breaking the Law of Valgus: the surprising and unexplained prevalence of medial patellofemoral cartilage damage. Ann Rheum Dis 2012;71(11):1827–32.
146. McAlindon T, Zhang Y, Hannan M, et al. Are risk factors for patellofemoral and tibiofemoral knee osteoarthritis different? J Rheumatol 1996;23(2):332–7.
147. Cicuttini FM, Spector T, Baker J. Risk factors for osteoarthritis in the tibiofemoral and patellofemoral joints of the knee. J Rheumatol 1997;24(6):1164–7.
148. Cooper C, McAlindon T, Snow S, et al. Mechanical and constitutional risk factors for symptomatic knee osteoarthritis: differences between medial tibiofemoral and patellofemoral disease. J Rheumatol 1994;21(2):307–13.
149. Hunter DJ, Zhang Y, Niu J, et al. Structural factors associated with malalignment in knee osteoarthritis: the Boston Osteoarthritis Knee Study. J Rheumatol 2005; 32(11):2192–9.
150. Zhang Y, Hunter DJ, Nevitt MC, et al. Association of squatting with increased prevalence of radiographic tibiofemoral knee osteoarthritis: the Beijing Osteoarthritis Study. Arthritis Rheum 2004;50(4):1187–92.

151. Englund M, Lohmander LS. Patellofemoral osteoarthritis coexistent with tibiofemoral osteoarthritis in a meniscectomy population. Ann Rheum Dis 2005;64(12): 1721–6.

152. Hunter DJ, Niu J, Zhang Y, et al. Knee height, knee pain, and knee osteoarthritis: the Beijing Osteoarthritis Study. Arthritis Rheum 2005;52(5):1418–23.

153. Baliunas AJ, Hurwitz DE, Ryals AB, et al. Increased knee joint loads during walking are present in subjects with knee osteoarthritis. Osteoarthritis Cartilage 2002;10(7):573–9.

154. Foroughi N, Smith R, Vanwanseele B. The association of external knee adduction moment with biomechanical variables in osteoarthritis: a systematic review. Knee 2009;16(5):303–9.

155. Mundermann A, Dyrby CO, Hurwitz DE, et al. Potential strategies to reduce medial compartment loading in patients with knee osteoarthritis of varying severity: reduced walking speed. Arthritis Rheum 2004;50(4):1172–8.

156. Maly MR, Robbins SM, Stratford PW, et al. Cumulative knee adductor load distinguishes between healthy and osteoarthritic knees-A proof of principle study. Gait Posture 2012. [Epub ahead of print].

157. Mundermann A, Dyrby CO, Andriacchi TP. Secondary gait changes in patients with medial compartment knee osteoarthritis: increased load at the ankle, knee, and hip during walking. Arthritis Rheum 2005;52(9):2835–44.

158. Astephen JL, Deluzio KJ, Caldwell GE, et al. Gait and neuromuscular pattern changes are associated with differences in knee osteoarthritis severity levels. J Biomech 2008;41(4):868–76.

159. Hurwitz DE, Hulet CH, Andriacchi TP, et al. Gait compensations in patients with osteoarthritis of the hip and their relationship to pain and passive hip motion. J Orthop Res 1997;15(4):629–35.

160. McGibbon CA, Krebs DE. Compensatory gait mechanics in patients with unilateral knee arthritis. J Rheumatol 2002;29(11):2410–9.

161. Chang A, Hayes K, Dunlop D, et al. Hip abduction moment and protection against medial tibiofemoral osteoarthritis progression. Arthritis Rheum 2005; 52(11):3515–9.

162. Shakoor N, Hurwitz DE, Block JA, et al. Asymmetric knee loading in advanced unilateral hip osteoarthritis. Arthritis Rheum 2003;48(6):1556–61.

163. Creaby MW, Bennell KL, Hunt MA. Gait differs between unilateral and bilateral knee osteoarthritis. Arch Phys Med Rehabil 2012;93(5):822–7.

164. Chang A, Hurwitz D, Dunlop D, et al. The relationship between toe-out angle during gait and progression of medial tibiofemoral osteoarthritis. Ann Rheum Dis 2007;66(10):1271–5.

165. Anderson DD, Marsh JL, Brown TD. The pathomechanical etiology of post-traumatic osteoarthritis following intraarticular fractures. Iowa Orthop J 2011; 31:1–20.

166. Lohmander LS, Englund PM, Dahl LL, et al. The long-term consequence of anterior cruciate ligament and meniscus injuries: osteoarthritis. Am J Sports Med 2007;35(10):1756–69.

167. Englund M, Joud A, Geborek P, et al. Prevalence and incidence of rheumatoid arthritis in southern Sweden 2008 and their relation to prescribed biologics. Rheumatology (Oxford) 2010;49(8):1563–9.

168. Crema MD, Roemer FW, Felson DT, et al. Factors associated with meniscal extrusion in knees with or at risk for osteoarthritis: the Multicenter Osteoarthritis Study. Radiology 2012;264(2):494–503.

169. Englund M, Felson DT, Guermazi A, et al. Risk factors for medial meniscal pathology on knee MRI in older US adults: a multicentre prospective cohort study. Ann Rheum Dis 2011;70(10):1733–9.
170. Englund M, Guermazi A, Gale D, et al. Incidental meniscal findings on knee MRI in middle-aged and elderly persons. N Engl J Med 2008;359(11):1108–15.
171. Englund M, Guermazi A, Roemer FW, et al. Meniscal pathology on MRI increases the risk for both incident and enlarging subchondral bone marrow lesions of the knee: the MOST Study. Ann Rheum Dis 2010;69(10):1796–802.
172. Lohmander LS, Felson D. Can we identify a 'high risk' patient profile to determine who will experience rapid progression of osteoarthritis? Osteoarthritis Cartilage 2004;12(Suppl A):S49–52.
173. von Porat A, Roos EM, Roos H. High prevalence of osteoarthritis 14 years after an anterior cruciate ligament tear in male soccer players: a study of radiographic and patient relevant outcomes. Ann Rheum Dis 2004;63(3):269–73.
174. Amin S, Guermazi A, Lavalley MP, et al. Complete anterior cruciate ligament tear and the risk for cartilage loss and progression of symptoms in men and women with knee osteoarthritis. Osteoarthritis Cartilage 2008;16(8):897–902.
175. Hernandez-Molina G, Guermazi A, Niu J, et al. Central bone marrow lesions in symptomatic knee osteoarthritis and their relationship to anterior cruciate ligament tears and cartilage loss. Arthritis Rheum 2008;58(1):130–6.
176. Chaudhari AM, Briant PL, Bevill SL, et al. Knee kinematics, cartilage morphology, and osteoarthritis after ACL injury. Med Sci Sports Exerc 2008;40(2):215–22.
177. Harris WH. Etiology of osteoarthritis of the hip. Clin Orthop 1986;(213):20–33.
178. Imam S, Khanduja V. Current concepts in the diagnosis and management of femoroacetabular impingement. Int Orthop 2011;35(10):1427–35.
179. Beck M, Kalhor M, Leunig M, et al. Hip morphology influences the pattern of damage to the acetabular cartilage: femoroacetabular impingement as a cause of early osteoarthritis of the hip. J Bone Joint Surg Br 2005;87(7):1012–8.
180. Beck M, Leunig M, Parvizi J, et al. Anterior femoroacetabular impingement: part II. Midterm results of surgical treatment. Clin Orthop 2004;(418):67–73.
181. Bardakos NV, Villar RN. Predictors of progression of osteoarthritis in femoroacetabular impingement: a radiological study with a minimum of ten years follow-up. J Bone Joint Surg Br 2009;91(2):162–9.
182. Pollard TC, McNally EG, Wilson DC, et al. Localized cartilage assessment with three-dimensional dGEMRIC in asymptomatic hips with normal morphology and cam deformity. J Bone Joint Surg Am 2010;92(15):2557–69.
183. Reichenbach S, Juni P, Werlen S, et al. Prevalence of cam-type deformity on hip magnetic resonance imaging in young males: a cross-sectional study. Arthritis Care Res (Hoboken) 2010;62(9):1319–27.
184. Laborie LB, Lehmann TG, Engesaeter IO, et al. Prevalence of radiographic findings thought to be associated with femoroacetabular impingement in a population-based cohort of 2081 healthy young adults. Radiology 2011;260(2): 494–502.
185. Coventry MB. Osteotomy of the upper portion of the tibia for degenerative arthritis of the knee. A preliminary report. J Bone Joint Surg Am 1965;47:984–90.
186. Wakabayashi S, Akizuki S, Takizawa T, et al. A comparison of the healing potential of fibrillated cartilage versus eburnated bone in osteoarthritic knees after high tibial osteotomy: an arthroscopic study with 1-year follow-up. Arthroscopy 2002;18(3):272–8.

187. Odenbring S, Egund N, Lindstrand A, et al. Cartilage regeneration after proximal tibial osteotomy for medial gonarthrosis. An arthroscopic, roentgenographic, and histologic study. Clin Orthop 1992;(277):210–6.

188. Ng VY, Arora N, Best TM, et al. Efficacy of surgery for femoroacetabular impingement: a systematic review. Am J Sports Med 2010;38(11):2337–45.

189. Clohisy JC, St John LC, Schutz AL. Surgical treatment of femoroacetabular impingement: a systematic review of the literature. Clin Orthop Relat Res 2010;468(2):555–64.

190. Reeves ND, Bowling FL. Conservative biomechanical strategies for knee osteoarthritis. Nat Rev Rheumatol 2011;7(2):113–22.

191. Rinonapoli E, Mancini GB, Corvaglia A, et al. Tibial osteotomy for varus gonarthrosis. A 10- to 21-year followup study. Clin Orthop 1998;(353):185–93.

192. W-Dahl A, Robertsson O, Lohmander LS. High tibial osteotomy in Sweden, 1998–2007: a population-based study of the use and rate of revision to knee arthroplasty. Acta Orthop 2012;83(3):244–8.

Diagnosis and Clinical Presentation of Osteoarthritis

A. Abhishek, MD, MRCP*, Michael Doherty, MD, FRCP

KEYWORDS

- Osteoarthritis • Clinical features • Differential diagnosis

KEY POINTS

- Osteoarthritis (OA) has a marked variability of clinical presentation and prognosis.
- OA targets specific joints (eg, knees, hips, finger IPJs, thumb bases, first metatarsophalangeal joints, and spinal facet joints).
- Frequent symptoms and signs include usage-related joint pain, morning-related or inactivity-related stiffness of short duration, locomotor restriction, coarse crepitus, bony enlargement, and joint-line tenderness.
- Rest pain, night pain, and deformity suggest severe OA.
- Painful periarticular soft tissue disorders frequently coexist with knee, hip, and first metatarsophalangeal OA.
- The diagnosis of OA may be reached without any laboratory or radiographic investigations in the at-risk population in the presence of typical signs and symptoms.
- Associated calcium pyrophosphate and basic calcium phosphate crystal deposition is common, especially in the elderly, and may be associated with inflammatory symptoms and signs.

INTRODUCTION

Osteoarthritis (OA) is a condition of synovial joints that represents failed repair of joint damage that results from stresses that may be initiated by an abnormality in any of the synovial joint tissues.[1] OA may be localized to 1 joint, to a few joints, or be generalized.[1] It is the commonest arthropathy, and presents with joint pain, locomotor restriction, and varying degrees of functional impairment.[2,3] It has a marked variability of phenotypic expression. The age of onset, pattern of joint involvement, and rate of progression vary from person to person and from site to site. For example, OA may be an asymptomatic incidental finding on clinical or radiographic examination, or be

Disclosures: None.
Academic Rheumatology, University of Nottingham, Nottingham, NG5 1PB, UK
* Corresponding author.
E-mail address: docabhishek@gmail.com

Rheum Dis Clin N Am 39 (2013) 45–66
http://dx.doi.org/10.1016/j.rdc.2012.10.007
0889-857X/13/$ – see front matter © 2013 Elsevier Inc. All rights reserved.

a progressive, painful, and disabling disorder at different joints in the same person. Thus there is an imperfect overlap between the disease OA (structural changes visualized on imaging) and the illness OA (patients' reported symptoms).[1] This article describes the clinical features of OA with an emphasis on symptoms and signs at the key target sites.

CLINICAL FEATURES

Pain, stiffness, and locomotor restriction are the main symptoms of OA (**Table 1**).[3] Other symptoms include crepitus, joint deformity, or joint swelling (caused by bony remodeling, excessive osteophytosis, or joint subluxation). These symptoms typically begin in just 1 or a few joints in a person of middle or older age.

Pain worse with joint use and relieved by rest (usage or mechanical pain) is often the most troublesome symptom. The origin of pain in OA is not completely understood. Pain may arise from the nociceptive fibers and mechanoreceptors in the synovium, subchondral bone, periosteum, capsule, tendons, or ligaments. Pain in large joint

Table 1 Principal manifestations of OA	
Symptoms	
Joint pain	Usually affects 1 to few joints at a time Insidious onset: slow progression over months to years Variable intensity throughout the day and the week May be intermittent and relapsing Increased by joint use and impact Relieved by rest Night pain may occur in severe OA
Stiffness	Short-lived (<30 min) early morning stiffness Short-lived inactivity-related stiffness (gelling)
Swelling	Some (eg, nodal OA) patients present with swelling and/or deformity
Age	>40 y[a]
Constitutional symptoms (eg, weight loss, sweats, fever)	Absent
Signs	
Appearance	Swelling (usually bony ± fluid/soft tissue) Resting position (attitude) Deformity Muscle wasting (global: all muscles acting over the joint)
Feel	Absence of warmth Swelling: bony or effusion Effusion if present is usually small and cool Joint-line tenderness Periarticular tenderness (especially knee, hip)
Movement	Coarse crepitus[b] Reduced range of movement Weak local muscles

[a] Major joint injury and certain rare conditions may predispose to OA before the age of 40 years.
[b] Audible crepitus may be a symptom of knee OA.
Adapted from Abhishek A, Doherty M. Disease diagnosis and clinical presentation. In: Henrotin Y, Hunter DJ, Kawaguchi H, editors. OARSI Online Primer. OARSI; 2011.

OA (eg, knee or hip) is also thought to arise from bone marrow lesions, and synovitis/ effusion by stimulation of nociceptive fibers and intra-articular hypertension, respectively,[4,5] and a similar mechanism may also operate in the small joints. However, hyaline cartilage is aneural, and is not a source of pain in OA. Whatever its source, both central and peripheral sensitization perpetuate and amplify pain in OA. Pain generally progresses through 3 stages (**Table 2**).[6] However, pain progression may be arrested at any stage, and not all patients go through 3 distinct stages.

Temporal and seasonal variations in OA pain have been reported as for other arthropathies. Pain in OA is reported to be worst on waking up in the morning, with an improvement in the next 2 hours.[7] It then worsens in the late afternoon/early evening to again reduce later in the evening.[7] However, night pain can be present in OA, which interferes with sleep and leads to fatigue, lack of well-being, and increased pain sensitivity. Such nonusage night pain is thought to arise largely from the subchondral bone. In some people, the pain has a burning (neuropathic) quality, is widespread around the joint, and associates with tenderness and paresthesiae.[6] Such features also suggest comorbid fibromyalgia, another common pain syndrome in older people.

Painful periarticular soft tissue lesions may coexist with large joint OA[8] (eg, pesanserine bursitis, greater trochanter pain syndrome) and it may be difficult to identify the cause of the pain. One solution to this problem is to ask the patient to point to the most painful area and then to map out the area that feels uncomfortable. Periarticular soft tissue lesions cause localized pain away from the joint line, whereas OA pain more commonly is most severe over the joint line except for proximal joints (hip, shoulder), which may have the maximal site of pain distal to the originating joint (radiated pain).

Stiffness is also common in OA. Stiffness may be thought of as a difficulty or discomfort during movement caused by a perceived inflexibility of the joint. Stiffness is usually most noticeable early in the morning, but may also occur later in the day, typically after periods of inactivity. Early morning stiffness is present both in classic inflammatory arthritis (eg, rheumatoid arthritis [RA]), and in OA. It can be considered an inflammatory symptom when prolonged and present for at least 30 minutes before maximal improvement. The morning stiffness in OA is typically short lived (usually a few minutes, but in general <30 minutes). Short-lived stiffness (gelling) may also be brought on by inactivity. In patients with OA, both morning and inactivity-related stiffness quickly improve and resolve with joint use, whereas the joint pain subsequently worsens with continued use.

Locomotor restriction and the resulting functional impairment depend on the site and severity of OA. For example, first carpometacarpal joint (CMCJ) OA may cause difficulty in gripping, whereas knee or hip OA may impair the ability to get up from a chair and walk. The resulting participation restriction depends on the individual's daily activities and occupational/recreational requirements.

Table 2	
Stages of pain in OA	
Stage 1 (Early)	Predictable sharp pain, usually brought on by a mechanical insult that eventually limits high-impact activities. There may only be a minimal effect on function.
Stage 2 (Mild-moderate)	Pain becomes a more regular feature, and begins to affect daily activities. There may be unpredictable episodes of stiffness.
Stage 3 (Advanced)	Constant dull/aching pain, punctuated by short episodes of often unpredictable intense, exhausting pain that results in severe functional limitations.

The main physical signs of OA are coarse crepitus, joint-line tenderness, bony swelling, deformity, and reduced range of movement.

Crepitus is a coarse crunching sensation or sound caused by friction between damaged articular cartilage and/or the bone. It may be more prominent during active movement than during passive movement during physical examination. It is often present throughout the range of movement.[9] Crepitus may be exacerbated by stressing the joint surfaces (eg, patellofemoral joint [PFJ] crepitus is increased by applying downward pressure on the patella with the examining hand during knee flexion).[10] Transmitted crepitus (felt on the adjacent periarticular bone) suggests a full-thickness cartilage defect on the affected side.[10]

Tenderness in and around the joint is common in OA. Joint-line tenderness suggests an articular disorder, whereas tenderness away from the joint line suggests a periarticular soft tissue disorder. Both joint-line and periarticular tenderness may be present simultaneously because of a high frequency of periarticular soft tissue disorders near joints with OA. Reduced range of movement (equal for both active and passive movements) mainly results from marginal osteophytosis and capsular thickening, but synovial hyperplasia and effusion also contribute. Fixed flexion deformities (the inability to fully extend the joint) occurs at the knees, hips, or elbows in advanced severe OA. Bony swelling, which may be evident in both small (eg, IPJ, first metatarsophalangeal) and large (eg, knee) joint OA, occurs because of a combination of bony remodeling, marginal osteophytosis, and joint subluxation. Deformity and instability are signs of marked joint damage. Muscle wasting suggests advanced OA.

HOLISTIC ASSESSMENT

Patients with OA should be assessed in a targeted manner for depression, sleep deprivation, hyperalgesia, central sensitization, and catastrophization.[11–14] Each of these has the potential to increase the pain severity. An attempt must similarly be made to assess the presence of joint pain at other sites as it increases pain severity at the index joint.[15] Mobility assessment and neuromuscular examination should be performed for patients with suspected hip or knee OA because these both associate with muscle weakness, impaired joint position sense, and falls.[16] The risk of falls may be further increased by postural hypotension, visual or vestibular impairment, and polypharmacy, which are common in the elderly. Fibromyalgia is another common comorbidity in the elderly and should be considered and sought (by examination for widespread hyperalgesic tender sites) in anyone presenting with musculoskeletal pain, especially if they report nonrestorative or nonrefreshing sleep. Adverse risk factors (**Box 1**) should be sought and considered in the management plan. In addition, illness perceptions regarding joint pain and OA should be explored and discussed with the patient because these may influence treatment adherence and outcome.[17]

ROLE OF INVESTIGATIONS

OA is a clinical diagnosis. It may be diagnosed without recourse to laboratory or radiographic investigations in the presence of typical symptoms and signs in the at-risk age group.[2,22,23] Peripheral joint OA may be diagnosed confidently on clinical grounds alone if there is:

- Persistent usage-related joint pain in 1 or a few joints
- Age ≥45 years
- Only brief morning stiffness (≤30 minutes).[2]

Box 1
Risk factors for poor prognosis in OA

Age

Obesity

Knee malalignment (varus-valgus), hindfoot malalignment

Lower limb length inequality ($\geq$1–2 cm)

Presence of OA in multiple joints (eg, generalized OA [GOA])

Excess or no joint use

Muscle wasting and weakness

Joint laxity

Poor mental health, lack of self-efficacy, and poor social support (for worsening symptoms only)

Data from Refs.[18–21]

Other features listed in **Table 1** add to the diagnostic certainty.[2] This approach to a clinical diagnosis of OA is supported by the poor correlation between radiographically assessed structural changes and symptoms in OA.[24] The American College of Rheumatology (ACR) clinical classification criteria for knee, hip, and hand OA have a high sensitivity, and at least a moderate to high specificity for discriminating OA from other rheumatic conditions in a hospital setting.[9,25,26] However, the ACR criteria are not diagnostic, and failure to meet the classification criteria does not exclude OA. They also have a low sensitivity and specificity for classifying mild-moderate OA in the community setting.[27] However, appropriate imaging and laboratory assessments should be performed:

- In younger individuals (ie, <45 years in age) in the absence of preceding major joint trauma,
- If symptoms and signs are atypical; for example, not usual target sites for OA, symptoms and signs of significant joint inflammation, marked rest and/or night pain, rapidly progressive pain,
- If there is weight loss or constitutional upset,
- If there is true locking at the knee, which suggests additional mechanical derangement.

Inflammatory markers (C-reactive protein, erythrocyte sedimentation rate, plasma viscosity) are normal or only minimally increased in OA, and may be useful in excluding other diagnoses. Radiographic examination may be used to support a clinical diagnosis of OA. However, patients with a clinically robust diagnosis of OA may have normal radiographs, and vice versa. Thus, radiographic examination should not be used to establish a diagnosis of OA by itself, and neither should a normal plain radiograph be used to refute a clinical diagnosis of OA; 86% of middle-aged community-dwelling residents (mean age 45 years) with knee pain for more than 3 months develop radiographic knee OA over the next 12 years, suggesting that knee pain may be the first sign of OA.[28] However, such patients should be examined carefully to exclude any other cause of joint pain, such as periarticular soft tissue lesions, before arriving at a diagnosis of OA and more sensitive examination of the joint (eg, ultrasound or magnetic resonance imaging) may be warranted. However, radiographic examination may have a role in defining the prognosis of patients with OA. In a prospective study of more than

1507 patients with knee OA, those with more severe joint space narrowing at baseline progressed more rapidly to complete joint space loss over time than those with no joint space narrowing at baseline.[29] Global OA severity had a similar but smaller role.[29] In summary, OA may be diagnosed on clinical grounds alone in the at-risk population, with radiographs being used more for prognostic than diagnostic purposes.

Synovial fluid examination is not routinely required to support a diagnosis of OA. However, joint aspiration and synovial fluid analysis are indicated if there is a suspicion of coexistent crystal deposition. Both monosodium urate and calcium pyrophosphate (CPP) crystal deposition (CPPD) associate with OA and may cause acute synovitis or more chronic inflammation in OA joints. Community-based studies suggest that coexistent self-reported gout and OA of the knee and hip occur in 1.1% and 0.8% of patients older than 25 years, respectively,[30] whereas coexistent knee chondrocalcinosis (a marker of CPPD) and knee OA occur in 2.4% of patients older than 40 years.[31] Basic calcium phosphate (BCP) crystal deposition is also common in OA but requires sophisticated techniques (eg, scanning electron microscopy) for accurate identification, and its presence is not sought routinely.

DISTRIBUTION OF JOINTS AFFECTED BY OA

OA can affect any synovial joint. However, it targets the knees, hips, first CMCJs, finger IPJs, first metatarsophalangeal (bunion) joints (first metatarsophalangeal joints [MTPJs]) and apophyseal (facet) joints of the lower cervical and lower lumbar spine (**Fig. 1**).[32]

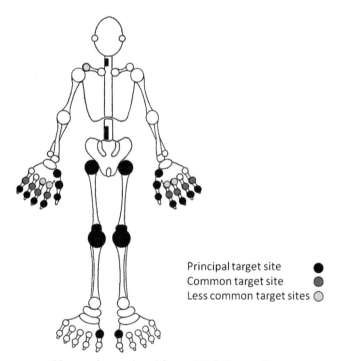

Principal target site ●
Common target site ◉
Less common target sites ○

Fig. 1. Joints targeted by OA. (*Reproduced from* Abhishek A, Doherty M. Disease diagnosis and clinical presentation. In: Henrotin Y, Hunter DJ, Kawaguchi H, editors. OARSI Online Primer. OARSI; 2011; with permission.)

CLASSIFICATION

OA can be classified according to the number of affected joints, presumed cause, age of onset, radiographic appearance (hypertrophic vs atrophic), presence of calcium crystals, and rate of progression. Several classification systems have been proposed. Each has its own strengths and weaknesses. We present a simplified system adapted from the original ACR classification[9] and that is possibly better suited for clinical use (**Box 2**).

Box 2
Simplified clinical approach to identifying OA subsets

1. Number of joints involved

   a. Localized: 1–2 joint regions involved only (specify location)

   b. GOA: ≥3 joint regions involved, with spine/hands being one of the regions affected (nodal GOA if nodes present)

2. Classic or atypical OA (atypical OA: unusual distribution, young age of onset [<45 years], rapid progression)

Causes of atypical OA include:

a. Prior trauma (common): mainly monoarticular or oligoarticular OA, young onset, often with a clear history of injury

b. Dysplasia:

   i. Localized (eg, hip): childhood or young adult onset

   ii. Polyarticular (eg, spondyloepiphysial dysplasia): young onset, short stature, morphologic features, and a positive family history may be present

c. Childhood arthropathy or derangement: eg, juvenile idiopathic arthritis, Perthes disease and slipped femoral epiphysis of hip, septic arthritis

d. Metabolic or endocrine diseases: eg, hemochromatosis, which mainly targets metacarpophalangeal joints (MCPJs), wrists, hips, and may be of young onset, mainly in men; acromegaly, which has typical signs of OA with little restriction in movements, hypermobility

e. Late avascular necrosis: predominantly hips, shoulders, and knees, more rapid progression, risk factors present (eg, steroid use)

f. Neuropathic joints: rapid clinical progression, marked joint disorganization

   i. Hindfoot, midfoot: diabetes mellitus

   ii. Shoulders, elbows, wrists: syringomyelia

g. Apatite-associated destructive arthritis: old age, rapid progression; targets hips, knees, and shoulders

3. Clinical joint inflammation: usually absent; if present, consider:

   a. Crystal deposition: CPPD and gout (OA encourages deposition of both crystal types)

   b. Coexistent inflammatory arthritis: eg, RA, seronegative spondyloarthropathy

   c. Erosive OA: targets hand IPJs

Modified from Abhishek A, Doherty M. Disease diagnosis and clinical presentation. In: Henrotin Y, Hunter DJ, Kawaguchi H, editors. OARSI Online Primer. OARSI; 2011.

GOA

Although it was recognized earlier, Kellgren and Moore[33] described a polyarticular subset of OA particularly involving the distal IPJs (DIPJs), thumb bases (first CMCJs and trapezioscaphoid joints), first MTPJs, facet joints, knees, and hips, and coined the term GOA for this subset. GOA is characterized by a slow accumulation of multiple joint involvement (compared with RA, which usually affects multiple joints synchronously). Symptoms usually commence in the hand joints around middle age and affect the knees and other joints over the next few decades. The clinical marker for GOA is the presence of multiple Heberden nodes, which are posterolateral hard swellings of the DIPJs, associated with underlying OA.[33] Heberden nodes are often accompanied by less well-defined posterolateral swellings of the proximal IPJs (PIPJs): so-called Bouchard nodes. A form of GOA showing identical joint targeting was subsequently identified in patients without Heberden nodes,[34] which led to GOA being classified as nodal and non-nodal forms,[34] the former being more common in women, and the latter mainly occurring in men.[35] There is no universal definition of the number of joints that must be affected before an individual can be diagnosed as having GOA. However, guidance from ACR and The European League Against Rheumatism suggests that GOA is present if there is OA at the spine or hand, and in at least 2 other joint regions.[9,23]

CLINICAL FEATURES AT THE MAIN SYMPTOMATIC SITES
Hands

Hand OA is usually bilaterally symmetric.[23,26] Symptoms affect just 1 or a few joints at a time.[23] Symptoms are often intermittent and occur at the target sites, namely DIPJs (~50%), thumb bases (~35%), PIPJs (~20%), and MCPJs (~10%), in descending order of frequency.[23,36] Individuals without pain may report a dull ache or stiffness.[26] The symptoms of hand OA deteriorate in half the patients over the next 6 years.[37] The predictors of a worse clinical outcome include a high level of functional impairment at baseline and a greater number of painful joints, with no correlation between clinical change and radiographic progression.[37]

Nodal OA

Heberden and/or Bouchard nodes plus underlying IPJ OA (defined clinically and/or radiologically) constitutes nodal OA.[23] It affects women more frequently than men, and familial predisposition is recognized. Symptoms usually start in middle age, often around the menopause, with pain, tenderness, and stiffness of 1 or a few DIPJs in the hands. There may be warmth and soft tissue swelling at the start. Over a period of months or years, involved IPJs usually become less painful and signs of inflammation subside, leaving behind firm to hard bony swellings on the posterolateral aspect of the IPJs, termed Heberden (DIPJ) and Bouchard (PIPJ) nodes (**Fig. 2**). Over the next decade or so, other IPJs go through the same process, in a monoarthritis multiplex manner. Established DIPJ (or PIPJ) nodes sometimes coalesce to form a single dorsal bar (see **Fig. 2**). In addition to bony swelling, the affected IPJs commonly deviate laterally (radial or ulnar, with most deviations pointing toward the middle finger) and have reduced range of movement. Lateral deviation at the IPJs without IPJ instability is a characteristic feature of nodal OA (**Fig. 3**). Nodal OA is most common at the index and middle fingers.[26] Fully evolved nodes are not painful, and usually associate with a good long-term functional outcome. However, some patients are concerned by the cosmetic aspect of these deformities.

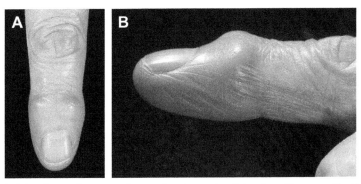

Fig. 2. (*A*) Heberden nodes appearing as discrete posterolateral swelling over the DIPJs, and (*B*) coalescing to form a single dorsal bar.

The thumb base, comprising the first CMCJ and trapezioscaphoid joint, is another target site for OA. Thumb base OA presents with pain on joint use at the thumb base area with some distal and proximal radiation. There may be radial subluxation of the metacarpal base or adduction at the thumb base, giving it a swollen, squared appearance (**Fig. 4**).[23,26] Unlike IPJ OA, thumb base OA associates with persistent symptoms and with greater functional impairment (occasionally requiring surgery), so the prognosis is generally worse.

OA mainly targets the second, third, and first MCPJs, in descending order of frequency, often causing bony enlargement without signs or symptoms of synovitis.[36] Isolated MCPJ OA sometimes occurs in elderly people who have had physically demanding occupations (Missouri arthritis).[38] Widespread MCPJ changes, especially with wrist arthropathy or chondrocalcinosis, suggest the possibility of hemochromatosis.

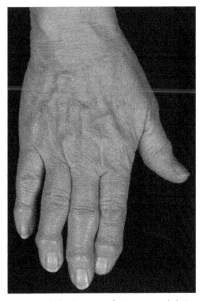

Fig. 3. Heberden nodes and lateral deviation of IPJs in nodal OA.

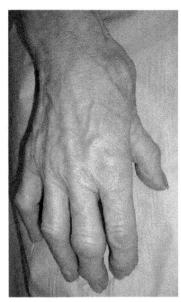

Fig. 4. Thumb base OA: squaring of the thumb base, caused by osteophytosis and subluxation at the first carpometacarpal joint.

Erosive OA

Erosive OA is an aggressive subset of hand OA. It presents with subacute or insidious onset of pain, stiffness, soft tissue swelling, and sometimes paresthesia affecting multiple IPJs (synchronous polyarticular onset).[23,39] Pain, tenderness, inflammation (warmth, soft tissue swelling, sometimes erythema) are more marked and prolonged compared with nodal hand OA[39,40] and there is no association with GOA. Erosive OA usually spares the thumb base and MCPJs[23] and targets DIPJs more commonly than PIPJs (**Fig. 5**).[40] Lateral instability and ankylosis at the IPJs are uncommon but characteristic clinical findings in erosive OA (**Fig. 6**). There may rarely be an opera-glass deformity,[40] and Heberden, and/or Bouchard nodes may coexist.[41] Erosive OA is defined radiographically by subchondral erosion, cortical destruction, marked bone and cartilage attrition, and subsequent reparative change that may include bony ankylosis. It has a worse outcome in terms of symptom persistence and functional impairment than nonerosive hand OA.[23] Although erosive OA as a clinical entity is rare, radiographic erosions are present in 1 or a few joints in up to 8.5% of patients with symptomatic hand OA.[42] The differential diagnosis for hand OA is wide, and includes:

- Psoriatic arthritis: targets DIPJs or affects just 1 ray
- RA: targets wrists, MCPJs, PIPJs
- Gout: may be superimposed on preexisting hand OA
- Hemochromatosis: mainly targets MCPJs, and wrists[23]

OA at Other Upper Limb Joints

OA may be present in the other upper limb joints, especially in the presence of occupational risk factors. For example, people with mechanically demanding jobs can develop elbow, shoulder, wrist, and acromioclavicular joint OA. Shoulder (glenohumeral joint) OA may also be a consequence of, or associate with, rotator cuff tear. The symptom at these joints is as for OA in other joints (see **Table 1**) and is most commonly unilateral.

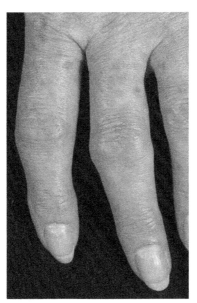

Fig. 5. Erosive OA: marked radial deviation and fixed flexion deformity in the left middle PIPJ, radial deviation with restriction in the index PIPJ, and bony swelling of both fingers. Note the absence of Heberden nodes. (*Reproduced from* Abhishek A, Doherty M. Disease diagnosis and clinical presentation. In: Henrotin Y, Hunter DJ, Kawaguchi H, editors. OARSI Online Primer. OARSI; 2011; with permission.)

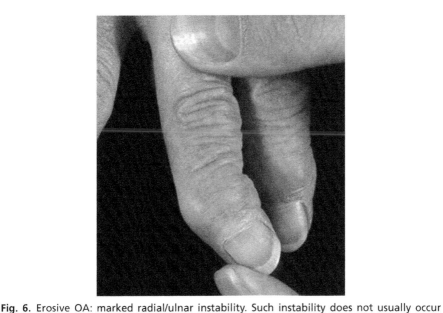

Fig. 6. Erosive OA: marked radial/ulnar instability. Such instability does not usually occur with the common hand OA. (*Reproduced from* Abhishek A, Doherty M. Disease diagnosis and clinical presentation. In: Henrotin Y, Hunter DJ, Kawaguchi H, editors. OARSI Online Primer. OARSI; 2011; with permission.)

Knee

The knee is an important target site for OA. Knee OA alone is the commonest cause of lower limb disability in elderly people. It is usually bilateral, although symptoms may be more pronounced on 1 side. Unilateral knee OA is more common in young men, and is often caused by prior knee injury or surgery. Most patients with knee OA have medial compartment tibiofemoral joint (TFJ) OA, PFJ OA, or a combination of both.[43,44]

Knee joint pain is felt anteriorly and the location and pattern of pain indicate the affected compartment(s). Pain is anteromedial in medial compartment TFJ OA, and anterior and behind the patella in PFJ OA.[45] Pain from PFJ OA is typically worsened by prolonged sitting, standing up from low chairs, and climbing stairs or inclines (coming down often being more painful than going up). Generalized knee pain with distal radiation suggests moderate to severe knee OA.[46] Persistent rest and night pain occur in advanced OA.[22] Knee OA symptoms usually do not cause posterior knee pain unless there is a complicating popliteal (Baker) cyst. Apart from pain, there may be a feeling of giving way (especially with PFJ OA and/or quadriceps weakness) and instability, both of which associate with falls.[22]

On examination, the findings are typical of OA (see **Table 1**). Tibiofemoral joint-line tenderness is felt anteriorly, on either side of the patella tendon with the knee flexed. Pain on patellofemoral compression, deformity (fixed flexion and/or varus; less commonly valgus deformity on weight bearing), quadriceps wasting and weakness, and hip muscle weakness may be present (**Fig. 7**).[22,47,48] Knee effusion is common, and increases in prevalence with the severity of knee OA. For example, in a study, 36% of patients with symptomatic knee OA (Kellgren and Lawrence [K&L] score $\geq$2) had a clinical knee effusion, whereas only 16% of symptomatic preradiographic knee OA (magnetic resonance imaging cartilage score $\geq$2, and K&L score $\leq$2) had clinically detectable knee effusion.[49]

Several painful periarticular soft tissue disorders coexist with knee OA and require careful assessment (**Table 3**).[8,50,51]

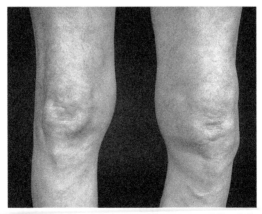

Fig. 7. Unilateral knee OA: swollen left knee with varus and fixed flexion deformities in a 63-year-old man with a history of knee trauma. On palpation there was marked crepitus, restricted flexion, bony swelling, and a small effusion. The cruciates were intact but there was minor varus/valgus instability on stress testing. (*Reproduced from* Abhishek A, Doherty M. Disease diagnosis and clinical presentation. In: Henrotin Y, Hunter DJ, Kawaguchi H, editors. OARSI Online Primer. OARSI; 2011; with permission.)

Table 3
Common periarticular lesions that coexist with knee OA

Soft Tissue Disorder	Signs and Symptoms
Anserine bursitis	Inferomedial knee pain, localized soft tissue swelling (rarely), tenderness over the upper medial tibia
Semimembranosus-tibial collateral ligament bursitis	Medial knee pain, tenderness closer to the joint line than in anserine bursitis
Medial collateral ligament (inferior insertion) enthesopathy	Medial knee pain, localized tenderness, and pain on stressing the medial ligament (valgus strain with knee unlocked)
Tender medial fat pad	Medial knee pain, tenderness over either the inferior or superior fat pad below or above the joint line
Iliotibial tract (band) syndrome	Lateral distal thigh and knee pain, and tenderness maximal over the lateral femoral condyle

Hip

Hip OA presents with pain, stiffness, and restricted movement. Pain caused by hip OA is usually maximal deep in the anterior groin, but may spread to the anteromedial or upper lateral thigh, and occasionally the buttocks. Distal radiation is common, and pain may predominate at the knee. Some people present with knee pain without any proximal pain; unlike knee-originated pain, such hip-referred pain is usually more generalized, involves the distal thigh, and may be improved by rubbing. Pain in hip OA is exacerbated by rising from a seated position, and during initial or midambulation.[25] It may be difficult to differentiate hip OA pain from referred spinal pain or concomitant knee OA,[25] and intra-articular local anesthetic injection may be required to resolve any diagnostic uncertainty.[52] Unlike knee OA, hip OA is often unilateral.[53]

Both active and passive hip movements may be painful.[25] Internal rotation with the hip flexed is frequently the earliest movement to be restricted, but movements may be globally restricted in severe disease (**Fig. 8**).[25] The typical end-stage deformity in hip OA is external rotation, adduction, and fixed flexion (**Fig. 9**). Wasting of thigh muscles, positive Trendelenburg test, antalgic gait, and shortening of the affected extremity may also be present.[25] However, such end-stage hip OA should be rare in modern clinical practice.

Hip OA may be subclassified largely according to radiographic features, specifically[54,55]:

1. Pattern of radiographic femoral head migration
   a. Superior: most usual pattern (especially in men), likely to be unilateral at presentation and to progress more rapidly
   b. Axial (along the axis of the femoral neck): progresses more slowly
   c. Medial: mainly in women, likely to be bilateral and associate with Heberden nodes
2. Bone response to joint space loss
   a. Atrophic: characterized by marked bone attrition and minimal osteophytosis, common in elderly, associated with chondrocalcinosis
   b. Hypertrophic: characterized by florid osteophytosis

In some patients, especially elderly women, hip OA can be rapidly progressive with a subacute onset of symptoms that progresses to joint destruction and instability in a matter of months rather than years. The radiographs may show paradoxic widening

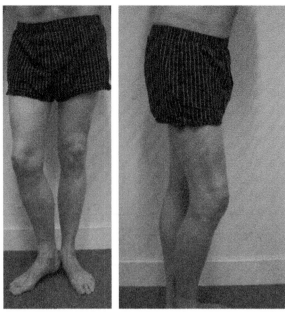

Fig. 8. Patient with right hip OA showing fixed flexion and external rotation deformity. (*Reproduced from* Abhishek A, Doherty M. Disease diagnosis and clinical presentation. In: Henrotin Y, Hunter DJ, Kawaguchi H, editors. OARSI Online Primer. OARSI; 2011; with permission.)

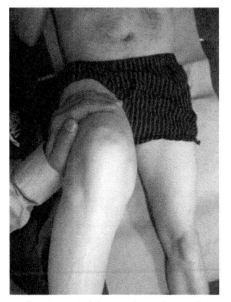

Fig. 9. Patient with hip OA, showing painful restriction in internal rotation in flexion: the tight-pack position for the hip and the first movement to be affected. (*Reproduced from* Abhishek A, Doherty M. Disease diagnosis and clinical presentation. In: Henrotin Y, Hunter DJ, Kawaguchi H, editors. OARSI Online Primer. OARSI; 2011; with permission.)

of joint space (although this is reduced or absent if standing or stressed films are taken), marked bone attrition, destruction of the femoral head, and paucity of osteo-phytosis (atrophic OA).[56] Such rapidly progressive destructive arthropathy has been associated with BCP (mainly hydroxyapatite) crystals, and termed apatite-associated destructive arthropathy (AADA).[57–59] Shoulders (Milwaukee shoulder)[60] and knees are other target sites for AADA. Muscle wasting, deformities, and moderate to large joint effusions with noninflammatory (viscous, occasionally hemorrhagic, low cell count) synovial fluid are common.

Several other disorders may lead to pain around the hip region.[61] For example, ante-rior groin pain may be caused by osteonecrosis (avascular necrosis) of the femoral head.[61] With this, pain is initially usually night predominant, well localized, unrelated to usage and progressive, becoming worse on usage and more widespread once the femoral bone and overlying cartilage collapse to result in arthropathy. Posterior hip and buttock pain may be caused by lumbar radiculopathy, iliolumbar ligament syndrome, sacroiliac joint pain, and hip extensor or rotator muscle strain.[61] Other peri-articular disorders that may coexist with hip OA are listed in **Table 4**.

Facet Joint OA

It is often difficult to attribute symptoms to facet joint OA because it commonly coex-ists with intervertebral disk degeneration. However, lumbar facet joint OA is thought to lead to localized lumbar pain, which may radiate unilaterally or bilaterally to the buttocks, groins, and thighs, typically ending above the knees.[62] Symptoms are worse in the morning and during periods of inactivity, and are increased by stress, exercise, lumbar spine extension, rotary motions, and when standing or sitting.[62] Lying flat and flexion of the lumbar spine lead to pain relief.[62] Cervical facet joint OA similarly may present with ipsilateral neck pain that does not radiate beyond the shoulder, and is worsened by neck rotation or extension.[63] The osteophytes in facet joint OA may also impinge on nerve roots and lead to radiculopathy.

First MTPJ OA

First MTPJ OA is usually bilateral, and when symptomatic, causes localized big toe pain mainly on standing and during ambulation. Bony enlargement of the first MTPJ may be present (**Fig. 11**). Hallux valgus (distal end of big toe points toward the midline of the foot), hallux rigidus (restricted flexion, and extension at the first MTPJ), and

Table 4	
Common periarticular lesions near the hip	
Soft Tissue Disorder	**Signs and Symptoms**
Trochanteric bursitis/gluteus medius tendinitis[a]	Lateral hip pain, worse on lying on that side at night and reproduced by pressure over the greater trochanter region
Iliopsoas bursitis	Anterior groin pain ± swelling. Frequently associates with other arthropathies
Ischiogluteal bursitis	Pain over the ischia, aggravated by local pressure brought on by sitting and lying. Local tenderness present
Adductor tendinitis	Medial groin pain aggravated by passive hip abduction and resisted active adduction

[a] Most common.

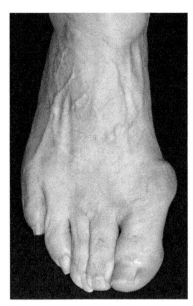

Fig. 10. First MTPJ OA with hallux valgus and an inflamed overlying superficial bursa ("bunion").

crossover toes are the other common deformities. Bony enlargement at the first MTPJ and hallux valgus frequently lead to the development of a complicating bursa with additional fibrous tissue reaction on the medial aspect of the first MTPJ (bunion; **Fig. 10**). This joint may get inflamed (eg, by rubbing against footwear) and cause medial big toe pain. Apart from the first MTPJ, OA also commonly targets the talonavicular joint in the midfoot (aggravated by pes planus; see **Fig. 11**), and sometimes the ankle and subtalar joints in the hindfoot (especially in those with previous trauma).

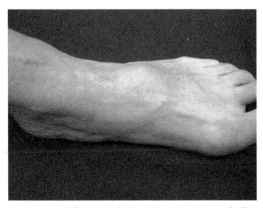

Fig. 11. Midfoot OA aggravated by pes planus. Note coexistent hallux valgus, suggesting first MTPJ OA.

OA WITH CPPD

OA with CPPD commonly occurs at the knee, radiocarpal joint, second to third MCPJs, shoulder joint, and elbow joint. Patients with OA plus CPPD are usually older than 60 years.[64,65] More than a quarter of patients with knee OA who require hospital referral, and more than half of those undergoing total knee replacement for OA, have CPPD.[44,66] The presence of CPPD may modify OA symptoms,[44,67] presumably because CPP crystals are hard, negatively charged particles that can exert both proinflammatory and adverse mechanical effects.[68] Compared with OA without CPPD, there may be a longer duration of early morning stiffness and more common and pronounced acute, intermittent, or low-grade and persistent synovitis (**Fig. 12**). Joint effusions are common, and may be hemorrhagic or turbid on aspiration. Large effusions, mainly at the knee or the shoulder, may leak into the surrounding soft tissues and lead to localized pain, swelling, and extensive bruising. Although studies give conflicting results, it is likely that OA with CPPD is not more rapidly progressive than OA alone.[66,69,70] However, there are anecdotal reports of patients with CPPD developing rapidly progressive destructive arthropathy at knees, shoulders, or hips. Some patients with OA with CPPD may have polyarticular arthropathy involving the knees, wrists, and the MCPJs that superficially mimics RA.

CLINICAL FEATURES INFLUENCE THE MANAGEMENT OF OA

Because OA has a diverse clinical presentation, it is important to target the therapeutic intervention to the patient, and to the symptoms. Patient education, appropriate advice concerning exercise and activity (ideally with physiotherapy and/or occupational therapy input), avoidance of adverse biomechanical factors, and adjunctive analgesia, are core to the management of OA. Oral paracetamol and topical analgesics (nonsteroidal antiinflamatory drugs, capsaicin) are recommended analgesics to try first, mainly based on their safety, but subsequent choice of analgesic depends on the clinical feature. For example, patients with pain and nonrestorative sleep

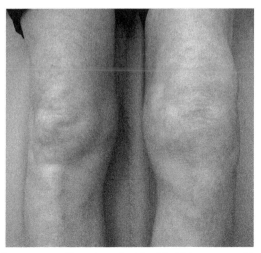

Fig. 12. Knee effusions are usually not marked in OA. This person with OA plus CPPD had a large left knee effusion expanding the suprapatellar pouch, giving a positive balloon sign (fluctuance) on palpation.

may benefit from amitriptyline, nortriptyline, or duloxetine,[71] whereas patients with neuropathic features to their pain may benefit from duloxetine, pregabalin, or amitriptyline.[72] Some patients who present with rapidly progressive severe OA of the knees or hips may warrant consideration for joint replacement surgery, whereas others who present with exacerbation of their joint symptoms may benefit from local intra-articular injections of corticosteroid to achieve short-term symptom control. The latter is especially true in those with thumb base, knee, and hip OA. Those with superadded acute CPP crystal arthritis may also derive rapid benefit from intra-articular corticosteroid injection and/or colchicine. In contrast, asymptomatic radiographic changes of OA in peripheral or spinal joints in the elderly require no further interventions apart from possibly modifying risk factors for the progression of OA (eg, obesity). The presence of comorbid fibromyalgia should be specifically sought and treated in patients who present with severe OA, and in those with symptomatic OA at several sites. Patients with GOA may have a worse prognosis than those without GOA, and should be targeted for risk factor modification (eg, patients with knee OA in the context of GOA are at higher risk of progression of their knee OA).[19]

SUMMARY

Usage-related pain, short-lived morning/inactivity stiffness, and locomotor restriction are the most common symptoms of OA. In patients with typical presentation at the target sites, clinical assessment alone is sufficient to allow a diagnosis of OA. Patients with OA should be assessed in a holistic manner, which should include a targeted examination for the associated comorbidities.

REFERENCES

1. Lane NE, Brandt K, Hawker G, et al. OARSI-FDA initiative: defining the disease state of osteoarthritis. Osteoarthritis Cartilage 2011;19(5):478–82.
2. National Institute for Health and Clinical Excellence. Osteoarthritis: the care and management of osteoarthritis in adults. [CG59]. London: National Institute for Health and Clinical Excellence; 2008.
3. Abhishek A, Doherty M. Disease diagnosis and clinical presentation. In: Henrotin Y, Hunter DJ, Kawaguchi H, editors. OARSI Online Primer. OARSI; 2011.
4. Yusuf E, Kortekaas MC, Watt I, et al. Do knee abnormalities visualised on MRI explain knee pain in knee osteoarthritis? A systematic review. Ann Rheum Dis 2011;70(1):60–7.
5. Goddard NJ, Gosling PT. Intra-articular fluid pressure and pain in osteoarthritis of the hip. J Bone Joint Surg Br 1988;70(1):52–5.
6. Hawker GA, Stewart L, French MR, et al. Understanding the pain experience in hip and knee osteoarthritis–an OARSI/OMERACT initiative. Osteoarthritis Cartilage 2008;16(4):415–22.
7. Allen KD, Coffman CJ, Golightly YM, et al. Daily pain variations among patients with hand, hip, and knee osteoarthritis. Osteoarthritis Cartilage 2009;17(10): 1275–82.
8. Hill CL, Gale DR, Chaisson CE, et al. Periarticular lesions detected on magnetic resonance imaging: prevalence in knees with and without symptoms. Arthritis Rheum 2003;48(10):2836–44.
9. Altman R, Asch E, Bloch D, et al. Development of criteria for the classification and reporting of osteoarthritis. Classification of osteoarthritis of the knee. Diagnostic and Therapeutic Criteria Committee of the American Rheumatism Association. Arthritis Rheum 1986;29(8):1039–49.

10. Ike R, O'Rourke KS. Compartment-directed physical examination of the knee can predict articular cartilage abnormalities disclosed by needle arthroscopy. Arthritis Rheum 1995;38(7):917–25.

11. Sale JE, Gignac M, Hawker G. The relationship between disease symptoms, life events, coping and treatment, and depression among older adults with osteoarthritis. J Rheumatol 2008;35(2):335–42.

12. Abad VC, Sarinas PS, Guilleminault C. Sleep and rheumatologic disorders. Sleep Med Rev 2008;12(3):211–28.

13. Imamura M, Imamura ST, Kaziyama HH, et al. Impact of nervous system hyperalgesia on pain, disability, and quality of life in patients with knee osteoarthritis: a controlled analysis. Arthritis Rheum 2008;59(10):1424–31.

14. Edwards RR, Bingham CO 3rd, Bathon J, et al. Catastrophizing and pain in arthritis, fibromyalgia, and other rheumatic diseases. Arthritis Rheum 2006; 55(2):325–32.

15. Suri P, Morgenroth DC, Kwoh CK, et al. Low back pain and other musculoskeletal pain comorbidities in individuals with symptomatic osteoarthritis of the knee: data from the osteoarthritis initiative. Arthritis Care Res (Hoboken) 2010;62(12): 1715–23.

16. Hurley MV, Scott DL, Rees J, et al. Sensorimotor changes and functional performance in patients with knee osteoarthritis. Ann Rheum Dis 1997;56(11):641–8.

17. Petrie KJ, Jago LA, Devcich DA. The role of illness perceptions in patients with medical conditions. Curr Opin Psychiatry 2007;20(2):163–7.

18. van Dijk GM, Dekker J, Veenhof C, et al. Course of functional status and pain in osteoarthritis of the hip or knee: a systematic review of the literature. Arthritis Rheum 2006;55(5):779–85.

19. Chapple CM, Nicholson H, Baxter GD, et al. Patient characteristics that predict progression of knee osteoarthritis: a systematic review of prognostic studies. Arthritis Care Res (Hoboken) 2011;63(8):1115–25.

20. Harvey WF, Yang M, Cooke TD, et al. Association of leg-length inequality with knee osteoarthritis: a cohort study. Ann Intern Med 2010;152(5):287–95.

21. Golightly YM, Allen KD, Helmick CG, et al. Hazard of incident and progressive knee and hip radiographic osteoarthritis and chronic joint symptoms in individuals with and without limb length inequality. J Rheumatol 2010;37(10): 2133–40.

22. Zhang W, Doherty M, Peat G, et al. EULAR evidence-based recommendations for the diagnosis of knee osteoarthritis. Ann Rheum Dis 2010;69(3):483–9.

23. Zhang W, Doherty M, Leeb BF, et al. EULAR evidence-based recommendations for the diagnosis of hand osteoarthritis: report of a task force of ESCISIT. Ann Rheum Dis 2009;68(1):8–17.

24. Bedson J, Croft PR. The discordance between clinical and radiographic knee osteoarthritis: a systematic search and summary of the literature. BMC Musculoskelet Disord 2008;9:116.

25. Altman R, Alarcon G, Appelrouth D, et al. The American College of Rheumatology criteria for the classification and reporting of osteoarthritis of the hip. Arthritis Rheum 1991;34(5):505–14.

26. Altman R, Alarcon G, Appelrouth D, et al. The American College of Rheumatology criteria for the classification and reporting of osteoarthritis of the hand. Arthritis Rheum 1990;33(11):1601–10.

27. Peat G, Thomas E, Duncan R, et al. Clinical classification criteria for knee osteoarthritis: performance in the general population and primary care. Ann Rheum Dis 2006;65(10):1363–7.

28. Thorstensson CA, Andersson ML, Jonsson H, et al. Natural course of knee osteoarthritis in middle-aged subjects with knee pain: 12-year follow-up using clinical and radiographic criteria. Ann Rheum Dis 2009;68(12):1890–3.

29. Wolfe F, Lane NE. The longterm outcome of osteoarthritis: rates and predictors of joint space narrowing in symptomatic patients with knee osteoarthritis. J Rheumatol 2002;29(1):139–46.

30. Picavet HS, Hazes JM. Prevalence of self reported musculoskeletal diseases is high. Ann Rheum Dis 2003;62(7):644–50.

31. Zhang W, Neame R, Doherty S, et al. Relative risk of knee chondrocalcinosis in siblings of index cases with pyrophosphate arthropathy. Ann Rheum Dis 2004; 63(8):969–73.

32. van Saase JL, van Romunde LK, Cats A, et al. Epidemiology of osteoarthritis: Zoetermeer survey. Comparison of radiological osteoarthritis in a Dutch population with that in 10 other populations. Ann Rheum Dis 1989;48(4):271–80.

33. Kellgren JH, Moore R. Generalized osteoarthritis and Heberden's nodes. Br Med J 1952;1(4751):181–7.

34. Kellgren JH, Lawrence JS, Bier F. Genetic factors in generalized osteo-arthrosis. Ann Rheum Dis 1963;22:237–55.

35. Lawrence JS. Generalized osteoarthrosis in a population sample. Am J Epidemiol 1969;90(5):381–9.

36. Dahaghin S, Bierma-Zeinstra SM, Ginai AZ, et al. Prevalence and pattern of radiographic hand osteoarthritis and association with pain and disability (the Rotterdam Study). Ann Rheum Dis 2005;64(5):682–7.

37. Bijsterbosch J, Watt I, Meulenbelt I, et al. Clinical and radiographic disease course of hand osteoarthritis and determinants of outcome after 6 years. Ann Rheum Dis 2011;70(1):68–73.

38. Williams WV, Cope R, Gaunt WD, et al. Metacarpophalangeal arthropathy associated with manual labor (Missouri metacarpal syndrome). Clinical radiographic, and pathologic characteristics of an unusual degeneration process. Arthritis Rheum 1987;30(12):1362–71.

39. Punzi L, Ramonda R, Sfriso P. Erosive osteoarthritis. Best Pract Res Clin Rheumatol 2004;18(5):739–58.

40. Punzi L, Frigato M, Frallonardo P, et al. Inflammatory osteoarthritis of the hand. Best Pract Res Clin Rheumatol 2010;24(3):301–12.

41. Bijsterbosch J, Watt I, Meulenbelt I, et al. Clinical burden of erosive hand osteoarthritis and its relationship to nodes. Ann Rheum Dis 2010;69(10):1784–8.

42. Cavasin F, Punzi L, Ramonda R, et al. Prevalence of erosive osteoarthritis of the hand in a population from Venetian area. Reumatismo 2004;56(1):46–50 [in Italian].

43. Duncan RC, Hay EM, Saklatvala J, et al. Prevalence of radiographic osteoarthritis–it all depends on your point of view. Rheumatology (Oxford) 2006;45(6): 757–60.

44. Ledingham J, Regan M, Jones A, et al. Radiographic patterns and associations of osteoarthritis of the knee in patients referred to hospital. Ann Rheum Dis 1993; 52(7):520–6.

45. Creamer P, Lethbridge-Cejku M, Hochberg MC. Where does it hurt? Pain localization in osteoarthritis of the knee. Osteoarthritis Cartilage 1998;6(5):318–23.

46. Wood LR, Peat G, Thomas E, et al. Knee osteoarthritis in community-dwelling older adults: are there characteristic patterns of pain location? Osteoarthritis Cartilage 2007;15(6):615–23.

47. Slemenda C, Brandt KD, Heilman DK, et al. Quadriceps weakness and osteoarthritis of the knee. Ann Intern Med 1997;127(2):97–104.

48. Hinman RS, Hunt MA, Creaby MW, et al. Hip muscle weakness in individuals with medial knee osteoarthritis. Arthritis Care Res (Hoboken) 2010;62(8):1190–3.
49. Cibere J, Zhang H, Thorne A, et al. Association of clinical findings with pre-radiographic and radiographic knee osteoarthritis in a population-based study. Arthritis Care Res (Hoboken) 2010;62(12):1691–8.
50. O'Reilly S, Doherty M. Signs, symptoms, and laboratory tests. In: Brandt KD, Doherty M, Lohmander LS, editors. Osteoarthritis. Oxford (England): Oxford; 2003. p. 197–210.
51. Rothstein CP, Laorr A, Helms CA, et al. Semimembranosus-tibial collateral ligament bursitis: MR imaging findings. AJR Am J Roentgenol 1996;166(4):875–7.
52. Crawford RW, Gie GA, Ling RS, et al. Diagnostic value of intra-articular anaesthetic in primary osteoarthritis of the hip. J Bone Joint Surg Br 1998;80(2):279–81.
53. Gofton JP. Studies in osteoarthritis of the hip. I. Classification. Can Med Assoc J 1971;104(8):679–83.
54. Ledingham J, Dawson S, Preston B, et al. Radiographic patterns and associations of osteoarthritis of the hip. Ann Rheum Dis 1992;51(10):1111–6.
55. Lanyon P, Muir K, Doherty S, et al. Influence of radiographic phenotype on risk of hip osteoarthritis within families. Ann Rheum Dis 2004;63(3):259–63.
56. Della Torre P, Picuti G, Di Filippo P. Rapidly progressive osteoarthritis of the hip. Ital J Orthop Traumatol 1987;13(2):187–200.
57. Dieppe PA, Crocker P, Huskisson EC, et al. Apatite deposition disease. A new arthropathy. Lancet 1976;1(7954):266–9.
58. Dieppe PA, Doherty M, Macfarlane DG, et al. Apatite associated destructive arthritis. Br J Rheumatol 1984;23(2):84–91.
59. Nuki G. Apatite associated arthritis. Br J Rheumatol 1984;23(2):81–3.
60. McCarty DJ, Halverson PB, Carrera GF, et al. "Milwaukee shoulder"–association of microspheroids containing hydroxyapatite crystals, active collagenase, and neutral protease with rotator cuff defects. I. Clinical aspects. Arthritis Rheum 1981;24(3):464–73.
61. Williams BS, Cohen SP. Greater trochanteric pain syndrome: a review of anatomy, diagnosis and treatment. Anesth Analg 2009;108(5):1662–70.
62. Kalichman L, Hunter DJ. Lumbar facet joint osteoarthritis: a review. Semin Arthritis Rheum 2007;37(2):69–80.
63. van Eerd M, Patijn J, Lataster A, et al. 5. Cervical facet pain. Pain Pract 2010;10(2):113–23.
64. Dieppe PA, Alexander GJ, Jones HE, et al. Pyrophosphate arthropathy: a clinical and radiological study of 105 cases. Ann Rheum Dis 1982;41(4):371–6.
65. Felson DT, Anderson JJ, Naimark A, et al. The prevalence of chondrocalcinosis in the elderly and its association with knee osteoarthritis: the Framingham Study. J Rheumatol 1989;16(9):1241–5.
66. Viriyavejkul P, Wilairatana V, Tanavalee A, et al. Comparison of characteristics of patients with and without calcium pyrophosphate dihydrate crystal deposition disease who underwent total knee replacement surgery for osteoarthritis. Osteoarthritis Cartilage 2007;15(2):232–5.
67. Pattrick M, Hamilton E, Wilson R, et al. Association of radiographic changes of osteoarthritis, symptoms, and synovial fluid particles in 300 knees. Ann Rheum Dis 1993;52(2):97–103.
68. Liu YZ, Jackson AP, Cosgrove SD. Contribution of calcium-containing crystals to cartilage degradation and synovial inflammation in osteoarthritis. Osteoarthritis Cartilage 2009;17(10):1333–40.

69. Ledingham J, Regan M, Jones A, et al. Factors affecting radiographic progression of knee osteoarthritis. Ann Rheum Dis 1995;54(1):53–8.
70. Neogi T, Nevitt M, Niu J, et al. Lack of association between chondrocalcinosis and increased risk of cartilage loss in knees with osteoarthritis: results of two prospective longitudinal magnetic resonance imaging studies. Arthritis Rheum 2006;54(6):1822–8.
71. Carville SF, Arendt-Nielsen S, Bliddal H, et al. EULAR evidence-based recommendations for the management of fibromyalgia syndrome. Ann Rheum Dis 2008;67(4):536–41.
72. National Institute for Health and Clinical Excellence. Neuropathic pain: the pharmacological management of neuropathic pain in adults in non-specialist settings. [CG96]. London: National Institute for Health and Clinical Excellence; 2010.

Imaging of Osteoarthritis

Ali Guermazi, MD, PhD[a],*, Daichi Hayashi, MD, PhD[a],
Felix Eckstein, MD[b], David J. Hunter, MBBS, MSc, PhD, FRACP[c],
Jeff Duryea, PhD[d], Frank W. Roemer, MD[a]

KEYWORDS

- Osteoarthritis • Imaging • Radiography • MR imaging • Ultrasound • CT • PET

KEY POINTS

- Although conventional radiography is still the most commonly used imaging modality for clinical management of patients with osteoarthritis, and loss of joint space width represents the only end point approved by the US Food and Drug Administration for structural disease progression in clinical trials, magnetic resonance (MR) imaging–based studies have revealed some of the limitations of radiography.
- The ability of MR to image the knee as a whole organ and to directly and three-dimensionally assess cartilage morphology and composition plays a crucial role in understanding the natural history of the disease and in the search for new therapies.
- MR imaging of osteoarthritis is classified into the following approaches: semiquantitative, quantitative, and compositional.
- Ultrasonography can also be useful to evaluate synovial disorders in osteoarthritis, particularly in the hand.

Disclosure: This article is an update to a review article (Guermazi A, Burstein D, Conaghan P, et al. Imaging in osteoarthritis. Rheum Dis Clin North Am 2008;34:645–687). As such, there are some contents that overlap and/or are reused from that article.

Competing interests: Dr Guermazi has received consultancies, speaking fees, and/or honoraria from Genzyme, Stryker, Merck Serono, Novartis, and Astra Zeneca and is the President of Boston Imaging Core Laboratory (BICL), a company providing image assessment services. He received a research grant from General Electric Health care. Dr Roemer is Chief Medical Officer and shareholder of BICL. Dr Roemer has received consultancies, speaking fees, and/or honoraria from Merck Serono and the National Institutes of Health. Dr Eckstein has received consultancies, speaking fees, and/or honoraria from Merck Serono, Sanofi, Novartis, Abbot, Medtronic, Bioclinica, and Synthes and is Chief Executive Officer and shareholder of Chondrometrics GmbH, a company providing image analysis services.

Funding sources: No funding received.

[a] Department of Radiology, Boston University School of Medicine, 820 Harrison Avenue, FGH Building 3rd Floor, Boston, MA 02118, USA; [b] Institute of Anatomy and Musculoskeletal Research, Paracelsus Medical University, Strubergasse 21, Salzburg 5020, Austria; [c] Department of Rheumatology, Royal North Shore Hospital and Northern Clinical School, University of Sydney, Sydney, New South Wales 2006, Australia; [d] Department of Radiology, Brigham and Women's Hospital, 75 Francis Street, Boston, MA 02115, USA
* Corresponding author.
E-mail address: guermazi@bu.edu

Rheum Dis Clin N Am 39 (2013) 67–105
http://dx.doi.org/10.1016/j.rdc.2012.10.003
0889-857X/13/$ – see front matter © 2013 Elsevier Inc. All rights reserved.

CONVENTIONAL RADIOGRAPHY
Overview

Radiography is the simplest and least expensive imaging technique. It can detect bony features associated with osteoarthritis (OA), including marginal osteophytes, subchondral sclerosis, and subchondral cysts.[1] Radiography can also determine joint space width (JSW), an indirect surrogate of cartilage thickness and meniscal integrity, but precise measurement of each of these articular structures is not possible with radiography.[2] Despite this drawback, slowing of radiographically detected joint space narrowing (JSN) is the only structural end point currently accepted by regulatory bodies in the United States (US Food and Drug Administration) to prove efficacy of disease-modifying OA drugs in phase-III clinical trials. OA is radiographically defined by the presence of osteophytes.[3] Progression of JSN is the most commonly used criterion for the assessment of OA progression and the complete loss of JSW characterized by bone-on-bone contact is one of the indicators for joint replacement.

However, previously held beliefs that JSN and its changes are the only visible evidence of cartilage damage have been shown to be incorrect. Recent studies have shown that alterations in the meniscus, such as meniscal extrusion or subluxation, also contribute to JSN.[2] The lack of sensitivity and specificity of radiography for the detection of articular tissue damage associated with OA, and its poor sensitivity to change at follow-up imaging, are inherent limitations of radiography.

Another limitation is the presence of variations in semiflexed knee positioning, which occur during image acquisition in trials and clinical practice despite standardization. Kinds and colleagues[4] showed that such variations have significant influence on the quantitative measurement of various radiographic parameters of OA including JSW. Thus, better standardization needs to be achieved during radiographic acquisition. Despite these limitations, radiography remains the gold standard for structural modification in clinical trials of knee OA.

Semiquantitative Assessments of Knee OA Features

The severity of OA can be estimated using semiquantitative scoring systems. Published atlases provide images that represent specific grades.[1] The Kellgren and Lawrence[5] (KL) grade is a widely accepted scheme used for defining the presence or absence of OA, usually using grade 2 disease as the threshold. However, KL grading has limitations; in particular, KL grade 3 includes all degrees of JSN, regardless of the extent. Felson and colleagues[6] suggested a modification of KL grading to improve the sensitivity to change in longitudinal knee OA studies. They recommend that OA be defined by a combination of joint space loss and definite osteophytes on radiography in a knee that did not have this combination on the previous radiographic assessment. For OA progression, they recommend a focus on JSN alone using either a semiquantitative[7] or a quantitative approach.

The Osteoarthritis Research Society International (OARSI) atlas[1] takes a different approach and grades tibiofemoral JSW and osteophytes separately for each compartment of the knee. This compartmental scoring seems to be more sensitive to longitudinal radiographic changes than KL grading. A recent study using data from the OA Initiative highlighted the importance of centralized radiographic assessment in regard to observer reliability, because even expert readers apply different thresholds when scoring JSN.[8]

Quantitative Assessments of JSW

Quantitative measures of JSW use a ruler, either a physical device or a software application, to measure the JSW as the distance between the projected femoral and tibial margins on the image (**Fig. 1**). The femoral margin is defined as the projected edge of the bone, whereas the software usually determines the tibial margin as a bright band corresponding with the projection of the X-ray beam through the radiodense cortical shell at the base of the tibial plateau. Quantification of JSW using image processing software requires a digital version of the image, which can be provided for plain films by a radiographic film digitizer, or files can be analyzed directly for fully digital modalities such as computed radiography and digital radiography. Minimum JSW is the standard metric, but some groups have investigated location-specific JSW as well.[9–14]

Studies using the software methods have shown improved precision compared with the manual method and semiquantitative scoring.[15,16] More recently, these methods have been evaluated using longitudinal knee radiographs to quantify the responsiveness to change.[11] Various degrees of responsiveness have been observed depending on the degree of OA severity, length of the follow-up, and the knee positioning protocol.[10,11,13,14,17,18]

Measurements of JSW obtained from radiographs of knee OA have been found to be reliable, especially when the study lasted longer than 2 years and when the radiographs were obtained with the knee in a standardized flexed position.[19] Studies of hip OA have shown conflicting results when correlating JSW and symptoms. However, several studies have shown that JSW can predict hip joint replacement.[20]

Recent Studies Using Radiographic Evaluation of OA and Associated Features

A prospective observational cohort study by Harvey and colleagues[21] associated leg length inequality of greater than or equal to 1 cm with prevalent radiographic and symptomatic OA in the shorter leg, and increased odds of progressive OA in the shorter leg over 30 months. This study showed that leg length inequality should be a modifiable risk factor for knee OA. Duryea and colleagues[18] compared the responsiveness of radiographic JSW using automated software with magnetic resonance (MR) imaging–derived measures of cartilage morphometry for OA progression.

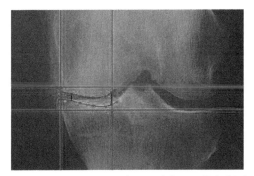

Fig. 1. Automated computer measurement of JSW of the medial tibial plateau of the knee. Minimum JSW is measured using software (Holy's software, Claude Bernard University, Lyon, France) in which the joint space contour is automatically delineated by the computer with the help of an edge-based algorithm. The area of measurement of minimum JSW is defined by 2 vertical lines and 2 horizontal lines obtained by a single click on the nonosteophytic outer edge of the medial femoral condyle and a single click on the inner edge of the medial tibial plateau close to the articular surface. Within these landmarks, the delineation of the bone edges of the medial femoral condyle and medial tibial plateau floor, in addition to the minimum JSW, are automatically obtained. (*From* Guermazi A, Burstein D, Conaghan P, et al. Imaging in osteoarthritis. Rheum Dis Clin North Am 2008;34:645–87.)

Measures of location-specific JSW, using a software analysis of digital knee radiographic images, were comparable with MR imaging in detecting OA progression. Although the limitations of radiography are known, the study showed that, when the lower cost and greater accessibility of radiography are compared with MR imaging, radiography still has a role to play in OA trials. A clinical trial by Mazzuca and colleagues[22] showed that varus malalignment of the lower limb negated the slowing of structural progression of medial JSN by doxycycline. It remains to be seen whether the same effect can be obtained on MR imaging–based evaluation of OA progression.

Using data from the Cohort Hip and Cohort Knee study, Kinds and colleagues[23] showed that measuring osteophyte area (odds ratio [OR] 7.0) and minimum JSW (OR 0.7), in addition to demographic and clinical characteristics, improved the prediction of radiographic OA occurring 5 years later (area under curve receiver operating characteristic 0.74 vs 0.64 without radiographic features) in patients with knee pain at baseline. A cross-sectional study based on the same cohort of patients showed that, in patients with early symptomatic knee OA, osteophytosis, bony enlargement, crepitus, pain, and higher body mass index (BMI) were associated with lower knee flexion.[24] JSN was associated with lower range of motion in all planes. In addition, osteophytosis, flattening of the femoral head, femoral buttressing, pain, morning stiffness, male gender, and higher BMI were found to be associated with poorer range of motion in the hip, in 2 planes.

Two publications from a large-scale Japanese population-based study showed that occupational activities involving kneeling and squatting,[25] as well as obesity, hypertension, and dyslipidemia,[26] were associated with lower medial minimum JSW compared with controls. Another cross-sectional study found that a low level of vitamin D was associated with knee pain but not radiographic OA.[27] A longitudinal study by the same group showed that accumulation of metabolic syndrome components (obesity, hypertension, dyslipidemia, and impaired glucose tolerance) is significantly related to occurrence and progression of radiographic knee OA.[28]

Two older methods (bone texture analysis and tomosynthesis) have experienced a revival lately. Bone texture analysis extracts information on two-dimensional trabecular bone texture from conventional radiography that directly relates to three-dimensional bone structure.[29,30] A recent study showed that bone texture may be a predictor of progression of tibiofemoral OA. Whether bone texture correlates with other changes of subchondral bone, such as MR imaging–detected bone marrow lesions (BMLs) or sclerosis, remains to be seen. Tomosynthesis generates an arbitrary number of section images from a single pass of the X-ray tube. It has been shown that digital tomosynthesis improves sensitivity for depicting lesions in the chest, the breast, and in rheumatoid arthritis.[31–34] However, Hayashi and colleagues[35] showed that tomosynthesis is more sensitive to detection of osteophytes and subchondral cysts than radiography, using 3-T MR imaging as the reference, in the context of knee OA. The clinical availability of these systems is currently limited, but the potential of this technique for OA research might be worth exploring.

MR IMAGING

Although not routinely used in clinical management of patients with OA, MR has become a key imaging tool for OA research[36–40] because of its ability to visualize disorders that are not detected on radiography (ie, articular cartilage, menisci, ligaments, synovium, capsular structures, fluid collections, and bone marrow; **Figs. 2–5**).[41–54] In addition, with MR imaging, OA can be classified into hypertrophic and atrophic phenotypes, according to the size of osteophytes.[55] Based on some of these

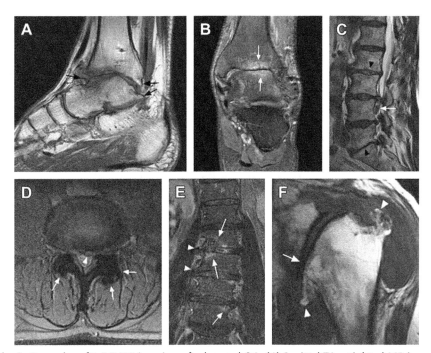

Fig. 2. Examples of 1.5-T MR imaging of advanced OA. (*A*) Sagittal T1-weighted MR image of posttraumatic ankle OA shows large periarticular osteophytes (*arrows*). (*B*) Coronal T2-weighted fat-suppressed MR image shows periarticular subchondral BMLs (*white arrows*). (*C*) Sagittal T2-weighted MR image of lumbar spine OA shows disc space narrowing at L2 to L3 and at L5 to S1 (*arrowheads*). There is an additional inferiorly displaced disc herniation at L3 to L4 (*white arrow*). (*D*) Axial T2-weighted gradient-echo MR image at the level of L3 to L4 shows hypertrophic facet joint OA (*white arrows*) and a small medial disc herniation (*arrowhead*). (*E*) Coronal short tau inversion recovery (STIR) MR image of the lumbar spine shows peridiscal edemalike lesions at L2 to L3 and at L4 to L5 (*arrows*). Note the peridiscal lateral osteophytes (*arrowheads*). (*F*) Sagittal T1-weighted MR image of advanced shoulder OA shows large humeral osteophytes (*arrowheads*) and severe JSN and cartilage loss (*arrow*). (*From* Guermazi A, Burstein D, Conaghan P, et al. Imaging in osteoarthritis. Rheum Dis Clin North Am 2008;34:645–87.)

pathologic features, an MR imaging–based definition of OA has recently been proposed.[56] Tibiofemoral OA on MR imaging is defined as either (1) the presence of both definite osteophyte formation and full-thickness cartilage loss, or (2) the presence of 1 of the features in (1) and 1 of the following: subchondral BML or cyst not associated with meniscal or ligamentous attachments; meniscal subluxation, maceration, or degenerative (horizontal) tear; partial thickness cartilage loss; and bone attrition.

With MR imaging, the following four things can be achieved:
- The joint can be evaluated as a whole organ
- Pathologic changes of preradiographic OA can be detected at an earlier stage of the disease
- Physiologic changes within joint tissues (eg, cartilage and menisci) can be assessed before morphologic changes become apparent
- Multiple tissue changes can be monitored simultaneously over several time points (**Fig. 6**)

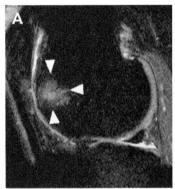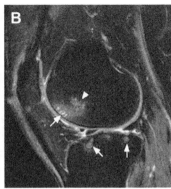

Fig. 3. Examples of 1.0-T and 3.0-T MR imaging of knee OA. (A) Sagittal proton density–weighted fat-suppressed 1.0-T MR image shows a subchondral BML in the anterior medial femur (arrowheads) associated with superficial cartilage damage. (B) Sagittal proton density–weighted fat-suppressed 3.0-T MR image shows a subchondral BML in the anterior lateral femur (arrowhead) and femoral and tibial subchondral cysts (arrows). (From Guermazi A, Burstein D, Conaghan P, et al. Imaging in osteoarthritis. Rheum Dis Clin North Am 2008;34:645–87.)

The use of MR imaging has led to significant findings about the association of pain with BMLs[57] and synovitis,[58] with implications for future OA clinical trials. Systematic reviews have shown that MR imaging biomarkers in OA have concurrent and predictive validity, with good responsiveness and reliability.[59,60] The Osteoarthritis Research Society International (OARSI)–US Food and Drug Administration working group now recommends MR imaging as a suitable imaging tool for cartilage morphology in clinical trials.[36]

Recent advances in the use of MR as an imaging tool in OA research are discussed later in this article. First, MR imaging–based semiquantitative OA scoring systems that

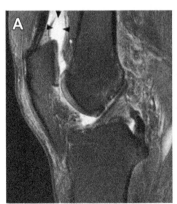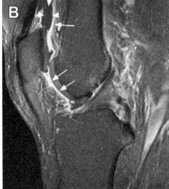

Fig. 4. Synovial activation in knee OA. (A) Sagittal proton density–weighted fat-suppressed MR image shows joint effusion depicted as fluid-equivalent signal in the articular cavity (black arrowheads). (B) Sagittal T1-weighted fat-suppressed contrast-enhanced MR image of the same knee shows joint effusion depicted as hypointense signal within the articular cavity (white arrowheads). Suprapatellar and infrapatellar synovial thickening is visualized (white arrows). Note that the extent of synovial thickening can only be appreciated on T1-weighted contrast-enhanced MR images. (From Guermazi A, Burstein D, Conaghan P, et al. Imaging in osteoarthritis. Rheum Dis Clin North Am 2008;34:645–87.)

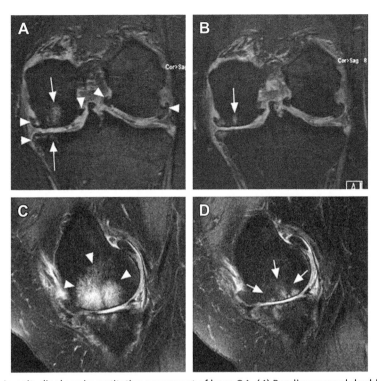

Fig. 5. Longitudinal semiquantitative assessment of knee OA. (*A*) Baseline coronal double-echo steady state MR image shows central osteophytes scored for the medial and lateral compartments (*arrowheads*). Subchondral BMLs are shown (*arrows*). (*B*) MR image at 12-month follow-up shows increasing cartilage loss in the medial compartment but a decrease of the periarticular BMLs (*arrow*). The size of the osteophytes has not changed. (*C*) Sagittal proton density–weighted fat-suppressed MR image shows a large BML in the central weight-bearing part of the medial femur (*arrowheads*). (*D*) MR image at 12-month follow-up shows a decrease in the size and signal intensity of the BML (*arrows*). Note that the BML is better depicted on the spin-echo images (*C, D*) than on the gradient-echo images (*A, B*). (*From* Guermazi A, Burstein D, Conaghan P, et al. Imaging in osteoarthritis. Rheum Dis Clin North Am 2008;34:645–87.)

were published after 2008 are reviewed. Second, research efforts in quantitative MR imaging techniques are described. Third, developments in compositional/physiologic MR imaging techniques are reviewed.

Semiquantitative MR Imaging Scoring Systems for Knee OA

In addition to the three well-established scoring systems (the Whole-organ Magnetic Resonance Imaging Score [WORMS],[61] the Knee Osteoarthritis Scoring System [KOSS],[62] and the Boston Leeds Osteoarthritis Knee Score [BLOKS])[63] a new scoring system called the MR Imaging Osteoarthritis Knee Score (MOAKS) has been added to the literature (**Tables 1** and **2**). Of these systems, WORMS and BLOKS have been widely disseminated and used, although only a limited number of studies have directly compared the two systems. Two recent studies by Lynch and colleagues[64] and Felson and colleagues[65] were helpful in identifying the relative strengths and weaknesses of the two systems in regard to certain features assumed to be most relevant to the natural history of the disease, including cartilage, meniscus, and BMLs. WORMS and BLOKS have weaknesses and it may be difficult for investigators to choose which

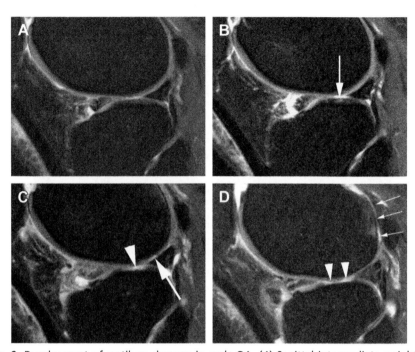

Fig. 6. Development of cartilage damage in early OA. (*A*) Sagittal intermediate-weighted fat-saturated image shows regular articular chondral surface without focal or diffuse cartilage damage. (*B*) Twelve-month follow-up image of the same knee at the identical section shows early intrachondral degeneration reflected as hyperintensity within the central weight-bearing region of the tibial cartilage but not altering the articular surface (*arrow*). (*C*) Twenty-four-month examination depicts focal full-thickness cartilage defect reaching the subchondral plateau at the same location (*arrowhead*). In addition, there is incident superficial cartilage damage at the central part of the lateral femoral condyle adjacent to the posterior horn of the lateral meniscus (arrow). (*D*) Thirty-six-month follow-up image shows progression to widespread full-thickness cartilage loss in the central weight-bearing part of the lateral tibia (*arrowheads*). In addition, there is incident full-thickness damage at the posterior aspect of the lateral femoral condyle (*thin arrows*). Note the presence of the adjacent BMLs, which often accompany cartilage damage as in this case. (*From* Guermazi A, Burstein D, Conaghan P, et al. Imaging in osteoarthritis. Rheum Dis Clin North Am 2008;34:645–87.)

is more suitable for the particular aims of the study they are planning. For instance, the WORMS meniscal scoring method mixes multiple constructs, whereas application of the BML scoring system in BLOKS is cumbersome and complex, and some of the scoring seems redundant. In addition, both of these systems have undergone unpublished modifications that make it difficult for general readers to determine the differences between the original description and how they have been applied in later research. The use of within-grade changes for longitudinal assessment of cartilage damage and BMLs is a good example.[66] Within-grade scoring describes progression or improvement of a lesion that does not meet the criteria of a full grade change but does represent a definite visual change. For example, in the original publication of WORMS, there was no mention of scoring of within-grade changes because the WORMS publication only used a cross-sectional dataset. It has become common practice to incorporate these within-grade changes whenever longitudinal cartilage

Table 1
Comparison of MR imaging features scored by the 4 semiquantitative MR imaging scoring systems

MR Imaging Features	BLOKS	WORMS	MOAKS	KOSS
Cartilage	Uses 2 scores Score 1: subregional approach (A) Percentage of any cartilage loss in subregion (B) Percentage of full-thickness cartilage loss in subregion Score 2: site-specific approach. Scoring of cartilage thickness at 11 specific locations (not subregions) from 0 (none) to 2 (full-thickness loss)	Subregional approach: scored from 0 to 6 depending on depth and extent of cartilage loss Intrachondral cartilage signal is scored as present or absent	Subregional approach: each articular cartilage region is graded from 0 to 3 for size of any cartilage loss as a percentage of surface area of each individual region surface, and percentage in this subregion that is full-thickness loss	Subregional approach: focal and diffuse defects are differentiated. Depth of lesions is scored from 0 to 3 Diameter of lesions is scored from 0 to 3 Osteochondral defects are scored separately
BMLs	Scoring of individual lesions 3 different aspects of BMLs are scored: (A) Size of BML scored from 0 to 3 concerning percentage of subregional bone volume (B) Percentage of surface area adjacent to subchondral plate (C) Percentage of BML that is noncystic	Summed BML size/volume for subregion from 0 to 3 based on percentage of subregional bone volume	Summed BML size/volume for subregion from 0 to 3 based on percentage of subregional bone volume Number of BMLs counted Percentage of each BML that is noncystic is graded from 0 to 3	Scoring of individual lesions from 0 to 3 based on maximum diameter of lesion
Subchondral cysts	Scored together with BMLs	Summed cyst size/volume for subregion from 0 to 3 in regard to percentage of subregional bone volume	Scored together with BMLs	Scoring of individual lesions from 0 to 3 based on maximum diameter of lesion

(continued on next page)

Table 1
(continued)

MR Imaging Features	BLOKS	WORMS	MOAKS	KOSS
Osteophytes	Scored from 0 to 3 at 12 sites	Scored from 0 to 7 at 16 sites	Same as BLOKS: scored from 0 to 3 at 12 sites	Scored from 0 to 3 Marginal intercondylar and central osteophytes are differentiated Locations/sites of osteophytes scoring not included
Bone attrition	Not scored	Scored from 0 to 3 in 14 subregions	Not scored	Not scored
Effusion	Scored from 0 to 3	Scored from 0 to 3	Scored from 0 to 3 (termed effusion synovitis)	Scored from 0 to 3
Synovitis	(A) Scoring of size of signal changes in Hoffa fat pad (B) Five additional sites scored as present or absent	Combined effusion/synovitis score	Scored from 0 to 3 (called Hoffa synovitis)	Synovial thickening scored as present or absent
Meniscal status	Intrasubstance signal changes in anterior horn, body, posterior horn scored separately in medial/lateral meniscus Presence/absence scored for the following: • Intrameniscal signal, vertical tear, horizontal tear, complex tear, root tear, maceration, meniscal cyst	Anterior horn, body, posterior horn scored separately in medial/lateral meniscus from 0 to 4: 1. Minor radial or parrot-beak tear 2. Nondisplaced tear or prior surgical repair 3. Displaced tear or partial resection 4. Complete maceration or destruction or complete resection	Same as BLOKS, plus additional scoring for meniscal hypertrophy, partial maceration, and progressive partial maceration	No subregional division of meniscus described. Presence or absence of tears: • Horizontal tear, vertical tear, radial tear, complex tear, bucket-handle tear Meniscal intrasubstance degeneration scored from 0 to 3

Meniscal extrusion	Scored as medial and lateral extrusion on coronal image, and anterior extrusion for medial or lateral meniscus on sagittal image from 0 to 3	Not scored	Same as BLOKS	Scored on coronal image from 0 to 3
Ligaments	Cruciate ligaments scored as normal or complete tear. Associated insertional BMLs are scored in tibia and in femur. Collateral ligaments not scored	Cruciate ligaments and collateral ligaments scored as intact or torn	Same as BLOKS	Not scored
Periarticular features	Features are scored as present or absent: • Patellar tendon signal, pes anserine bursitis, iliotibial band signal, popliteal cyst, infrapatellar bursa, prepatellar bursa, ganglion cysts of the tibiofibular joint, meniscus, anterior and posterior cruciate ligaments, semimembranosus, semitendinosus, other	Popliteal cysts, anserine bursitis, semimembranosus bursa, meniscal cyst, infrapatellar bursitis, prepatellar bursitis, tibiofibular cyst scored from 0 to 3	Same as BLOKS	Popliteal cysts only, scored from 0 to 3
Loose bodies	Scored as present or absent	Scored from 0 to 3 depending on number of loose bodies	Same as BLOKS	Not scored

Table 2
Comparison of technical aspects of each scoring system and their reliabilities

	BLOKS	WORMS	MOAKS	KOSS
MR imaging system used	1.5-T system	1.5-T system	3-T system	1.5-T system
MR imaging protocol of original publication	For reliability exercise (10 knees): sagittal/coronal T2-weighted fat-suppressed, sagittal T1-weighted spin-echo, axial/coronal 3D FLASH. For validity of BML assessment (71 knees): sagittal proton density weighted/T2 weighted, axial/coronal proton density weighted/T2 weighted fat suppressed	Axial T1-weighted spin echo, coronal T1-weighted spin echo, sagittal T1-weighted spin echo, sagittal T2-weighted fat-suppressed, sagittal 3D SPGR	Coronal intermediate-weighted 2D turbo spin echo, sagittal 3D DESS with axial/coronal reformation, sagittal intermediate-weighted fat-suppressed fast spin echo	Coronal/sagittal T2-weighted and proton density–weighted, sagittal 3D SPGR, axial proton density–weighted and axial T2-weighted fat suppressed
Subregional division of knee	9 subregions: medial/lateral patella, medial/lateral trochlea, medial/lateral weight-bearing femur, medial/lateral weight-bearing tibia, subspinous tibia	15 subregions: medial/lateral patella, medial/lateral femur (anterior/central/posterior), medial/lateral tibia (anterior/central/posterior), subspinous tibia	15 subregions: medial/lateral patella, medial/lateral femur (trochlea/central/posterior), medial/lateral tibia (anterior/central/posterior), subspinous tibia	9 subregions: medial patella, patellar crest, lateral patella, medial/lateral trochlea, medial/lateral femoral condyle, medial/lateral tibial plateau

Inter-reader reliability	Based on 10 knees Weighted κ between 0.51 (meniscal extrusion) and 0.79 (meniscal tear)	Based on 19 knees ICC between 0.74 (bone marrow abnormalities and synovitis/effusion) and 0.99 (cartilage)	Based on 20 knees Weighted κ between 0.36 (tibial cartilage area) and 1.00 (patellar BML percentage cyst) Agreement between 55% (tibial osteophytes) and 100% (patellar BML percentage cyst)	Based on 25 knees Weighted κ between 0.57 (osteochondral defects) and 0.88 (bone marrow edema)
Intrareader reliability	Not presented	Not presented	Based on 20 knees Weighted κ between 0.42 (Hoffa synovitis) and 1.00 (patellar BML size and medial meniscal morphology) Agreement between 55% (Hoffa synovitis) and 100% (patellar BML size and medial meniscal morphology)	Based on 25 knees Weighted κ between 0.56 (intrasubstance meniscal degeneration) and 0.91 (bone marrow edema and Baker cyst)

Abbreviations: DESS, dual-echo steady state; FLASH, fast low-angle shot; ICC, Intraclass correlation coefficient; SPGR, spoiled gradient echo; 2D, two dimensional; 3D, three dimensional.

assessment is contemplated. A recent study by Roemer and colleagues[66] showed that within-grade changes in semiquantitative MR imaging assessment of cartilage and BMLs are valid and their use may increase the sensitivity of semiquantitative readings in detecting longitudinal changes in these structures.

There has never been a published correction or an addendum to the original WORMS publication. The effort to evolve semiquantitative scoring methods that circumvent the limitations of WORMS and BLOKS led to the development of MOAKS. By integrating expert readers' experience with all of the available scoring tools and the published data comparing different scoring systems, MOAKS refined the scoring of BMLs, added subregional assessment, omitted some redundancy in cartilage and BML scoring, and refined elements of meniscal morphology.

For BML size assessment, the threshold for grading in terms of percentage of subregional volume was modified. Also, rather than a lesion-based approach, the subregion-based approach of WORMS was incorporated. The number of lesions is counted, but the percentage of BML in the area of the adjacent subchondral plate is no longer recorded. There is only one cartilage score using a WORMS-like subregional approach. Synovitis as detected in the form of high signal intensity in the Hoffa fat pad is now called Hoffa synovitis. Effusion was renamed effusion synovitis, because high signal within the joint cavity on T2-weighted images incorporates both joint fluid (ie, effusion) and synovial thickening (ie, synovitis). A detailed differentiation of the different types of meniscal tears, meniscal hypertrophy, partial maceration, and progressive partial maceration has been incorporated, allowing detailed assessment of meniscal damage over time (**Fig. 7**). The scoring of noncystic BML percentage, osteophytes, meniscal extrusion and signal, ligaments, and periarticular features remain unchanged from BLOKS.

The MOAKS system is currently being deployed in the Meniscal Tear in Osteoarthritis Research (MeTeOR) trial[67] and the Pivotal Osteoarthritis Initiative Magnetic Resonance Imaging Analyses (POMA).[68] However, it is a new scoring system and needs more data to show its validity and reliability when applied to OA studies.

Synovitis is an important feature of OA, with a demonstrated association with pain.[58,69] Although synovitis can be evaluated with non–contrast-enhanced MR imaging by using the presence of signal changes in Hoffa fat pad or joint effusion as an indirect marker of synovitis, only contrast-enhanced MR imaging can reveal the extent of synovial inflammation (see **Fig. 4**).[70] **Table 3** summarizes two comprehensive scoring systems for synovitis in knee OA based on contrast-enhanced MR imaging. These scoring systems could potentially be used in clinical trials of new OA drugs that target synovitis.[58,69]

Semiquantitative MR Imaging Whole-organ Scoring System for Hand OA

Conventional radiography is still the imaging modality of choice clinically for OA of the hand, but the use of more sensitive imaging techniques such as ultrasonography and MR imaging is becoming more common, especially for research purposes. However, the literature concerning MR imaging of pathologic features of hand OA is still sparse, and studies have been performed without applying standardized methods.[71–77] In 2011, Haugen and colleagues[78] proposed a semiquantitative MR imaging scoring system for hand OA features, called the Oslo Hand OA MR Imaging Score: it incorporates osteophyte presence and JSN (0–3 scale) and malalignment (absence/presence) in analog to the OARSI atlas.[1] Cysts and collateral ligament disorders are also recorded as absent or present. These features are assessed at 8 locations (distal interphalangeal [DIP] and proximal interphalangeal [PIP]) joints of the second, third, fourth, and fifth fingers) of the dominant hand using an extremity 1.0-T MR system. An atlas is included in the publication to facilitate scoring. Each MR image feature was analyzed

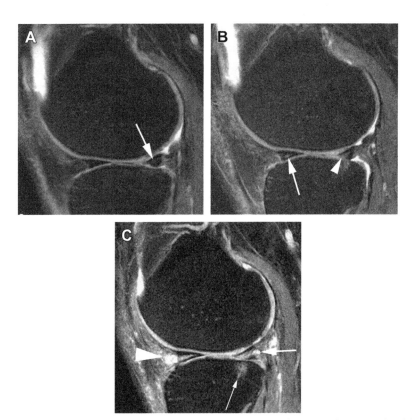

Fig. 7. Progression of meniscal damage over time. (*A*) Sagittal intermediate-weighted fat-saturated image shows intrameniscal high signal representing mucoid degeneration (*arrow*) in the posterior horn of the medial meniscus that does not reach the meniscal surface. No tear is seen and there is no signal change in the anterior horn. (*B*) Twelve-month follow-up examination depicts development of the horizontal-oblique tear in the posterior horn. Meniscal hyperintensity now reaches the meniscal undersurface (*arrowhead*). In addition, there is incident mucoid degeneration in the anterior horn (*arrow*). (*C*) At 36-month follow-up, an incident horizontal tear in the anterior horn is seen. In addition, meniscal cysts communicating with horizontal tears of the anterior horn (*arrowhead*) and posterior horn (*thick arrow*) are visible. Note the subchondral BML adjacent to the full-thickness cartilage damage in the posterior aspect of the lateral tibial plateau (*thin arrow*).

and stratified for joint groups and as aggregated scores (ie, DIP and PIP). Key features such as synovitis, flexor tenosynovitis, erosions, osteophytes, JSN, and BMLs showed good to very good intrareader and inter-reader reliability.[79]

Using this scoring system, Haugen and colleagues[80] showed that MR imaging could detect approximately twice as many joints with erosions and osteophytes as conventional radiography (*P*<.001), but identification of JSN, cysts, and malalignment was similar. The prevalence of most MR imaging features increased with radiographic severity, but synovitis was more frequent in joints with mild OA than with moderate/severe OA. The same group of investigators also showed in another study that MR imaging–assessed moderate/severe synovitis, BMLs, erosions, attrition, and osteophytes were associated with joint tenderness independently of each other.[81] Weaker associations were found between the sum score of MR imaging–defined attrition and

Table 3
Summary of contrast-enhanced MR imaging–based semiquantitative scoring systems for synovitis in knee osteoarthritis

Scoring system	Modified Rhodes et al (used in Baker et al,[69] 2010)	Guermazi et al[58]
MRI system used (T)	1.5	1.5
Number of knees	454	400
MRI sequence	Axial/sagittal T1-weighted fat-suppressed postcontrast	Axial/sagittal T1-weighted fat-suppressed
Sites of synovitis evaluation	6 sites: Medial and lateral parapatellar recess, suprapatellar pouch, and infrapatellar fat pad (graded 0–3); Medial and lateral posterior condyle (scored 0 or 1)	11 sites: Medial and lateral parapatellar recess, suprapatellar, infrapatellar, intercondylar, medial and lateral perimeniscal, and adjacent to anterior and posterior cruciate ligaments, adjacent to loose bodies, within Baker cyst
Contrast administration	Gd-DTPA 0.2 mL (0.1 mmol)/kg body weight Postcontrast axial image acquired 2 min after injection, immediately followed by sagittal image	Gd-DTPA 0.2 mL (0.1 mmol)/kg body weight Postcontrast axial image acquired 2 min after injection, immediately followed by sagittal image
Grades	0, normal; 1, diffuse even thickening; 2, nodular thickening; 3, gross nodular thickening	0, maximal synovial thickness <2 mm; 1, 2–4 mm; 2, greater than 4 mm
Analysis approach	Synovitis categories: 1, normal or questionable (<4 sites scored as 1 and all other sites scored as 0); 2, some (≥4 sites scored as 1 and/or ≤1 site scored as 2); 3, a lot (≥2 sites scored as 2 and no score of 3); 4, extensive (>1 site scored as 3)	Whole-knee synovitis scores of 11 sites were summed and categorized: 0–4, normal or equivocal; 5–8, mild synovitis; 9–12, moderate synovitis; ≥13, severe synovitis
Reliability	Inter-reader: weighted κ 0.80 Intrareader: weighted κ 0.58	For each site: Inter-reader, weighted κ 0.67–0.92; intrareader, weighted κ 0.67–1.00 (rater 1), 0.60–1.00 (rater 2) For summed score: inter-reader, ICC 0.94; intrareader, ICC 0.98 (reader 1), 0.96 (reader 2)

Abbreviations: DTPA, diethylene triamine pentaacetic acid; Gd, gadolinium; ICC, intraclass correlation coefficient.

the Functional Index of Hand Osteoarthritis (FIHOA), and between the sum score of osteophytes and grip strength.[81] These studies showed that some of the semiquanti-tatively assessed MR imaging features of hand OA may be potential targets for ther-apeutic interventions.

Semiquantitative MR Imaging Whole-organ Scoring System for Hip OA

Compared with knee OA, few studies have focused on the hip joint, and only 1 used an approach similar to the whole-organ evaluation of knee OA.[82,83] The hip joint has a spherical structure and its thin covering of articular hyaline cartilage makes MR imaging assessment of the hip more challenging than the knee.[84] Patients with OA of the hip often have to be followed for a long time to assess the natural course of joint disorders, or to evaluate surgical or pharmacologic treatment effects. Noninvasive follow-up methods are necessary, and surrogate markers based on MR imaging would be useful. A novel tool for use in observational studies and clinical trials of hip joints, a whole-organ semiquantitative multi-feature scoring method called the Hip Osteoarthritis MRI Scoring System (HOAMS), was therefore introduced by Roemer and colleagues[85] in 2011.

In HOAMS, 14 articular features are assessed: cartilage morphology, subchondral BMLs, subchondral cysts, osteophytes, acetabular labrum, synovitis (only scored when contrast-enhanced sequences were available), joint effusion, loose bodies, attri-tion, dysplasia, trochanteric bursitis/insertional tendonitis of the greater trochanter, lab-ral hypertrophy, paralabral cysts, and herniation pits at the superolateral femoral neck. Cartilage and osteophytes are scored on a scale from 0 to 4: BMLs, subchondral cysts, and labral disorders are graded 0 to 3; synovitis and effusion are graded 0 to 2; and all other lesions are scored 0 (absent) or 1 (present). Cartilage morphology is scored in 9 subregions, and BMLs and subchondral cysts in 15 subregions for acetabular and femoral subchondral bone marrow assessment. MR imaging sequences acquired in the protocol include coronal and axial non–fat-suppressed T1-weighted spin echo, coronal and sagittal proton density–weighted fat-suppressed fast spin echo, and, where indicated, coronal and axial contrast-enhanced T1-weighted sequences.

Whether this scoring tool is similarly applicable to longitudinal studies, particularly with regard to its responsiveness and predictive validity, remains to be seen. HOAMS showed satisfactory reliability and good agreement concerning intraobserver and interobserver assessment, but further validation, assessment of responsiveness, and iterative refinement of the scoring system are still needed to maximize its useful-ness in clinical trials and epidemiologic studies.

Quantitative Cartilage Morphometry

Quantitative measurement of cartilage morphology segments the cartilage image (**Figs. 8** and **9**) and exploits the three-dimensional nature of MR imaging data sets to evaluate tissue dimensions (such as thickness and volume) or signal as continuous variables. Examples of nomenclature for MR imaging–based cartilage measures were proposed by Eckstein and colleagues[86]: dAB, denuded area of subchondral bone; tAB, total area of subchondral bone; ThCtAB.Me, mean cartilage thickness over the tAB; VC, cartilage volume. Because many of these measures are strongly related, Buck and colleagues[87] identified an efficient subset of core measures (tAB and dAB) that can provide a comprehensive description of cartilage morphology and its longitudinal changes in knees with or without OA. The same group also proposed a strategy (the ordered values approach) for more efficiently analyzing longitudinal changes in (subregional) cartilage thickness[88] and found that determining the magni-tude of subregional cartilage thickness changes independent of anatomic location

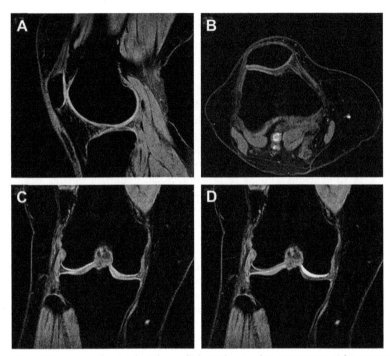

Fig. 8. Knee MR image obtained with spoiled gradient-echo sequences with water excitation, in the same person. (*A*) Sagittal image; (*B*) axial image; (*C*) coronal image; (*D*) same coronal image with the medial tibial cartilage marked (segmented) blue, medial femoral cartilage marked yellow, lateral tibial cartilage marked green, and lateral femoral cartilage marked red. (*From* Guermazi A, Burstein D, Conaghan P, et al. Imaging in osteoarthritis. Rheum Dis Clin North Am 2008;34:645–87.)

provided improved discrimination between OA participants and healthy subjects longitudinally. Further, the ordered values approach was found to be superior in detecting risk factors of OA progression.[89] Wirth and colleagues[90] proposed an extended ordered values approach with better discrimination of cartilage thickness changes in KL grade 2 versus KL grade 3 knees than measures of total plate and subregional cartilage thickness or changes in radiographic JSW.

Quantitative measurements of cartilage volume and thickness have been used in several intervention studies. Ding and colleagues[91] examined the associations between nonsteroidal antiinflammatory drugs (NSAIDs) and changes in knee cartilage volume. Comparing users of cyclooxygenase-2 inhibitors with NSAIDs users, the latter had more knee cartilage volume loss. After evaluating the effect of celecoxib on cartilage volume loss over 1 year in knee OA, Raynauld and colleagues[92] found that the drug did not show a protective effect on knee cartilage loss. Wei and colleagues[93] conducted a cross-sectional study of middle-aged and elderly women and showed that parity, but not use of hormone replacement therapy or oral contraceptives, was independently associated with lower cartilage volume primarily in the tibial compartment. Joint distraction was effective in regenerating cartilage by increasing its thickness and decreasing denuded areas of subchondral bone, and the effects lasted for months after the intervention.[94]

Bennell and colleagues[95] showed that increased dynamic medial knee load was associated with a greater loss of medial cartilage volume over 1 year. Eckstein and

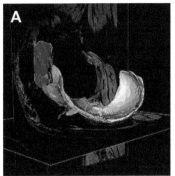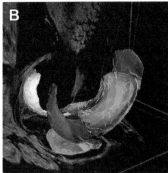

Fig. 9. (*A, B*) Three-dimensional reconstruction and visualization of knee cartilage plates from a sagittal MR imaging data set: blue, medial tibial cartilage; yellow, medial femoral cartilage; green, lateral tibial cartilage; red, lateral femoral cartilage; turquoise, femoral trochlear cartilage; magenta, patellar cartilage. (*From* Guermazi A, Burstein D, Conaghan P, et al. Imaging in osteoarthritis. Rheum Dis Clin North Am 2008;34:645–87.)

colleagues[96] compared knees with frequent pain with knees without pain, and found higher rates of (medial femorotibial) cartilage loss over 1 year in the painful knees compared with the painless knees. Adjustment or stratification for radiographic disease stage did not affect this association. The investigators concluded that enrolling participants with frequent knee pain in clinical trials could increase the observed rate of structural progression. The same group also showed that radiographic and MR cartilage morphometry features suggesting advanced OA (high KL grade) seem to be associated with greater cartilage thickness loss.[97,98] Knees with early radiographic OA (KL grade 2) display thicker cartilage than healthy reference knees or the contralateral knees without radiographic findings of OA, specifically in the external femoral subregions.[99,100]

Quantitative measures of articular cartilage structure, such as cartilage thickness loss and denuded areas of subchondral bone, have been shown to predict an important clinical outcome: knee replacement.[101] However, long-term observations are needed to achieve robust results on tibiofemoral cartilage thickness loss in individual knees in observational OA studies, by comparing 1-year with 2-year and 4-year rates of change in OA knees.[102] Further, investigators intending to use the quantitative morphometry approach in a multicenter study should be aware of at least 1 pitfall: quantitative data collected from different segmentation teams cannot be pooled unless equivalence is shown for the cartilage metrics of interest. Schneider and colleagues[103] showed that segmentation team differences dominated measurement variability in most cartilage regions for all image series.

Functional studies in healthy subjects reported nocturnal changes of cartilage thickness, with more morning postexercise deformation than evening postexercise deformation.[104] Osteoarthritic cartilage tended to show more deformation on loading than healthy cartilage, suggesting that knee OA affects the mechanical properties of cartilage, and the pattern of in vivo deformation indicated that cartilage loss in OA progression is mechanically driven.[105] A correlation between changes in cartilage thickness and those in a molecular serum marker (ie, cartilage oligomeric matrix protein) after drop landing was also reported.[106]

Quantitative MR Imaging Analysis of Tissues Other than Cartilage

Several investigators have reported studies using MR imaging to quantitatively evaluate the menisci. Wirth and colleagues[107] presented a technique for three-dimensional and quantitative analysis of meniscal shape, position, and signal intensity, which displayed adequate interobserver and intraobserver precision.[108,109] When examining healthy reference subjects using these techniques, the investigators reported that meniscus surface area strongly corresponds with (ipsilateral) tibial plateau area across both sexes, and that tibial coverage by the meniscus is similar between men and women.

Swanson and colleagues[110] developed an algorithm to semiautomatically segment the meniscus in a series of MR images. Their method produced accurate and consistent segmentations of the meniscus compared with the manual segmentations. Wenger and colleagues[111] described an association between knee pain and meniscal extrusion using a between-knee, intraperson comparison using three-dimensional measures of extrusion.

Other than menisci, investigators have used quantitative MR imaging to assess BMLs,[112,113] synovitis,[114] and joint effusion.[115] However, using segmentation approaches for ill-defined lesions such as BMLs is more challenging than segmentation of clearly delineated structures such as cartilage, menisci, and effusion.[40]

Compositional MR Imaging of Cartilage and Menisci

Compositional MR imaging can assess the biochemical properties of different joint tissues and thus is sensitive to early, premorphologic changes that cannot be seen on conventional MR imaging. Most studies applying compositional MR imaging have focused on cartilage, although the technique can also be used to assess other tissues such as the meniscus or ligaments. Compositional imaging of cartilage matrix changes can be performed using advanced MR imaging techniques such as delayed gadolinium-enhanced MR imaging of cartilage (dGEMRIC; **Fig. 10**), T1 rho, and T2

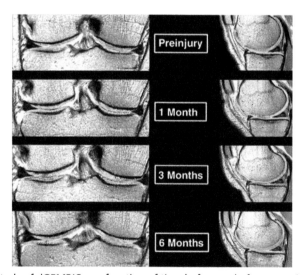

Fig. 10. Case study of dGEMRIC as a function of time before and after posterior cruciate ligament injury. A decline in the dGEMRIC index is apparent at 1 month, with a further decrease at 3 months and recovery at 6 months. These data show the potential for biochemical monitoring of cartilage to demonstrate degeneration and recovery of the tissue from a traumatic injury. Similar studies might be used to monitor cartilage status improvement with other mechanical, surgical, or pharmaceutical interventions. (*From* Young AA, Stanwell P, Williams A, et al. Glycosaminoglycan content of knee cartilage following posterior cruciate ligament rupture demonstrated by delayed gadolinium-enhanced magnetic resonance imaging of cartilage (dGEMRIC). A case report. J Bone Joint Surg Am 2005;87(12):2765; with permission.)

mapping (**Fig. 11**). For detailed descriptions of these techniques, readers are referred to the published review articles.[42,116]

In a placebo-controlled double-blind pilot trial of collagen hydrolysate for mild knee OA, McAlindon and colleagues[117] showed that the dGEMRIC score increased in tibial cartilage regions of interest in subjects receiving collagen hydrolysate, and decreased in the placebo group. A significant difference was observed at 24 weeks. It will be of interest to see whether macroscopic cartilage changes are associated with those dGEMRIC findings in future studies. Another study[118] showed an increase in dGEMRIC indices of knee cartilage in asymptomatic untrained women who were enrolled in a 10-week running program, compared with sedentary controls. Souza and colleagues[119] showed that acute loading of the knee joint resulted in a significant decrease in T1 rho and T2 relaxation times of the medial tibiofemoral compartment, and especially in cartilage regions with small focal defects. These data suggest that changes of T1 rho values under mechanical loading may be related to the biomechanical and structural properties of cartilage.

Hovis and colleagues[120] reported that light exercise was associated with low cartilage T2 values but moderate and strenuous exercise were associated with high T2 values in women, suggesting that activity levels can affect cartilage composition. Another study of the normal control group at baseline and 2 years later found a high

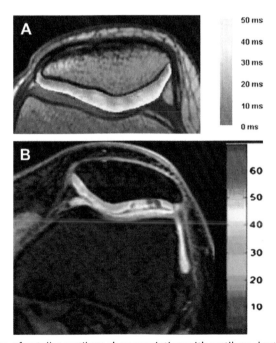

Fig. 11. (*A*) T2 map of patellar cartilage shows variation with cartilage depth. (B) T1 rho map of patellar cartilage shows a lesion in cartilage that is morphologically thick and intact. The variation and lesions apparent in maps of these parameters across morphologically intact cartilage enable monitoring of biochemical changes in cartilage before morphologic changes become apparent. (*From* [A] Maier CF, Tan SG, Hariharan H, et al. T2 quantitation of articular cartilage at 1.5 T. J Magn Reson Imaging 2003;17(3):363, with permission; and [B] Borthakur A, Mellon E, Niyogi S, et al. Sodium and T1 rho MRI for molecular and diagnostic imaging of articular cartilage. NMR Biomed 2006;19(7):799, with permission.)

prevalence of structural abnormalities and a significant increase in cartilage T2 values in the tibiofemoral, but not the patellofemoral, joint.[121] In an interventional study assessing the effect of weight loss on articular cartilage, Anandacoomarasamy and colleagues[122] reported that improved articular cartilage quality was reflected as an increase in the dGEMRIC index over 1 year for the medial, but not the lateral, compartment. This finding highlights the role of weight loss in possible clinical and structural improvement.

Williams and colleagues[123] described intrameniscal biochemical alterations using ultrashort echo time–enhanced T2* mapping. The investigators found significant increases of ultrashort echo time–enhanced T2* values in the menisci of subjects with anterior cruciate ligament injuries but who showed no clinical evidence of subsurface meniscal abnormality.

Novel compositional techniques have been explored further. Raya and colleagues[124] found that in vivo diffusion tensor imaging with a 7-T MR system could distinguish OA knees from non-OA knees better than T2 mapping. Other work on 7-T systems reported on the reproducibility of the method in vivo.[125,126] Another compositional technique that might reward further exploration is T2* mapping of cartilage.[127] These techniques show promise, but they need to be practical and deployable using standard MR imaging systems before they can be widely used as research or a clinical diagnostic tools.

ULTRASONOGRAPHY

Ultrasound imaging allows multiplanar and real-time imaging without radiation exposure at low cost. It can offer reliable assessment of OA-associated features, including inflammatory and structural abnormalities, without contrast administration.[128] Limitations of ultrasonography include that it is an operator-dependent technique and that the physical properties of sound limit its ability to assess deeper articular structures and the subchondral bone (**Fig. 12**).

Ultrasonography is useful for evaluation of cortical erosive changes and synovitis in inflammatory arthritis.[129] In OA, the ability to detect synovial disorders is the major advantage ultrasonography has compared with conventional radiography. Current ultrasound technology can detect synovial disorders including hypertrophy, increased vascularity, and the presence of synovial fluid in joints affected by arthritis (**Fig. 13**).[128]

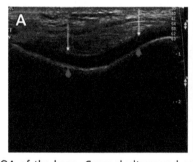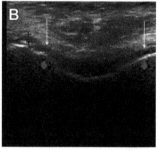

Fig. 12. OA of the knee. Coronal ultrasound scans through the distal femur of a normal knee (*A*) and an osteoarthritic knee (*B*) show the intracondylar notch. The red arrows indicate the cortical surface of the femur, and the yellow arrows indicate the superficial surface of the cartilage. Note that, compared with the normal knee, the cartilage in the osteoarthritic knee is more echoic, there is loss of definition of the margins, and it seems thinner laterally. (*From* Guermazi A, Burstein D, Conaghan P, et al. Imaging in osteoarthritis. Rheum Dis Clin North Am 2008;34:645–87.)

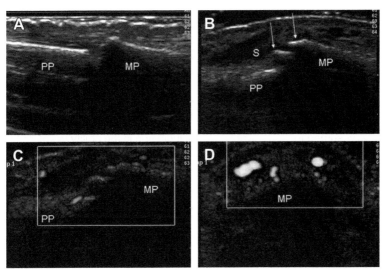

Fig. 13. OA of the PIP joint. (*A*) Dorsal longitudinal ultrasound image of a normal PIP joint, with smooth cortical outlines. (*B*) Dorsal longitudinal ultrasound scan of osteoarthritic PIP joint shows proximal and distal dorsal osteophytes (*yellow arrows*) and synovial hypertrophy (dark area indicated by an S). Dorsal longitudinal (*C*) and transverse (*D*) ultrasound scans of the PIP joint shown in *B*, with power Doppler function added, show Doppler signal within the hypoechoic synovial hypertrophy. PP, proximal phalanx; MP, middle phalanx. (*From* Guermazi A, Burstein D, Conaghan P, et al. Imaging in osteoarthritis. Rheum Dis Clin North Am 2008;34:645–87.)

The Outcome Measures in Rheumatoid Arthritis Clinical Trials (OMERACT) Ultrasonography Taskforce reported an ultrasonography definition of synovial hypertrophy as, "abnormal hypoechoic (relative to subdermal fat, but sometimes may be isoechoic or hyperechoic) intra-articular tissue that is non-displaceable and poorly compressible and which may exhibit Doppler."[130] Although this definition was developed for use in rheumatoid arthritis, it may also be applied to OA because the difference in synovial inflammation between OA and rheumatoid arthritis is quantitative rather than qualitative.[128]

A preliminary ultrasonographic scoring system for features of hand OA was published recently.[131] This scoring system included evaluation of gray-scale synovitis and power Doppler signal in 15 joints of the hand. These features were assessed for their presence/absence and, if present, were scored semiquantitatively using a scale from 1 to 3. Overall, the reliability exercise showed moderately good intra-reader and inter-reader reliability. This study showed that an ultrasonography outcome measure suitable for multicenter trials assessing hand OA is feasible and likely to be reliable, and has provided a foundation for further development.

Ultrasonography has been increasingly used for assessment of OA of the hand (see **Fig. 13**). Kortekaas and colleagues[132] showed that ultrasonography-detected osteophytes and JSN are associated with hand pain. In a more recent study, the same group of investigators showed that signs of inflammation appear more frequently on ultrasonography in hands with erosive OA than in hands without erosive OA, not only in erosive joints but also in nonerosive joints.[133] This finding suggests the presence of an underlying systemic cause for erosive evolution. Klauser and colleagues[134] evaluated the efficacy of weekly ultrasonography-guided intra-articular injections of hyaluronic acid. A decrease in pain correlated with a decrease in synovial thickening and power Doppler ultrasonography score between baseline and the end of therapy. To take advantage of ultrasound and MR imaging, lagnocco and colleagues[75] performed integrated MR imaging and ultrasound real-time fusion imaging in hand and wrist OA, and found a high concordance of the bony profile visualization at the level of osteophytes.

Evaluation of synovitis in OA of the knee has also been documented (**Fig. 14**).[100] A cross-sectional, multicenter European study supported by The European League Against Rheumatism (EULAR) analyzed 600 patients with painful knee OA, and found that ultrasonography-detected synovitis correlated with advanced radiographic OA and clinical signs and symptoms suggesting an inflammatory flare.[135] However, ultrasonography-detected synovitis was not a predictor of subsequent joint replacement. In addition, ultrasonography signs of synovitis were found to be reflected metabolically by markers of joint tissue metabolism.[136] Saarakkala and colleagues[137] evaluated the diagnostic performance of knee ultrasonography for the detection of degenerative changes of articular cartilage, using arthroscopic findings as the reference. They found that positive ultrasonography findings were strong indicators of cartilage degeneration, but negative findings did not exclude cartilage degeneration. Kawaguchi and colleagues[138] used ultrasonography to study medial radial displacement of the meniscus in the supine weight-bearing positions. They showed the medial meniscus was significantly displaced radially by weight bearing in control knees and in those with KL grades 1 to 3. Significant differences were noted between knees of KL grade greater than or equal to 2 and controls in the supine and the standing positions, and displacement increased in all weight-bearing knees at 1-year follow-up, except for KL grade 4 knees.

Chao and colleagues[139] assessed whether inflammation on ultrasonography can predict clinical response to intra-articular corticosteroid injections in patients with knee OA. There was a significantly greater improvement in pain among noninflammatory patients than among inflammatory patients 12 weeks after injection. A small

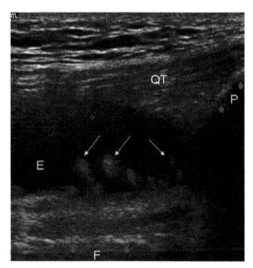

Fig. 14. OA in the knee. A longitudinal ultrasound image through the suprapatellar pouch shows synovial hypertrophy with villi formation (*yellow arrows*) and an effusion (E). The cortical surface of the femur (F) and patella (P) are indicated by the red arrows, and the quadriceps tendon (QT) is also shown. (*From* Guermazi A, Burstein D, Conaghan P, et al. Imaging in osteoarthritis. Rheum Dis Clin North Am 2008;34:645–87.)

sample size, a lack of power Doppler imaging, and imaging only of the suprapatellar pouch could have led to these unexpected results. Wu and colleagues[140] investigated the association of ultrasonography features with pain and the functional scores in patients with equal radiographic grades of OA in both knees. Ultrasonography-detected inflammatory features, including suprapatellar effusion and medial compartment synovitis, were positively and linearly associated with knee pain in motion. Medial compartment synovitis was also degree-dependently associated with pain at rest and with the presence of medial knee pain. These findings confirmed the association between synovitis and knee pain, which has also been reported in MR imaging-based studies.[58]

NUCLEAR MEDICINE

Use of technetium 99m (99mTc) hydroxymethane diphosphonate (HDP) scintigraphy and 2-^{18}F-fluoro-2-deoxy–D-glucose (18-FDG) or 18F-fluoride (18-F$^-$) positron emission tomography (PET) for assessing OA have been described in the literature (**Figs. 15** and **16**).[141] Bone scintigraphy is a simple examination that can provide a full-body survey that helps to discriminate between soft tissues and bone origins of pain, and to locate the site of pain in patients with complex symptoms.[141] 18-FDG-PET can show the site of synovitis and BMLs associated with OA.[142] 18-F$^-$ PET can be used for bone imaging; the amount of tracer uptake depends on the regional blood flow and bone remodeling conditions. An animal study by Umemoto and colleagues[143] using a rat OA model showed that uptake of 18-F$^-$ was significantly higher in knees that had undergone anterior cruciate ligament transection than in sham-operated knees, and was higher in all the compartments of the tibiofemoral joint

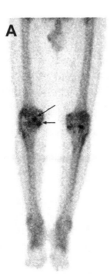
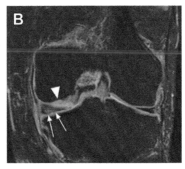

Fig. 15. Scintigraphy. (*A*) Radionuclide accumulation is observed in the medial compartment of the left knee (*black arrows*) in a patient who has prostate cancer and a high risk for bone metastases. This appearance is nonspecific and more likely secondary to degenerative disease. (*B*) Coronal T2-weighted fat-suppressed MR image of the same knee shows meniscal degeneration (*white arrows*) and cartilage damage (*arrowhead*). The image confirms normal bone marrow without metastatic deposits. (*Courtesy of* G. Mercier, MD, PhD, Boston, MA; and *From* Guermazi A, Burstein D, Conaghan P, et al. Imaging in osteoarthritis. Rheum Dis Clin North Am 2008;34:645–87.)

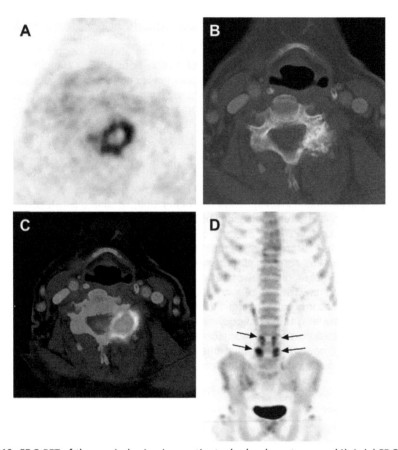

Fig. 16. FDG-PET of the cervical spine in a patient who has breast cancer. (*A*) Axial FDG-PET shows inflammatory facet joint of the cervical spine OA with strong glucose accumulation around the left facet joint. Note the low spatial resolution of PET. (*B*) Axial CT shows hypertrophic left-sided facet joint and confirms the osteoarthritic nature of the lesion. (*C*) Fused PET-CT image superiorly shows the correlation between metabolic changes depicted by PET and spatial localization by CT. (*D*) Coronal FDG-PET in the same patients shows bilateral facet joint OA at L4 to L5 and L5 to S1 (*arrows*). (*Courtesy of* G. Mercier, MD, PhD, Boston, MA; and *From* Guermazi A, Burstein D, Conaghan P, et al. Imaging in osteoarthritis. Rheum Dis Clin North Am 2008;34:645–87.)

8 weeks after surgery. An in vivo study by Temmerman and colleagues[144] showed a significant increase in bone metabolism in the proximal femur of patients with symptomatic hip OA. These studies showed that $18\text{-}F^-$ PET is a potentially useful technique for early detection of OA changes.

Another imaging technique in the nuclear medicine category is single-photon emission computed tomography (SPECT). Researchers are searching for a cartilage-specific radiopharmaceutical agent that can be applied to OA imaging. A recent ex vivo study by Cachin and colleagues[145] using 99mTc-N-triethylammonium-3-proyl-[15]ane-N5 (NTP 15-5), which binds to cartilage, quantified the uptake by human articular cartilage relative to bone 99mTc-HDP radiotracer. Visual analysis of fused SPECT-computed tomography (CT) slices showed selective, intense 99mTc-NTP 15-5 accumulation in articular cartilage, whereas 99mTc-HDP binding was low. A cartilage defect visualized on CT was associated with focal decreased uptake of 99mTc-NTP 15-5. Thus, it is hoped this agent may be applied to human cartilage molecular imaging and clinical applications in OA staging and monitoring.

Limitations of radioisotope methods include poor anatomic resolution and the use of ionizing radiation. However, there are ways to overcome these issues. Hybrid technologies such as PET-CT and PET-MR imaging combine functional imaging with high-resolution anatomic imaging. A study by Moon and colleagues[146] showed that PET-CT could detect active inflammation in patients with OA of the shoulder. Techniques to achieve the optimum registration of PET and MR images are being developed.[147] Moreover, PET scanners have been developed that image small parts of the body.[148] Although originally developed for breast imaging, these small-part scanners may be useful for imaging of joints.[141] The small-part PET scanners have the advantages of lower operating costs and lower radiation exposure while retaining high spatial resolution and sensitivity for detection of lesions.

CT

CT is more useful than MR imaging for depicting cortical bone and soft tissue calcifications. It has an established role in assessing facet joint OA of the spine in both clinical and research settings.[149] Using a CT-based semiquantitative grading system of facet joint OA, a population-based study by Kalichman and colleagues[150] showed a high prevalence of facet joint OA and that the prevalence of facet joint OA increases with age, with the highest prevalence at the L4 to L5 spinal level. Also, in the same cohort of subjects, several associations were observed: self-reported back pain with spinal stenosis[151]; abdominal aortic calcification with facet joint OA[152]; obesity with higher prevalence of facet joint OA[153]; and increasing age with higher prevalence of disc narrowing, facet joint OA, and degenerative spondylolisthesis.[153] A recent animal study by Kim and colleagues[154] used micro-CT to assess the cartilage alterations in the facet joint of rats, and showed that monosodium iodoacetate injection into facet joints provided a useful model for the study of OA changes in the facet joint and indicated that facet joint degeneration is a major cause of low back pain.

CT AND MR ARTHROGRAPHY

Arthrography using CT or MR imaging enables evaluation of damage to articular cartilage with a high anatomic resolution in multiple planes. CT arthrography can be performed using a single (iodine alone) or double-contrast (iodine and air) technique.[141] In general, the single-contrast technique is considered easier to perform and to cause less pain to patients.[155] To avoid beam-hardening artifacts, the contrast material can be diluted with saline or local anesthetics.[141] For MR arthrography, gadolinium–diethylene triamine pentaacetic acid (DTPA) is injected intra-articularly to delineate superficial cartilage defects. The optimum concentration of gadolinium-DTPA varies depending on the magnetic field strength of the MR system.[156] It has been shown that iodine-based and gadolinium-based contrast agents can be mixed, enabling combined MR arthrography and CT arthrography examinations.[157] These arthrographic examinations have a low risk of infection from the intra-articular injection.[158] Other risks include pain and vasovagal reactions, and systemic allergic reactions. CT arthrography exposes patients to radiation but MR arthrography does not.

At present, CT arthrography is the most accurate method for evaluating cartilage thickness. It offers high spatial resolution and high contrast between the low-attenuating cartilage and high-attenuating superficial (contrast material filling the joint space) and deep (subchondral bone) boundaries.[141] Cadaveric studies have shown that CT arthrography is more accurate than MR imaging[159] or MR arthrography.[160] However, a more recent study showed that evaluation of hip cartilage thickness in the coronal plane by MR arthrography has similar accuracy to CT arthrography (**Fig. 17**).[161] For other planes, CT arthrography showed better diagnostic performance than MR arthrography.

Superficial focal cartilage lesions are well delineated by both arthrographic techniques and appear as areas filled with the intra-articular contrast agent. Again, CT arthrography offers higher spatial resolution as well as higher contrast between the cartilage and the intra-articular contrast agent filling the joint space, leading to a high degree of confidence in depicting these lesions with a higher inter-reader reproducibility.[162]

Regarding subchondral changes, MR arthrography is the only technique that allows delineation of subchondral BMLs on the fluid-sensitive sequences with fat suppression.[141] CT arthrography is better than MR arthrography at depicting subchondral bone sclerosis and osteophytes. Both techniques enable visualization of central osteophytes, which are associated with more severe changes of OA than marginal osteophytes.[163]

Because of the high cost (caused by the use of contrast agents), invasive nature, and potential, albeit low, risk associated with intra-articular injection, arthrographic examinations are rarely used in large-scale clinical or epidemiologic OA studies. However, arthrography has been used in a small-scale clinical study of posttraumatic OA.[164] Tamura and colleagues[165] used high-resolution CT arthrography to examine the three-dimensional progression pattern of early acetabular cartilage damage in

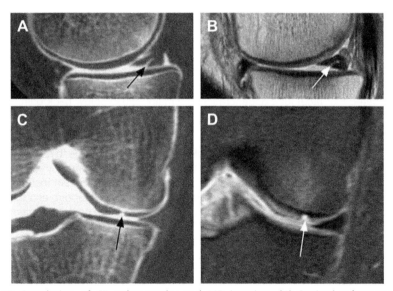

Fig. 17. Correlation of CT arthrography and MR imaging. (*A*) Sagittal reformatted CT arthrography of the medial knee compartment shows posterior horn meniscal tear (*arrow*). Note superficial cartilage thinning at the femoral condyle adjacent to the meniscus. (*B*) Sagittal proton density–weighted MR image of the same knee shows the posterior horn meniscal tear (*arrow*). (*C*) Coronal reformatted CT arthrography of the medial compartment shows focal cartilage defect in the central femoral condyle (*arrow*). (*D*) Coronal fat-suppressed T2-weighted MR image shows the same defect (*arrow*). (*Courtesy of* B. Van de Berg, MD, PhD, Brussels, Belgium; and *From* Guermazi A, Burstein D, Conaghan P, et al. Imaging in osteoarthritis. Rheum Dis Clin North Am 2008;34:645–87.)

32 patients with hip dysplasia. They found that the lateral/medial ratio, which was defined as cartilage thickness in the lateral zone divided by that in the medial zone, may be a sensitive index for quantifying early cartilage damage associated with extent of labral disorders.

SUMMARY

Since publication of the previous edition of this review article in 2008, OA imaging has been driven by publically available images and analyses from the Osteoarthritis Initiative (OAI). OAI study design, image archive, and available image analyses and science have been recently summarized.[37] In a research setting, conventional radiography is still commonly used to semiquantitatively and quantitatively evaluate structural OA features such as osteophytes and JSN. Radiographic JSW measurement is still a recommended option for trials of structural modification, with the understanding that the concept of JSW represents several disorders, including cartilage and meniscal damage, and trial duration may be long. MR imaging is currently the most important imaging modality for research into OA, and investigators may select from semiquantitative, quantitative, and compositional techniques, depending on the aims of the study. Ultrasonography is commonly used in hand OA studies and is particularly useful for evaluation of synovitis. Nuclear medicine, CT, and CT-MR arthrography can also be used for evaluation of OA features, but they are rarely used in large-scale clinical or epidemiologic studies.

ACKNOWLEDGMENTS

We thank those who are not listed as authors in this article, but who were coauthors of the previous edition (Deborah Burstein, Philip Conaghan, Marie-Pierre Hellio Le Graverand-Gastineau, and Helen Keen).

REFERENCES

1. Altman RD, Gold GE. Atlas of individual radiographic features in osteoarthritis, revised. Osteoarthritis Cartilage 2007;15(Suppl A):A1–56.
2. Hunter DJ, Zhang YQ, Tu X, et al. Change in joint space width: hyaline articular cartilage loss or alteration in meniscus? Arthritis Rheum 2006;54:2488–95.
3. Altman R, Asch E, Bloch D, et al. Development of criteria for the classification and reporting of osteoarthritis. Classification of osteoarthritis of the knee. Diagnostic and Therapeutic Criteria Committee of the American Rheumatism Association. Arthritis Rheum 1986;29:1039–49.
4. Kinds MB, Vincken KL, Hoppinga TN, et al. Influence of variation in semiflexed knee positioning during image acquisition on separate quantitative radiographic parameters of osteoarthritis, measured by knee images digital analysis. Osteoarthritis Cartilage 2012;20:997–1003.
5. Kellgren JH, Lawrence JS. Radiological assessment of osteo-arthrosis. Ann Rheum Dis 1957;16:494–502.
6. Felson DT, Niu J, Guermazi A, et al. Defining radiographic incidence and progression of knee osteoarthritis: suggested modifications of the Kellgren and Lawrence scale. Ann Rheum Dis 2011;70:1884–6.
7. Felson DT, Nevitt MC, Yang M, et al. A new approach yields high rates of radiographic progression in knee osteoarthritis. J Rheumatol 2008;35:2047–54.
8. Guermazi A, Hunter DJ, Li L, et al. Different thresholds for detecting osteophytes and joint space narrowing exist between the site investigators and the

centralized reader in a multicenter knee osteoarthritis study–data from the Osteoarthritis Initiative. Skeletal Radiol 2012;41:179–86.

9. Duryea J, Zaim S, Genant HK. New radiographic-based surrogate outcome measures for osteoarthritis of the knee. Osteoarthritis Cartilage 2003;11:102–10.

10. Chu E, DiCarlo JC, Peterfy C, et al. Fixed-location joint space width measurement increases sensitivity to change in osteoarthritis. Osteoarthritis Cartilage 2007;15:S192.

11. Neumann G, Hunter D, Nevitt M, et al. Location specific radiographic joint space width for osteoarthritis progression. Osteoarthritis Cartilage 2009;17:761–5.

12. Beattie KA, Duryea J, Pui M, et al. Minimum joint space width and tibial cartilage morphology in the knees of healthy individuals: a cross-sectional study. BMC Musculoskelet Disord 2008;9:119.

13. Duryea J, Hunter DJ, Nevitt MC, et al. Study of location specific lateral compartment radiographic joint space width for knee osteoarthritis progression: analysis of longitudinal data from the Osteoarthritis Initiative (OAI). Osteoarthritis Cartilage 2008;16:S168.

14. Nevitt MC, Peterfy C, Guermazi A, et al. Longitudinal performance evaluation and validation of fixed-flexion radiography of the knee for detection of joint space loss. Arthritis Rheum 2007;56:1512–20.

15. Duryea J, Li J, Peterfy CG, et al. Trainable rule-based algorithm for the measurement of joint space width in digital radiographic images of the knee. Med Phys 2000;27:580–91.

16. Marijnissen AC, Vincken KL, Vos PA, et al. Knee Images Digital Analysis (KIDA): a novel method to quantify individual radiographic features of knee osteoarthritis in detail. Osteoarthritis Cartilage 2008;16:234–43.

17. Benichou OD, Hunter DJ, Nelson DR, et al. One-year change in radiographic joint space width in patients with unilateral joint space narrowing: data from the Osteoarthritis Initiative. Arthritis Care Res (Hoboken) 2010;62:924–31.

18. Duryea J, Neumann G, Niu J, et al. Comparison of radiographic joint space width with magnetic resonance imaging cartilage morphometry: analysis of longitudinal data from the Osteoarthritis Initiative. Arthritis Care Res (Hoboken) 2010;62:932–7.

19. Reichmann WM, Maillefert JF, Hunter DJ, et al. Responsiveness to change and reliability of measurement of radiographic joint space width in osteoarthritis of the knee: a systematic review. Osteoarthritis Cartilage 2011;19:550–6.

20. Chu Miow Lin D, Reichmann WM, Gossec L, et al. Validity and responsiveness of radiographic joint space width metric measurement in hip osteoarthritis: a systematic review. Osteoarthritis Cartilage 2011;19:543–9.

21. Harvey WF, Yang M, Cooke TD, et al. Association of leg-length inequality with knee osteoarthritis: a cohort study. Ann Intern Med 2010;152:287–95.

22. Mazzuca SA, Brandt KD, Chakr R, et al. Varus malalignment negates the structure-modifying benefits of doxycycline in obese women with knee osteoarthritis. Osteoarthritis Cartilage 2010;18:1008–11.

23. Kinds MB, Marijnissen AC, Vincken KL, et al. Evaluation of separate quantitative radiographic features adds to the prediction of incident radiographic osteoarthritis in individuals with recent onset of knee pain: 5-year follow-up in the CHECK cohort. Osteoarthritis Cartilage 2012;20:548–56.

24. Holla JF, Steultjens MP, van der Leeden M, et al. Determinants of range of joint motion in patients with early symptomatic osteoarthritis of the hip and/or knee: an exploratory study in the CHECK cohort. Osteoarthritis Cartilage 2011;19:411–9.

25. Muraki S, Oka H, Akune T, et al. Association of occupational activity with joint space narrowing and osteophytosis in the medial compartment of the knee: the ROAD study (OAC5914R2). Osteoarthritis Cartilage 2011;19:840–6.

26. Yoshimura N, Muraki S, Oka H, et al. Association of knee osteoarthritis with the accumulation of metabolic risk factors such as overweight, hypertension, dyslipidemia, and impaired glucose tolerance in Japanese men and women: the ROAD study. J Rheumatol 2011;38:921–30.

27. Muraki S, Dennison E, Jameson K, et al. Association of vitamin D status with knee pain and radiographic knee osteoarthritis. Osteoarthritis Cartilage 2011; 19:1301–6.

28. Yoshimura N, Muraki S, Oka H, et al. Accumulation of metabolic risk factors such as overweight, hypertension, dyslipidaemia, and impaired glucose tolerance raises the risk of occurrence and progression of knee osteoarthritis: a 3-year follow-up of the ROAD study. Osteoarthritis Cartilage 2012;20:1217–26.

29. Pothuaud L, Benhamou CL, Porion P, et al. Fractal dimension of trabecular bone projection texture is related to three-dimensional microarchitecture. J Bone Miner Res 2000;15:691–9.

30. Apostol L, Boudousq V, Basset O, et al. Relevance of 2D radiographic texture analysis for the assessment of 3D bone micro-architecture. Med Phys 2006; 33:3546–56.

31. Dobbins JT 3rd, McAdams HP. Chest tomosynthesis: technical principles and clinical update. Eur J Radiol 2009;72:244–51.

32. Stevens GM, Birdwell RL, Beaulieu CF, et al. Circular tomosynthesis: potential in imaging of breast and upper cervical spine—preliminary phantom and in vitro study. Radiology 2003;228:569–75.

33. Canella C, Philippe P, Pansini V, et al. Use of tomosynthesis for erosion evaluation in rheumatoid arthritic hands and wrists. Radiology 2011;258:199–205.

34. Duryea J, Dobbins JT, Lynch JA. Digital tomosynthesis of hand joints for arthritis assessment. Med Phys 2003;30:325–33.

35. Hayashi D, Xu L, Roemer FW, et al. Detection of osteophytes and subchondral cysts in the knee with use of tomosynthesis. Radiology 2012;263:206–15.

36. Conaghan PG, Hunter DJ, Maillefert JF, et al. Summary and recommendations of the OARSI FDA osteoarthritis Assessment of Structural Change Working Group. Osteoarthritis Cartilage 2011;19:606–10.

37. Eckstein F, Wirth W, Nevitt MC. Recent advances in osteoarthritis imaging-the Osteoarthritis Initiative. Nat Rev Rheumatol 2012;8:622–30.

38. Hayashi D, Guermazi A, Hunter DJ. Osteoarthritis year 2010 in review: imaging. Osteoarthritis Cartilage 2011;19:354–60.

39. Hayashi D, Roemer FW, Guermazi A. Osteoarthritis year 2011 in review: imaging in OA - a radiologists' perspective. Osteoarthritis Cartilage 2012;20: 207–14.

40. Roemer FW, Guermazi A. Osteoarthritis year 2012 in review: imaging. Osteoarthritis Cartilage 2012;20(12):1440–6.

41. Guermazi A, Niu J, Hayashi D, et al. Prevalence of abnormalities in knees detected by MRI in adults without knee osteoarthritis: population based observational study (Framingham Osteoarthritis Study). BMJ 2012;345:e5339.

42. Crema MD, Roemer FW, Marra MD, et al. Articular cartilage in the knee: current MR imaging techniques and applications in clinical practice and research. Radiographics 2011;31:37–61.

43. Hayashi D, Roemer FW, Katur A, et al. Imaging of synovitis in osteoarthritis: current status and outlook. Semin Arthritis Rheum 2011;41:116–30.

44. Roemer FW, Crema MD, Trattnig S, et al. Advances in imaging of osteoarthritis and cartilage. Radiology 2011;260:332–54.

45. Xu L, Hayashi D, Roemer FW, et al. Magnetic resonance imaging of subchondral bone marrow lesions in association with osteoarthritis. Semin Arthritis Rheum 2012;42(2):105–18.

46. Englund M, Roemer FW, Hayashi D, et al. Meniscus pathology, osteoarthritis and the treatment controversy. Nat Rev Rheumatol 2012;8:412–9.

47. Hayashi D, Roemer FW, Dhina Z, et al. Longitudinal assessment of cyst-like lesions of the knee and their relation to radiographic osteoarthritis and MRI-detected effusion and synovitis in patients with knee pain. Arthritis Res Ther 2010;12:R172.

48. Hayashi D, Guermazi A, Kwoh CK, et al. Semiquantitative assessment of subchondral bone marrow edema-like lesions and subchondral cysts of the knee at 3T MRI: a comparison between intermediate-weighted fat-suppressed spin echo and dual echo steady state sequences. BMC Musculoskelet Disord 2011;12:198.

49. Hayashi D, Englund M, Roemer FW, et al. Knee malalignment is associated with an increased risk for incident and enlarging bone marrow lesions in the more loaded compartments: the MOST study. Osteoarthritis Cartilage 2012;20:1227–33.

50. Roemer FW, Felson DT, Wang K, et al. Co-localisation of non-cartilaginous articular pathology increases risk of cartilage loss in the tibiofemoral joint–the MOST study. Ann Rheum Dis 2012. [Epub ahead of print].

51. Crema MD, Roemer FW, Felson DT, et al. Factors associated with meniscal extrusion in knees with or at risk for osteoarthritis: the Multicenter Osteoarthritis study. Radiology 2012;264:494–503.

52. Roemer FW, Guermazi A, Felson DT, et al. Presence of MRI-detected joint effusion and synovitis increases the risk of cartilage loss in knees without osteoarthritis at 30-month follow-up: the MOST study. Arthritis Rheum 2012;64:1888–98.

53. Roemer FW, Guermazi A, Felson DT, et al. Presence of MRI-detected joint effusion and synovitis increases the risk of cartilage loss in knees without osteoarthritis at 30-month follow-up: the MOST study. Ann Rheum Dis 2011;70:1804–9.

54. Englund M, Felson DT, Guermazi A, et al. Risk factors for medial meniscal pathology on knee MRI in older US adults: a multicentre prospective cohort study. Ann Rheum Dis 2011;70:1733–9.

55. Roemer FW, Guermazi A, Niu J, et al. Prevalence of magnetic resonance imaging-defined atrophic and hypertrophic phenotypes of knee osteoarthritis in a population-based cohort. Arthritis Rheum 2012;64:429–37.

56. Hunter DJ, Arden N, Conaghan P, et al. Definition of osteoarthritis on MRI: results of a Delphi exercise. Osteoarthritis Cartilage 2011;19:963–9.

57. Zhang Y, Nevitt M, Niu J, et al. Fluctuation of knee pain and changes in bone marrow lesions, effusions, and synovitis on magnetic resonance imaging. Arthritis Rheum 2011;63:691–9.

58. Guermazi A, Roemer FW, Hayashi D, et al. Assessment of synovitis with contrast-enhanced MRI using a whole-joint semiquantitative scoring system in people with, or at high risk of, knee osteoarthritis: the MOST study. Ann Rheum Dis 2011;70:805–11.

59. Hunter DJ, Zhang W, Conaghan PG, et al. Systematic review of the concurrent and predictive validity of MRI biomarkers in OA. Osteoarthritis Cartilage 2011; 19:557–88.

60. Hunter DJ, Zhang W, Conaghan PG, et al. Responsiveness and reliability of MRI in knee osteoarthritis: a meta-analysis of published evidence. Osteoarthritis Cartilage 2011;19:589–605.

61. Peterfy CG, Guermazi A, Zaim S, et al. Whole-Organ Magnetic Resonance Imaging Score (WORMS) of the knee in osteoarthritis. Osteoarthritis Cartilage 2004;12:177–90.
62. Kornaat PR, Ceulemans RY, Kroon HM, et al. MRI assessment of knee osteoarthritis: Knee Osteoarthritis Scoring System (KOSS)–inter-observer and intraobserver reproducibility of a compartment-based scoring system. Skeletal Radiol 2005;34:95–102.
63. Hunter DJ, Lo GH, Gale D, et al. The reliability of a new scoring system for knee osteoarthritis MRI and the validity of bone marrow lesion assessment: BLOKS (Boston Leeds Osteoarthritis Knee Score). Ann Rheum Dis 2008;67:206–11.
64. Lynch JA, Roemer FW, Nevitt MC, et al. Comparison of BLOKS and WORMS scoring systems part I. Cross sectional comparison of methods to assess cartilage morphology, meniscal damage and bone marrow lesions on knee MRI: data from the osteoarthritis initiative. Osteoarthritis Cartilage 2010;18: 1393–401.
65. Felson DT, Lynch J, Guermazi A, et al. Comparison of BLOKS and WORMS scoring systems part II. Longitudinal assessment of knee MRIs for osteoarthritis and suggested approach based on their performance: data from the Osteoarthritis Initiative. Osteoarthritis Cartilage 2010;18:1402–7.
66. Roemer FW, Nevitt MC, Felson DT, et al. Predictive validity of within-grade scoring of longitudinal changes of MRI-based cartilage morphology and bone marrow lesion assessment in the tibio-femoral joint - the MOST Study. Osteoarthritis Cartilage 2012;20(11):1391–8.
67. Katz JN, Chaisson CE, Cole B, et al. The MeTeOR Trial (Meniscal Tear in Osteoarthritis Research): rationale and design features. Contemp Clin Trials 2012; 33(6):1189–96.
68. Pivotal osteoarthritis initiative magnetic resonance imaging analyses (POMA). Available at: http://www.niams.nih.gov/Funding/Funded_Research/Osteoarthritis_ Initiative/pivotal_mri.asp. Accessed October 5, 2012.
69. Baker K, Grainger A, Niu J, et al. Relation of synovitis to knee pain using contrast-enhanced MRIs. Ann Rheum Dis 2010;69:1779–83.
70. Loeuille D, Sauliere N, Champigneulle J, et al. Comparing non-enhanced and enhanced sequences in the assessment of effusion and synovitis in knee OA: associations with clinical, macroscopic and microscopic features. Osteoarthritis Cartilage 2011;19:1433–9.
71. Grainger AJ, Farrant JM, O'Connor PJ, et al. MR imaging of erosions in interphalangeal joint osteoarthritis: is all osteoarthritis erosive? Skeletal Radiol 2007;36: 737–45.
72. Tan AL, Grainger AJ, Tanner SF, et al. A high-resolution magnetic resonance imaging study of distal interphalangeal joint arthropathy in psoriatic arthritis and osteoarthritis: are they the same? Arthritis Rheum 2006;54:1328–33.
73. Tan AL, Grainger AJ, Tanner SF, et al. High-resolution magnetic resonance imaging for the assessment of hand osteoarthritis. Arthritis Rheum 2005;52: 2355–65.
74. Tan AL, Toumi H, Benjamin M, et al. Combined high-resolution magnetic resonance imaging and histological examination to explore the role of ligaments and tendons in the phenotypic expression of early hand osteoarthritis. Ann Rheum Dis 2006;65:1267–72.
75. Iagnocco A, Perella C, D'Agostino MA, et al. Magnetic resonance and ultrasonography real-time fusion imaging of the hand and wrist in osteoarthritis and rheumatoid arthritis. Rheumatology (Oxford) 2011;50:1409–13.

76. Schraml C, Schwenzer NF, Martirosian P, et al. Assessment of synovitis in erosive osteoarthritis of the hand using DCE-MRI and comparison with that in its major mimic, the psoriatic arthritis. Acad Radiol 2011;18:804–9.

77. Wittoek R, Jans L, Lambrecht V, et al. Reliability and construct validity of ultrasonography of soft tissue and destructive changes in erosive osteoarthritis of the interphalangeal finger joints: a comparison with MRI. Ann Rheum Dis 2011;70:278–83.

78. Haugen IK, Lillegraven S, Slatkowsky-Christensen B, et al. Hand osteoarthritis and MRI: development and first validation step of the proposed Oslo Hand Osteoarthritis MRI score. Ann Rheum Dis 2011;70:1033–8.

79. Slatkowsky-Christensen B, Mowinckel P, Loge JH, et al. Health-related quality of life in women with symptomatic hand osteoarthritis: a comparison with rheumatoid arthritis patients, healthy controls, and normative data. Arthritis Rheum 2007;57:1404–9.

80. Haugen IK, Boyesen P, Slatkowsky-Christensen B, et al. Comparison of features by MRI and radiographs of the interphalangeal finger joints in patients with hand osteoarthritis. Ann Rheum Dis 2012;71:345–50.

81. Haugen IK, Boyesen P, Slatkowsky-Christensen B, et al. Associations between MRI-defined synovitis, bone marrow lesions and structural features and measures of pain and physical function in hand osteoarthritis. Ann Rheum Dis 2012;71:899–904.

82. Neumann G, Mendicuti AD, Zou KH, et al. Prevalence of labral tears and cartilage loss in patients with mechanical symptoms of the hip: evaluation using MR arthrography. Osteoarthritis Cartilage 2007;15:909–17.

83. Reichenbach S, Leunig M, Werlen S, et al. Association between cam-type deformities and magnetic resonance imaging-detected structural hip damage: a cross sectional study in young men. Arthritis Rheum 2011;63:4023–30.

84. Potter HG, Schachar J. High resolution noncontrast MRI of the hip. J Magn Reson Imaging 2010;31:268–78.

85. Roemer FW, Hunter DJ, Winterstein A, et al. Hip Osteoarthritis MRI Scoring System (HOAMS): reliability and associations with radiographic and clinical findings. Osteoarthritis Cartilage 2011;19:946–62.

86. Eckstein F, Ateshian G, Burgkart R, et al. Proposal for a nomenclature for magnetic resonance imaging based measures of articular cartilage in osteoarthritis. Osteoarthritis Cartilage 2006;14:974–83.

87. Buck RJ, Wyman BT, Le Graverand MP, et al. An efficient subset of morphological measures for articular cartilage in the healthy and diseased human knee. Magn Reson Med 2010;63:680–90.

88. Buck RJ, Wyman BT, Le Graverand MP, et al. Does the use of ordered values of subregional change in cartilage thickness improve the detection of disease progression in longitudinal studies of osteoarthritis? Arthritis Rheum 2009;61:917–24.

89. Buck RJ, Wyman BT, Hellio Le Graverand MP, et al. Using ordered values of subregional cartilage thickness change increases sensitivity in detecting risk factors for osteoarthritis progression. Osteoarthritis Cartilage 2011;19:302–8.

90. Wirth W, Buck R, Nevitt M, et al. MRI-based extended ordered values more efficiently differentiate cartilage loss in knees with and without joint space narrowing than region-specific approaches using MRI or radiography–data from the OA initiative. Osteoarthritis Cartilage 2011;19:689–99.

91. Ding C, Cicuttini F, Jones G. Do NSAIDs affect longitudinal changes in knee cartilage volume and knee cartilage defects in older adults? Am J Med 2009; 122:836–42.

92. Raynauld JP, Martel-Pelletier J, Beaulieu A, et al. An open-label pilot study evaluating by magnetic resonance imaging the potential for a disease-modifying effect of celecoxib compared to a modelized historical control cohort in the treatment of knee osteoarthritis. Semin Arthritis Rheum 2010;40(3):185–92.

93. Wei S, Venn A, Ding C, et al. The associations between parity, other reproductive factors and cartilage in women aged 50-80 years. Osteoarthritis Cartilage 2011; 19:1307–13.

94. Intema F, Van Roermund PM, Marijnissen AC, et al. Tissue structure modification in knee osteoarthritis by use of joint distraction: an open 1-year pilot study. Ann Rheum Dis 2011;70:1441–6.

95. Bennell KL, Bowles KA, Wang Y, et al. Higher dynamic medial knee load predicts greater cartilage loss over 12 months in medial knee osteoarthritis. Ann Rheum Dis 2011;70:1770–4.

96. Eckstein F, Cotofana S, Wirth W, et al. Greater rates of cartilage loss in painful knees than in pain-free knees after adjustment for radiographic disease stage: data from the osteoarthritis initiative. Arthritis Rheum 2011;63:2257–67.

97. Eckstein F, Wirth W, Hudelmaier MI, et al. Relationship of compartment-specific structural knee status at baseline with change in cartilage morphology: a prospective observational study using data from the osteoarthritis initiative. Arthritis Res Ther 2009;11:R90.

98. Eckstein F, Nevitt M, Gimona A, et al. Rates of change and sensitivity to change in cartilage morphology in healthy knees and in knees with mild, moderate, and end-stage radiographic osteoarthritis: results from 831 participants from the Osteoarthritis Initiative. Arthritis Care Res (Hoboken) 2011;63:311–9.

99. Cotofana S, Buck R, Wirth W, et al. Cartilage thickening in early radiographic human knee osteoarthritis - within-person, between-knee comparison. Arthritis Care Res (Hoboken) 2012;64:1681–90.

100. Frobell RB, Nevitt MC, Hudelmaier M, et al. Femorotibial subchondral bone area and regional cartilage thickness: a cross-sectional description in healthy reference cases and various radiographic stages of osteoarthritis in 1,003 knees from the Osteoarthritis Initiative. Arthritis Care Res (Hoboken) 2010;62:1612–23.

101. Eckstein F, Kwoh CK, Boudreau RM, et al. Quantitative MRI measures of cartilage predict knee replacement: a case-control study from the Osteoarthritis Initiative. Ann Rheum Dis 2012. [Epub ahead of print].

102. Eckstein F, Mc Culloch CE, Lynch JA, et al. How do short-term rates of femorotibial cartilage change compare to long-term changes? Four year follow-up data from the osteoarthritis initiative. Osteoarthritis Cartilage 2012;20:1250–7.

103. Schneider E, Nevitt M, McCulloch C, et al. Equivalence and precision of knee cartilage morphometry between different segmentation teams, cartilage regions, and MR acquisitions. Osteoarthritis Cartilage 2012;20:869–79.

104. Sitoci KH, Hudelmaier M, Eckstein F. Nocturnal changes in knee cartilage thickness in young healthy adults. Cells Tissues Organs 2012;196:189–94.

105. Cotofana S, Eckstein F, Wirth W, et al. In vivo measures of cartilage deformation: patterns in healthy and osteoarthritic female knees using 3T MR imaging. Eur Radiol 2011;21:1127–35.

106. Niehoff A, Müller M, Brüggemann L, et al. Deformational behaviour of knee cartilage and changes in serum cartilage oligomeric matrix protein (COMP) after running and drop landing. Osteoarthritis Cartilage 2011;19:1003–10.

107. Wirth W, Frobell RB, Souza RB, et al. A three-dimensional quantitative method to measure meniscus shape, position, and signal intensity using MR images: a pilot study and preliminary results in knee osteoarthritis. Magn Reson Med 2010;63: 1162–71.

108. Siorpaes K, Wenger A, Bloecker K, et al. Interobserver reproducibility of quantitative meniscus analysis using coronal multiplanar DESS and IWTSE MR imaging. Magn Reson Med 2012;67:1419–26.

109. Bloecker K, Englund M, Wirth W, et al. Size and position of the healthy meniscus, and its correlation with sex, height, weight, and bone area- a cross-sectional study. BMC Musculoskelet Disord 2011;28(12):248.

110. Swanson MS, Prescott JW, Best TM, et al. Semi-automated segmentation to assess the lateral meniscus in normal and osteoarthritic knees. Osteoarthritis Cartilage 2010;18:344–53.

111. Wenger A, Englund M, Wirth W, et al. Relationship of 3D meniscal morphology and position with knee pain in subjects with knee osteoarthritis: a pilot study. Eur Radiol 2012;22:211–20.

112. Roemer FW, Khrad H, Hayashi D, et al. Volumetric and semiquantitative assessment of MRI-detected subchondral bone marrow lesions in knee osteoarthritis: a comparison of contrast-enhanced and non-enhanced imaging. Osteoarthritis Cartilage 2010;18:1062–6.

113. Driban JB, Lo GH, Lee JY, et al. Quantitative bone marrow lesion size in osteoarthritic knees correlates with cartilage damage and predicts longitudinal cartilage loss. BMC Musculoskelet Disord 2011;12:217.

114. Fotinos-Hoyer AK, Guermazi A, Jara H, et al. Assessment of synovitis in the osteoarthritic knee: Comparison between manual segmentation, semi-automated segmentation and semiquantitative assessment using contrast-enhanced fat-suppressed T1-weighted MRI. Magn Reson Med 2010;64:604–9.

115. Habib S, Guermazi A, Ozonoff A, et al. MRI-based volumetric assessment of joint effusion in knee osteoarthritis using proton density-weighted fat-suppressed and T1-weighted contrast-enhanced fat-suppressed sequences. Skeletal Radiol 2011;40:1581–5.

116. Burstein D, Gray M, Mosher T, et al. Measures of molecular composition and structure in osteoarthritis. Radiol Clin North Am 2009;47:675–86.

117. McAlindon TE, Nuite M, Krishnan N, et al. Change in knee osteoarthritis cartilage detected by delayed gadolinium enhanced magnetic resonance imaging following treatment with collagen hydrolysate: a pilot randomized controlled trial. Osteoarthritis Cartilage 2011;19:399–405.

118. Van Ginckel A, Baelde N, Almqvist KM, et al. Functional adaptation of knee cartilage in asymptomatic female novice runners compared to sedentary controls. A longitudinal analysis using delayed gadolinium enhanced magnetic resonance imaging of cartilage (dGEMRIC). Osteoarthritis Cartilage 2010;18: 1564–9.

119. Souza RB, Stehling C, Wyman BT, et al. The effects of acute loading on T1rho and T2 relaxation times of tibiofemoral articular cartilage. Osteoarthritis Cartilage 2010;18:1557–63.

120. Hovis KK, Stehling C, Souza RB, et al. Physical activity is associated with magnetic resonance imaging-based knee cartilage T2 measurements in asymptomatic subjects with and those without osteoarthritis risk factors. Arthritis Rheum 2011;63:2248–56.

121. Pan J, Pialat JB, Joseph T, et al. Knee cartilage T2 characteristics and evolution in relation to morphologic abnormalities detected at 3-T MR imaging: a longitudinal

study of the normal control cohort from the Osteoarthritis Initiative. Radiology 2011;261:507–15.

122. Anandacoomarasamy A, Leibman S, Smith G, et al. Weight loss in obese people has structure-modifying effects on medial but not on lateral knee articular cartilage. Ann Rheum Dis 2012;71:26–32.

123. Williams A, Qian Y, Golla S, et al. UTE-T2* mapping detects sub-clinical meniscus injury after anterior cruciate ligament tear. Osteoarthritis Cartilage 2012;20:486–94.

124. Raya JG, Horng A, Dietrich O, et al. Articular cartilage: in vivo diffusion-tensor imaging. Radiology 2012;262:550–9.

125. Madelin G, Babb JS, Xia D, et al. Reproducibility and repeatability of quantitative sodium magnetic resonance imaging in vivo in articular cartilage at 3 T and 7 T. Magn Reson Med 2012;68:841–9.

126. Newbould RD, Miller SR, Tielbeek JA, et al. Reproducibility of sodium MRI measures of articular cartilage of the knee in osteoarthritis. Osteoarthritis Cartilage 2012;20:29–35.

127. Newbould RD, Miller SR, Toms LD, et al. T2* measurement of the knee articular cartilage in osteoarthritis at 3T. J Magn Reson Imaging 2012;35:1422–9.

128. Keen HI, Conaghan PG. Ultrasonography in osteoarthritis. Radiol Clin North Am 2009;47:581–94.

129. Wakefield RJ, Gibbon WW, Conaghan PG, et al. The value of sonography in the detection of bone erosions in patients with rheumatoid arthritis: a comparison with conventional radiography. Arthritis Rheum 2000;43:2762–70.

130. Wakefield RJ, Balint P, Szkudlarek M, et al. Musculoskeletal ultrasound including definitions for ultrasonographic pathology. J Rheumatol 2005;32:2485–7.

131. Keen HI, Lavie F, Wakefield RJ, et al. The development of a preliminary ultrasonographic scoring system for features of hand osteoarthritis. Ann Rheum Dis 2008;67:651–5.

132. Kortekaas MC, Kwok WY, Reijnierse M, et al. Ostephytes and joint space narrowing are independently associated with pain in finger joints in hand osteoarthritis. Ann Rheum Dis 2011;70:1835–7.

133. Kortekaas MC, Kwok WY, Reijnierse M, et al. In erosive hand osteoarthritis more inflammatory signs on ultrasound are found than in the rest of hand osteoarthritis. Ann Rheum Dis 2012. [Epub ahead of print].

134. Klauser AS, Faschingbauer R, Kupferthaler K, et al. Sonographic criteria for therapy follow-up in the course of ultrasound-guided intra-articular injections of hyaluronic acid in hand osteoarthritis. Eur J Radiol 2012;81:1607–11.

135. Conaghan PG, D'Agostino MA, Le Bars M, et al. Clinical and ultrasonographic predictors of joint replacement for knee osteoarthritis: results from a large, 3-year, prospective EULAR study. Ann Rheum Dis 2010;69:644–7.

136. Kumm J, Tamm A, Lintrop M, et al. Association between ultrasonographic findings and bone/cartilage biomarkers in patients with early-stage knee osteoarthritis. Calcif Tissue Int 2009;85:514–22.

137. Saarakkala S, Waris P, Waris V, et al. Diagnostic performance of knee ultrasonography for detecting degenerative changes of articular cartilage. Osteoarthritis Cartilage 2012;20:376–81.

138. Kawaguchi K, Enokida M, Otsuki R, et al. Ultrasonographic evaluation of medial radial displacement of the medial meniscus in knee osteoarthritis. Arthritis Rheum 2012;64:173–80.

139. Chao J, Wu C, Sun B, et al. Inflammatory characteristics on ultrasound predict poorer longterm response to intraarticular corticosteroid injections in knee osteoarthritis. J Rheumatol 2010;37:650–5.

140. Wu PT, Shao CJ, Wu KC, et al. Pain in patients with equal radiographic grades of osteoarthritis in both knees: the value of gray scale ultrasound. Osteoarthritis Cartilage 2012;20(12):1507–13.

141. Omoumi P, Mercier GA, Lecouvet F, et al. CT arthrography, MR arthrography, PET and scintigraphy in osteoarthritis. Radiol Clin North Am 2009;47: 595–615.

142. Nakamura H, Masuko K, Yudoh K, et al. Positron emission tomography with 18F-FDG in osteoarthritic knee. Osteoarthritis Cartilage 2007;15:673–81.

143. Umemoto Y, Oka T, Inoue T, et al. Imaging of a rat osteoarthritis model using (18) F-fluoride positron emission tomography. Ann Nucl Med 2010;24:663–9.

144. Temmerman OP, Raijmakers PG, Kloet R, et al. In vivo measurements of blood flow and bone metabolism in osteoarthritis. Rheumatol Int 2012. [Epub ahead of print].

145. Cachin F, Boisgard S, Vidal A, et al. First ex vivo study demonstrating that 99mTc-NTP 15-5 radiotracer binds to human articular cartilage. Eur J Nucl Med Mol Imaging 2011;38:2077–82.

146. Moon YL, Lee SH, Park SY, et al. Evaluation of shoulder disorders by 2-[F-18]-fluoro-2-deoxy-D-glucose positron emission tomography and computed tomography. Clin Orthop Surg 2010;2:167–72.

147. Magee D, Tanner SF, Waller M, et al. Combining variational and model-based techniques to register PET and MR images in hand osteoarthritis. Phys Med Biol 2010;55:4755–69.

148. Naviscan. Naviscan high-resolution PET scanner. Available at: http://www.naviscan.com/products/product-overview/product-overview. Accessed October 1, 2012.

149. Hechelhammer L, Pfirmann CW, Zanetti M, et al. Imaging findings predicting the outcome of cervical facet joint blocks. Eur Radiol 2007;17:959–64.

150. Kalichman L, Li L, Kim DH, et al. Facet joint osteoarthritis and low back pain in the community-based population. Spine 2008;33:2560–5.

151. Kalichman L, Kim DH, Li L, et al. Computed tomography evaluated features of spinal degeneration: prevalence, intercorrelation, and association with self-reported low back pain. Spine 2010;10:200–8.

152. Suri P, Katz JN, Rainville J, et al. Vascular disease is associated with facet joint osteoarthritis. Osteoarthritis Cartilage 2010;18:1127–32.

153. Kalichman L, Guermazi A, Li L, et al. Association between age, sex, BMI and CT-evaluated spinal degeneration features. J Back Musculoskeletal Rehabil 2009;22:189–95.

154. Kim JS, Kroin JS, Buvanendran A, et al. Characterization of a new animal model for evaluation and treatment of back pain due to lumbar facet joint osteoarthritis. Arthritis Rheum 2011;63:2966–73.

155. Hall FM, Goldberg RP, Wyshak G, et al. Shoulder arthrography: comparison of morbidity after use of various contrast media. Radiology 1985;154:339–41.

156. Andreisek G, Froehlich JM, Hodler J, et al. Direct MR arthrography at 1.5 and 3.0 T: signal dependence on gadolinium and iodine concentrations–phantom study. Radiology 2008;247:706–16.

157. Brown RR, Clarke DW, Daffner RH. Is a mixture of gadolinium and iodinated contrast material safe during MR arthrography? AJR Am J Roentgenol 2000; 175:1087–90.

158. Berquist TH. Imaging of articular pathology: MRI, CT, arthrography. Clin Anat 1997;10:1–13.

159. El-Khoury GY, Alliman KJ, Lundberg HJ, et al. Cartilage thickness in cadaveric ankles: measurement with double-contrast multi-detector row CT arthrography versus MR imaging. Radiology 2004;233:768–73.

160. Wyler A, Bousson V, Bergot C, et al. Hyaline cartilage thickness in radiographically normal cadaveric hips: comparison of spiral CT arthrographic and macroscopic measurements. Radiology 2007;242:441–9.
161. Wyler A, Bousson V, Bergot C, et al. Comparison of MR-arthrography and CT arthrography in hyaline cartilage-thickness measurement in radiographically normal cadaver hips with anatomy as gold standard. Osteoarthritis Cartilage 2009;17:19–25.
162. Schmid MR, Pfirrmann CW, Hodler J, et al. Cartilage lesions in the ankle joint: comparison of MR arthrography and CT arthrography. Skeletal Radiol 2003; 32:259–65.
163. McCauley TR, Kornaat PR, Jee WH. Central osteophytes in the knee: prevalence and association with cartilage defects on MR imaging. AJR Am J Roentgenol 2001;176:359–64.
164. Kraniotis P, Maragkos S, Tyllianakis M, et al. Ankle posttraumatic osteoarthritis: a CT arthrography study in patients with bi- and trimalleolar fractures. Skeletal Radiol 2012;41:803–9.
165. Tamura S, Nishii T, Shiomi T, et al. Three-dimensional patterns of early acetabular cartilage damage in hip dysplasia; a high-resolutional CT arthrography study. Osteoarthritis Cartilage 2012;20:646–52.

The Health and Structural Consequences of Acute Knee Injuries Involving Rupture of the Anterior Cruciate Ligament

Edward A. Riordan, BSc[a], Richard B. Frobell, PhD[b],
Frank W. Roemer, MD[c], David J. Hunter, MBBS, MSc, PhD, FRACP[d],*

KEYWORDS

- Knee injury • Anterior cruciate ligament • Prevention • Management

KEY POINTS

- Evidence suggests that the associated joint damage incurred during – and immediately after – rupture of the anterior cruciate ligament (ACL) may be predictive of the subsequent development of knee osteoarthritis (OA).
- The mechanism of this increased susceptibility to OA is not yet clear, but trauma to the osteochondral unit, the immediate biochemical response, loss of the protective function of the menisci and biomechanics-related cartilage damage are likely to be factors.
- Reconstructive surgery has not yet been shown to reduce the rate of OA development, and the most effective current management for ACL injuries appears to be prevention of the initial rupture through training programs.
- Future treatments will likely focus on halting the early pattern of joint damage by addressing the immediate biochemical response and short-term cartilage changes.

INTRODUCTION

Despite the recent introduction of biomechanical training initiatives in school and college athletics programs aimed at preventing knee injuries, the knee remains the most commonly injured joint.[1] Although the overall annual rate of injuries stands at 2.29 per 1000 individuals, the rate of injuries within the 15-year-old to 24-year-old age group is almost 70% higher, with organized sporting and recreational activities accounting for most of the injuries.[1,2]

[a] School of Medicine, University of Sydney, Sydney, New South Wales, Australia; [b] Department of Orthopedics, Clinical Sciences Lund, Lund University Hospital, Lund SE-22185, Sweden; [c] Department of Radiology, Klinikum Augsburg, Stenglinstr. 2, Augsburg 86156, Germany; [d] Department of Rheumatology, Royal North Shore Hospital and Northern Clinical School, University of Sydney, Sydney, Reserve road, St Leonards, New South Wales 2065, Australia
* Corresponding author.
E-mail address: David.Hunter@sydney.edu.au

Rheum Dis Clin N Am 39 (2013) 107–122
http://dx.doi.org/10.1016/j.rdc.2012.10.002   rheumatic.theclinics.com
0889-857X/13/$ – see front matter © 2013 Elsevier Inc. All rights reserved.

Of particular interest (in the context of osteoarthritis) are knee injuries resulting in rupture of the acute anterior cruciate ligament (ACL), often accompanied by damage to the chondral articular surface, menisci, subchondral bone, and collateral ligaments. Most ACL tears occur in young, active individuals, and require a prolonged layoff from sport regardless of treatment choice. Standard treatment options include early ligament reconstruction or extensive rehabilitation with the possibility of delayed surgical repair in the event of clinically relevant instability.[3] They are, therefore, potentially expensive injuries, with the cost of surgical reconstruction and rehabilitation estimated to be approximately US $17,000 per patient, in addition to the loss of income related to the short-term functional disability.[2,4] ACL rupture is also strongly linked to the subsequent development of osteoarthritis, with a substantial percentage of patients showing osteoarthritic changes and related functional disability as early as 10 to 15 years after the initial injury.[5,6] The possibility of early interventions targeting the structural changes that take place within the knee after ACL rupture may therefore have significant economic and long-term health implications.

This article outlines the pattern of joint damage that accompanies an ACL rupture and the long-term structural changes that predispose the injured knee to the development of osteoarthritis. The current evidence for the efficacy and cost-effectiveness of surgical and nonsurgical treatment strategies is also reviewed.

MECHANISMS OF ACL INJURY

ACL rupture is believed to be a result of postural readjustments that simultaneously produce a valgus force and internal or external rotation.[3] This dynamic loading in multiple planes of motion can produce sufficient tension to rupture the ACL.[7] The archetypal scenario in sport is one in which the participant attempts to change direction at the time of landing on the foot, and hence generates a rotational force in addition to the considerable load resulting from decelerating on landing.[8,9]

Most tears therefore occur in sports that involve rapid changes of direction or sudden deceleration.[10] Heavy-contact sports like American football and rugby do not have particularly high injury rates (approximately 0.08 per 1000 exposures), because most injuries occur in the absence of direct contact.[11] Less contact-based sports like basketball (0.29 per 1000 exposures for women and 0.08 for men), soccer (0.32 for women and 0.12 for men) and skiing (0.40) have markedly higher injury rates.[12-14] Basketball and soccer account for the largest number of injuries in the United States because of their superior participation rates.[10,15]

The increased female/male injury ratio has been a consistent finding across numerous studies and sports, and is a particularly well-studied phenomenon.[3,10] Despite this finding, the reason for the higher incidence of ACL tears in women has yet to be elucidated, although it is likely that several factors contribute to the finding (most notably, differences in quadriceps activation, muscle stiffness, movement patterns during landing, and hormone-dependent knee laxity).[3,16,17]

ASSOCIATED INJURIES

Knee injuries resulting in ACL tears are often associated with a range of additional structural joint damage. Posttraumatic bone lesions (with or without associated osteochondral injury), meniscal damage, and collateral ligament injuries are particularly common, and have all been linked with long-term damage to the synovial joint.[18-21] These associated injuries are therefore worth discussing because of their potential role in the development of osteoarthritic changes.

Posttraumatic Bone Marrow Lesions

Posttraumatic bone marrow lesions (BMLs, also called bone bruises or contusions) are observed on magnetic resonance imaging as regions of diffuse signal abnormality in the subchondral bone marrow.[22] These contusions are a result of the impaction forces between the anterolateral femur and the posterolateral tibia that occur during the initial trauma (kissing lesions), and are present in virtually all knees with complete ACL rupture.[18,23] Most of these BMLs occur in the lateral compartment, most notably on the lateral femoral condyle and the posterior lateral tibial plateau as a result of the valgus distribution of force usually experienced during the injury (**Fig. 1**).[18,24] A recent study by Boks and colleagues[25] suggests that, contrary to expectations, reticular posttraumatic BMLs are not associated with increased pain severity in posttraumatic knees. Simple posttraumatic BMLs without involvement of the articular surface are thus likely to be benign occurrences.[26,27] Posttraumatic BMLs generally resolve without sequelae within 6 to 12 months after the injury, although new BMLs have been shown to develop in approximately one-third of ACL-injured knees over the first 2 years after injury.[26–28]

In contrast, BMLs that are accompanied by disruption to the articular surface are predictive of long-term osteochondral sequelae.[29–31] Johnson and colleagues[32] found significant proteoglycan loss, chondrocyte injury, and matrix degeneration in the articular cartilage adjacent to a geographic BML, as well as osteocyte necrosis within the affected bone marrow. A separate follow-up study by Theologis and colleagues[18] found that the matrix composition in cartilage overlying bruises in the lateral tibia was still abnormal 1 year after injury, despite most of the original osteochondral lesions healing almost completely within 2 weeks to 6 months. This finding indicates that the initial cartilage injury accompanying geographic bone bruises, osteochondral defects, and cortical impactions may lead to sustained cartilage trauma, and could therefore play a role in long-term osteoarthritic changes.[22]

Large BML volumes have also been shown to be associated with the presence of cortical depression fractures, which are likely to be of greater short-term clinical relevance than the presence of a simple BML.[23,33] A recent study published by Kijowski and colleagues[33] reported that patients with cortical depression fractures had lower International Knee Documentation Committee clinical outcome scores 1 year after injury and higher rates of meniscal tears.

Meniscal Injury

Damage to the menisci is observed in approximately 65% to 75% of ACL-ruptured knees during arthroscopy.[19,34] Traumatic longitudinal tears in the posterior and middle one-third of the medial menisci account for most lesions, although damage to the posterior-middle portion of the lateral meniscus is also common (**Fig. 2**).[20] It is still unclear whether this meniscal damage occurs primarily as a result of trauma during the initial injury or is secondary to the initial trauma and occurs between ACL rupture and arthroscopy. Retrospective observational studies have suggested that increased time between ACL injury and ligament reconstruction may result in higher rates of meniscal tears, but the fact that most of these reports are confounded by indication makes it difficult to interpret their findings.[35–39]

Numerous studies have shown that meniscal damage in ACL-insufficient knees is associated with cartilage damage. Murrel and colleagues[34] found that patients with meniscal injury had a 3-fold increase in cartilage damage 2 years after injury, and partial or complete menisectomies have long been linked to cartilage damage and earlier-onset osteoarthritic changes.[40,41] This finding may indicate that the role of

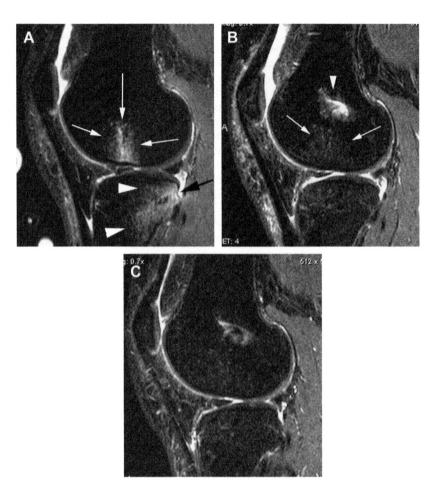

Fig. 1. Characteristic traumatic BMLs without associated osteochondral injury after rotational trauma. A 28-year-old patient suffered complete ACL disruption. (*A*) The most common locations of traumatic bone changes in conjunction with ACL disruption are the central lateral femoral condyle (*white arrows*) and the posterior lateral tibial plateau (*arrowheads*). Bone contusions are characterized by signal hyperintensity on fat-suppressed water-sensitive sequences. In addition, there is a subchondral fracture of the posterior lateral tibial plateau (*black arrow*). (*B*) At 4-month follow-up, there is almost complete resolution of BMLs. Only minimal residual hyperintensity is still observed in the central lateral femur. Note susceptibility artifact caused by femoral metallic screw after ACL reconstruction, which may be mistaken as a posttraumatic bone marrow edemalike lesion (*arrowhead*). (*C*) At 12-month follow-up, there is complete resolution of subchondral bone changes. Cortical depression of lateral tibial plateau is persistently observed.

the menisci in reducing contact stresses and friction within the joint is protective of articular cartilage, and therefore the development of osteoarthritis. However, it is as yet unclear whether the loss of the meniscal function causes articular cartilage damage, or is merely a concurrent destructive occurrence.[34]

Direct Articular Cartilage Damage

Nearly half of knee injuries that result in an ACL rupture also cause direct articular cartilage damage, particularly on the medial (41%–43%) and lateral (20%) femoral condyles

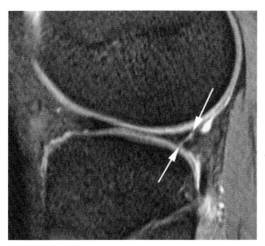

Fig. 2. Sagittal dual echo at steady state image shows a longitudinal meniscal tear of the posterior horn of the lateral meniscus in conjunction with a complete ACL disruption. Tear is characterized by a longitudinal hyperintense line extending from the meniscal upper surface to the undersurface (*arrows*).

(**Fig. 3**).[20,42] Direct cartilage damage is associated with short-term matrix disruption, chondrocyte necrosis, and proteoglycan loss.[32] Although it is not yet known whether these changes are reversible, or become irreversible if a certain amount of damage is sustained, it is possible that the initial trauma plays a role in instigating the well-described progressive cartilage loss that is characteristic of osteoarthritis.[18,32]

A recent study by Frobell[28] using data from the longitudinal Knee Anterior cruciate ligament NON-operative vs. operative treatment (KANON) trial reported that 2 years after injury, significant cartilage thickening was observed in the central medial aspect of the femur, whereas marked thinning had occurred in the femoral trochlea and the posterior aspects of both the medial and lateral aspects of the femur. These findings were particularly interesting in the context of osteoarthritis, given that osteoarthritis occurs predominantly in the medial compartment and that animal models have shown that cartilage hypertrophy precedes the characteristic cartilage breakdown.[43]

ACL INJURY AND OSTEOARTHRITIS
How Strong is the Link?

As noted by Oiestad and colleagues[44] in a systematic review in 2009, most studies assessing the long-term link between ACL rupture and osteoarthritis made use of inconsistent radiologic classification methods and heterogeneous populations with respect to treatment, previous activity levels, and the presence of concurrent injuries. It is therefore difficult to draw firm figures from the literature on the prevalence of osteoarthritis after ACL injuries, with reported rates ranging from 10% to 90% at 10 to 15 years after injury.[5]

In their 2009 review, Oiestad and colleagues suggested that the lack of a consistent radiologic classification system (7 distinct classification systems were identified in the articles included in the analysis) has resulted in the prevalence of knee osteoarthritis after isolated ACL ruptures being greatly overestimated (**Fig. 4**). Oiestad and colleagues conducted a methodological quality assessment of 31 studies and found that the highest-rated studies reported a prevalence for knee osteoarthritis of 0% to

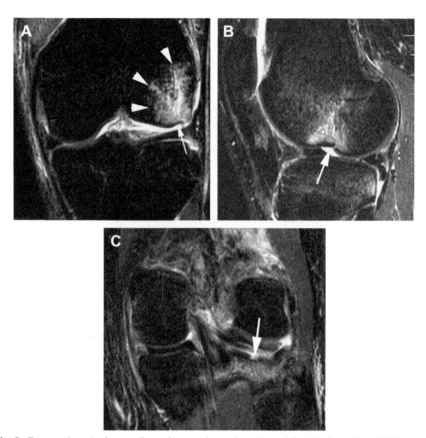

Fig. 3. Traumatic articular cartilage damage in conjunction with ACL disruption. (*A*) Coronal T2-weighted fat-suppressed image shows a traumatic BML in the lateral femoral condyle (*arrowheads*) and an osteochondral depression (*arrow*). (*B*) Corresponding sagittal image shows depression and disruption of the articular surface (*arrow*). (*C*) Coronal short-tau inversion recovery image of different patient shows an example of a traumatic focal cartilage defect in the posterior lateral tibial plateau (*arrow*). Note subchondral traumatic BML adjacent to defect reflected as hyperintensity in the subchondral bone marrow.

13% after isolated rupture of the ACL; significantly less than the 50% to 70% prevalence rate often quoted in the literature.[45–47] However, combined injuries involving ACL rupture and meniscal damage resulted in a higher prevalence of osteoarthritis of 21% to 48%. As discussed earlier, both meniscal injury and direct articular cartilage trauma are linked to long-term cartilage damage after a knee injury and are predictive of long-term tibiofemoral and patellofemoral osteoarthritis.[48] Given that isolated rupture of the ACL is rare, and most ACL ruptures are accompanied by meniscal and chondral damage, the overall rate of osteoarthritis after an injury resulting in an ACL rupture is likely to be closer to the quoted combined injury rate than that reported for isolated injuries.[19,20,34]

Why the Increased Prevalence of Osteoarthritis After ACL Rupture?

It has long been suggested that osteochondral damage and intra-articular bleeding experienced during the initial trauma may induce a cascade of biochemical events within the joint that result in the development of osteoarthritis.[49] Recent studies seem to support this idea, with Sward and colleagues[50] reporting that an acute knee injury

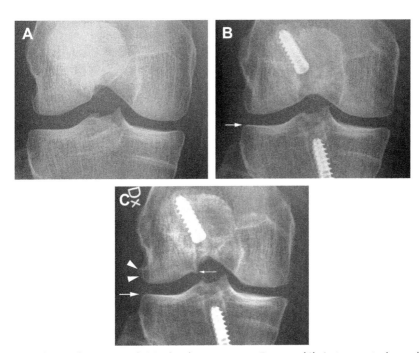

Fig. 4. Radiographic osteoarthritis development over 5 years. (A) Anteroposterior radiograph at baseline obtained directly after trauma shows no signs of radiographic osteoarthritis. Normal medial and lateral joint space width and absence of osteophytes are observed. (B) Two-year follow-up image shows metallic screws in the femur and tibia after ACL reconstruction. Normal joint space width is observed. There is a tiny equivocal marginal osteophyte at the lateral tibial plateau. (C) At 5-year follow-up, definite osteophytes are observed at the lateral femoral condyle (*arrowheads*) and tibial plateau (*large arrow*), representing radiographic osteoarthritis grade 2 according to the Kellgren-Lawrence classification scheme. In addition, there is a prominent notch osteophyte at the lateral femoral condyle, potentially causing ligament impingement (*small arrow*).

is associated with an immediate local biochemical response, potentially affecting the adjacent cartilage and bone in addition to inducing inflammation. However, little is known about the relationship between the immediate release of traumatic factors and subsequent osteoarthritis development, although the area is gaining increasing interest.

Recurrent episodes of instability may also play a role in initiating the pathologic changes to the articular cartilage observed after injury. It has previously been postulated that frequent episodes of instability or pivot shifting could result in sustained damage to both the articular cartilage and menisci that results in loss of the cartilage.[51] The extent to which cartilage must be damaged in the initial trauma before structural damage becomes irreversible is not yet known, but it is possible that the regular occurrence of instability-related trauma and altered biomechanical loading could overwhelm the limited restorative capacity of the joint and lead to longer-term osteoarthritic changes.[32] Concurrent injury to the menisci and the corresponding loss of its protective function would merely serve to exacerbate the damage to articular cartilage.[34]

Although reconstructive surgery can partially restore joint stability after ACL rupture, it is unlikely that surgery fully restores normal biomechanical loading across the knee.[45,52–54] An altered loading pattern causes a shift in compressive and tension load bearing to unconditioned regions, and reduces loads in conditioned regions.[55,56] Numerous studies have described adaptations by cartilage to altered loading: chondrocyte metabolism and volume/aspect ratio, proteoglycan production, collagen fiber orientation, and matrix metalloproteinase expression are all altered during the cartilage response.[57,58] It has therefore been suggested that early changes in cartilage may be partially explained by the altered biomechanics of the knee after injury.[55]

Surgical Versus Nonsurgical Treatment

Despite a paucity of evidence that ACL reconstruction is the most effective treatment of an ACL rupture, more than 200,000 procedures are performed each year in the United States alone.[59–61] Allografts, ipsilateral bone-patellar tendon-bone autografts and quadruple hamstring tendon (HT) autografts are the most commonly used procedures.[62,63] Recent meta-analyses have suggested that although the 3 procedures produce similar long-term functional outcomes, allografts and HT autografts may be associated with lower rates of anterior knee pain.[63–66]

The short-term benefits of surgical intervention in relation to nonsurgical treatments are still unclear, and several recent studies have reported that surgery and rehabilitation alone may produce comparable functionality.[61] Frobell and colleagues[61] conducted a randomized trial in which patients were assigned to receive either structured rehabilitation and early reconstruction or structured rehabilitation alone (with the option of delayed ACL reconstruction). These investigators reported that although early surgical treatment was associated with greater measured stability in Lachman and pivot-shift tests, after 2 years there were no significant differences between the treatment groups with respect to patient-relevant outcomes, knee-related adverse events, or return to preinjury activity levels. Similarly, a prospective cohort study by Moknes and Risberg[67] found no difference in performance-based outcomes and the number of patients returning to preinjury activity levels between nonoperatively and operatively treated groups. In a case-control study, Meuffels and colleagues[68] also found no statistical difference in activity levels or subjective and objective functional outcomes at 10 years after injury between patients treated conservatively or operatively.

ACL reconstructions are commonly advocated on the basis that they are protective against secondary meniscal injury and thereby reduce the risk of osteoarthritis development. Numerous retrospective studies have suggested that an increased time between injury and reconstruction is associated with higher rates of chondral and meniscal injuries.[69,70] However, the studies are largely confounded by indication, because the fact that patients have symptomatic meniscal or cartilage injuries means they are more likely to undergo surgery. A long-term follow-up of a previous randomized controlled trial showed that, although the rate of secondary meniscal surgery was higher after nonsurgical treatment, there was no statistical difference in terms of radiographic osteoarthritis.[45] A systematic review in 2007[5] had similar findings, reporting that no treatment-related differences in osteoarthritis could be found within the literature.

It is similarly unclear whether ACL reconstruction decreases the incidence of osteoarthritis development over the long-term. That osteoarthritis still develops in a substantial portion of patients treated with surgical repair is beyond doubt, but virtually no high-quality randomized studies comparing nonoperative treatment and reconstructive surgery have been conducted.[5,6,71] A case-control study by Meuffels and colleagues found no statistical difference in prevalence of radiographic osteoarthritis between the operatively and nonsurgically treated groups.[68] In 2007, Meunier and colleagues[45] published the results of a 15-year-long trial in which 2 groups were allocated to receive either surgical treatment or conservative nonsurgical treatment by their year of birth (odd or even), and no statistically significant differences in osteoarthritis development were identified between the 2 groups. However, the investigators did note that there were several major problems with the randomization procedures used when the study was initiated in the early 1980s, most notably the exclusion of some patients from the surgical group because their injuries were not deemed to be amenable to surgical treatment, and the markedly different rehabilitation protocols used across the groups. This finding is symptomatic of the difficulties faced in attempting a meta-analysis, with the available studies all being of poor methodological quality or of insufficient length to allow a proper evaluation of osteoarthritis development.[5,64] As noted in a recent Cochrane review,[72] there is therefore a need for long-term randomized trials comparing surgical reconstruction and nonsurgical treatment to establish the efficacy of surgical repair in reducing the incidence of osteoarthritis.

However, from the limited evidence available, there is little to suggest that surgical intervention is significantly superior to conservative rehabilitation in terms of decreasing the rate of osteoarthritis.[5,61]

ECONOMICS OF ACL RUPTURE

Given the initially debilitating nature of the injury, an ACL tear necessarily produces an array of indirect costs: personal loss of income because of time away from work; government-funded injury leave (in certain countries); absence from school or university; and the loss of conditioning resulting from reduced activity.[3] It is difficult to adequately measure these indirect costs, but they must be considered when devising an appropriate patient-oriented treatment strategy.[73] An athlete's desire to return to sport within the shortest possible time frame, to avoid deconditioning and subsequent disruption to their sporting career, may increase a physician's willingness to recommend surgical reconstruction. One of the primary indications for reconstructive surgery is the need for the patient to quickly resume sporting activities,[74,75] although a recent meta-analysis of 5770 individuals who underwent reconstruction found that only 44% had returned to competitive sport at a mean follow-up of 41.5 months after injury.[76] This finding must also be balanced against the risk of reinjury that accompanies an early return to sport. The asymmetrical limb loading observed in patients up to 15 months after surgery has been shown to significantly increase the risk of a new ipsilateral or contralateral ACL injury, suggesting that a longer period of rehabilitation than typically advocated may be required for a successful long-term return to sport.[75,77–79] A conservative, nonsurgical rehabilitation plan may suffice for a patient for whom the indirect cost of an extended layoff from sport is less, because it is likely that their long-term functional outcome does not differ greatly from that of the surgically reconstructed patient, and the direct costs of treatment are significantly less.[61,67] The indirect costs incurred by the patient as a result of the injury or particular treatment protocol are therefore worthy of consideration.

The direct costs associated with ACL rupture are considerable, with the cost of reconstructions alone estimated to be US $3 billion annually in the United States.[80] On an individual level, expected health care costs with operative treatment are between US $11,000 and US $17,000, with the main contributors being the surgery itself and the subsequent in-hospital stay.[2,4,81,82] Modeling studies by Gottlob and colleagues[81] and Farshad and colleagues[83] calculated that the cost of nonoperative treatment (largely because of physician services and structured rehabilitation) would be closer to US $2000 to US $2500. Although both studies found ACL reconstruction to be slightly more cost-effective than conservative treatment because of the lower cost per quality-adjusted life year (US $20,612 vs US $23,391), the investigators acknowledged that this was largely based on the assumption that surgical repair significantly reduces the rate of sequelae such as osteoarthritis, an assumption that lacks any firm evidence. The general assumption that ACL reconstruction is a cost-effective procedure could therefore be questioned, and further randomized controlled trials need to be conducted to properly assess the cost-effectiveness of both surgical and conservative treatment protocols.

FUTURE TREATMENTS
Prevention

Given the high risk of knee osteoarthritis after ACL rupture, and the apparent inefficacy of current treatment regimens in reducing rates of osteoarthritis, prevention of the injury must be afforded a high priority. Several studies have attempted to assess the effectiveness of prevention programs in reducing the incidence of ACL ruptures, with most reporting a moderately successful outcome.[84–88] The forms of intervention have varied widely, with neuromuscular training, strengthening activities, aerobic conditioning, plyometrics, resistance training, speed training, and education among the more common methods used within the program.[3,89] A recent systematic review by Gagnier and colleagues[89] of 8 cohort studies and 6 randomized trials found a reduction in the rate of ACL ruptures by approximately 50% in the training groups across the 14 studies. Meta-analyses conducted by Hewett and colleagues[90] and Grindstaff and colleagues[91] reported similar results, with fixed-effect estimates of 0.40 and 0.30, respectively. The heterogeneity and complexity of the training programs meant that it was not possible to determine which particular components of the programs were effective, so future studies comparing isolated training techniques are required.[89] Despite this situation, it is encouraging that training programs have demonstrated the capacity to reduce ACL tear rates. Although such programs are expensive, the prevention of a substantial portion of annual ACL tears would undoubtedly bring about considerable savings in terms of treatment costs and long-term osteoarthritis-related disability.[92]

Early Intervention

The possibility that the initial biochemical response to the trauma incurred during ACL rupture may be involved in initiating the series of events that culminates in osteoarthritis implies that prevention or moderation of this acute response may have a significant impact on disease progression.[49] Given that this biochemical response is still poorly understood, the means to alter it are some time away, but will undoubtedly be of considerable interest in the future.

The observations that early changes in the articular cartilage and menisci are associated with the long-term development of osteoarthritis seems to suggest that an intervention to correct these initial changes would also be protective against future osteoarthritis.[41,48] However, meniscal repair and surgical reconstruction do not seem to reduce the risk, raising the possibilities that interventions must occur earlier (ie, irreparable damage has already occurred by the time that surgery takes place) or must focus on the articular cartilage and ensuing synovitis itself.[5,93] It would be interesting to investigate whether prevention of the initial cartilage change described in numerous studies would alter the subsequent pattern of joint damage.[28] Although it is likely that the means to implement any such intervention are still years away, it is probable that halting the early articular changes would have a significant impact on long-term disease progression.

SUMMARY

There is considerable evidence to suggest that the associated joint damage incurred during (and immediately after) the initial ACL rupture may be predictive of the subsequent development of osteoarthritis. Although the mechanism of this increased susceptibility is not yet clear, initial trauma to the osteochondral unit, the immediate biochemical response, loss of the protective function of the menisci, and biomechanics-related cartilage damage are likely to be significant factors. Reconstructive surgery has not yet been shown to reduce the rate of development of osteoarthritis, and it is probable that a successful preventative treatment must be delivered rapidly after injury to address the early pattern of joint damage changes. The most effective current treatment of ACL injuries, therefore, seems to be prevention of the initial ACL rupture, with several large studies showing success in reducing ACL tear rates.

REFERENCES

1. Gage B, McIlvain N, Collins C, et al. Epidemiology of 6.6 million knee injuries presenting to United States emergency departments from 1999 through 2008. Acad Emerg Med 2012;19:378–85.
2. Parkkari J, Pasanen K, Mattila V, et al. The risk of cruciate ligament injury of the knee in adolescents and young adults: a population-based cohort study of 46500 people with a 9 year follow-up. Br J Sports Med 2008;42:422–6.
3. Griffin L, Albohm M, Arendt E. Understanding and preventing noncontact anterior cruciate ligament injuries. Am J Sports Med 2005;34:1512–32.
4. Gianotti S, Marshall S, Hume P, et al. Incidence of anterior cruciate ligament injury and other knee ligament injuries: a national population-based study. J Sci Med Sport 2009;12:622–7.
5. Lohmander L, Englund M, Dahl L, et al. The long-term consequences of anterior cruciate ligament and meniscus injuries: osteoarthritis. Am J Sports Med 2007; 35:1756–69.
6. Lohmander L, Ostenberg A, Englund M, et al. High prevalence of knee osteoarthritis, pain and functional limitations in female soccer players twelve years after anterior cruciate ligament injury. Arthritis Rheum 2004;50:3145–52.
7. Shimokochi Y, Shultz S. Mechanisms of noncontact anterior cruciate ligament injury. J Athl Train 2008;43:396–408.
8. Arnold J, Coker T, Heaton L, et al. Natural history of anterior cruciate tears. Am J Sports Med 1979;7:305–13.
9. Gray J, Taunton J, McKenzie D, et al. A survey of injuries to the anterior cruciate ligament of the knee in female basketball players. Int J Sports Med 1985;6:314–6.
10. Chadwick P, Han Y, Rogowski J, et al. A meta-analysis of the incidence of anterior cruciate ligament tears as a function of gender, sport and a knee injury-reduction regimen. Arthroscopy 2007;23:1320–5.
11. Scranton PJ, Whitesel J, Powell JW. A review of selected non-contact anterior cruciate ligament injuries in the national football league. Foot Ankle Int 1997;18: 772–6.
12. Agel J, Arendt E, Bershadsky B. Anterior cruciate ligament injury in national collegiate athletic association basketball and soccer. Am J Sports Med 2005;33: 524–31.
13. Mihata L, Beutler A, Boden B. Comparing the incidence of anterior cruciate ligament injury in collegiate lacrosse, soccer, and basketball players. Am J Sports Med 2006;34:899–904.

14. Deibert M, Aronsson D, Johnson R. Skiing injuries in children, adolescents, and adults. J Bone Joint Surg Am 1998;80:25–32.

15. Ryan T. SGMA study. Business Source Premier 2011;44:18–20.

16. Slauterbeck J, Clevenger C, Lundberg W, et al. Estrogen level alters the failure load of the rabbit anterior cruciate ligament. J Orthop Res 1999;17:405–8.

17. White K, Lee S, Cutuk A, et al. EMG power spectra of intercollegiate athletes and anterior cruciate ligament injury risk in females. Med Sci Sports Exerc 2003;35: 371–6.

18. Theologis A, Kuo D, Cheng J, et al. Evaluation of bone bruises and associated cartilage in anterior cruciate ligament-injured and -reconstructed knees using quantitative T1p magnetic resonance imaging: 1-year cohort study. Arthroscopy 2011;27:65–76.

19. Slauterbeck J, Kousa P, Clifton B, et al. Geographic mapping of meniscus and cartilage lesions associated with anterior cruciate ligament injuries. J Bone Joint Surg Am 2009;91:2094–103.

20. Tandogan R, Taser O, Kayaalp A, et al. Analysis of meniscal and chondral lesions accompanying anterior cruciate ligament tears: relationship with age, time from injury and level of sport. Knee Surg Sports Traumatol Arthrosc 2004;12:262–70.

21. Yoon K, Yoo J, Kim K. Bone contusion and associated meniscal and medial collateral ligament injury in patients with anterior cruciate ligament rupture. J Bone Joint Surg Am 2011;93:1510–8.

22. Boks S, Vroegindeweij D, Koes B, et al. Follow-up of occult bone lesions detected at MR imaging. Radiology 2006;238:853–63.

23. Frobell R, Roos H, Roos E, et al. The acutely ACL injured knee assessed by MRI: are large volume traumatic bone marrow lesions a sign of severe compression injury? Osteoarthritis Cartilage 2008;16:829–36.

24. Stevens K, Dragoo J. Anterior cruciate ligament tears and associated injuries. Top Magn Reson Imaging 2006;17:347–62.

25. Boks S, Vroegindeweij D, Koes B, et al. Clinical consequences of posttraumatic bone bruise in the knee. Am J Sports Med 2007;35:990–5.

26. Bretlau T, Tuxoe J, Larsen L, et al. Bone bruise in the acutely injured knee. Knee Surg Sports Traumatol Arthrosc 2002;10:96–101.

27. Miller M, Osborne J, Gordon W, et al. The natural history of bone bruises: a prospective study of magnetic resonance imaging-detected trabecular micro-fractures in patients with isolated medial collateral ligament injuries. Am J Sports Med 1998;26:15–9.

28. Frobell R. Change in cartilage thickness, posttraumatic bone marrow lesions and joint fluid volumes after acute ACL disruption. J Bone Joint Surg Am 2011;93: 1096–103.

29. Vellet A, Marks P, Fowler P, et al. Occult posttraumatic osteochondral lesions of the knee: prevalence, classification, and short-term sequelae evaluated with MR imaging. Radiology 1991;178:271–6.

30. Costa-Paz M, Muscolo D, Ayerza M, et al. Magnetic resonance imaging follow-up study of bone bruises associated with anterior cruciate ligament ruptures. Arthroscopy 2001;17:445–9.

31. Lahm A, Erggelet C, Steinwachs M, et al. Articular and osseous lesions in recent ligament tears: arthroscopic changes compared with magnetic resonance imaging findings. Arthroscopy 1998;14:597–604.

32. Johnson D, Urban W Jr, Caborn D, et al. Articular cartilage changes seen with magnetic resonance imaging-detected bone bruises associated with acute anterior cruciate ligament rupture. Am J Sports Med 1998;26:409–16.

33. Kijowski R, Sanogo M, Lee K, et al. Short-term clinical importance of osseous injuries diagnosed at MR imaging in patients with anterior cruciate ligament tear. Radiology 2012;264:531–41.
34. Murrell G, Maddali S, Horovitz L, et al. The effects of time course after anterior cruciate ligament injury in correlation with meniscal and cartilage loss. Am J Sports Med 2001;29:9–14.
35. Shelbourne K, Gray T, Haro M. Incidence of subsequent injury to either knee within 5 years after anterior cruciate ligament reconstruction with patellar tendon autograft. Am J Sports Med 2009;37:246–51.
36. Church S, Keating J. Reconstruction of the anterior cruciate ligament: timing of surgery and the incidence of meniscal tears and degenerative change. J Bone Joint Surg Am 2005;87:1639–42.
37. Granan L, Bahr R, Lie S, et al. Timing of anterior cruciate ligament reconstructive surgery and risk of cartilage lesions and meniscal tears: a cohort study based on the Norwegian National Knee Ligament Registry. Am J Sports Med 2009;37: 955–61.
38. Tayton E, Verma R, Higgins B, et al. A correlation of time with meniscal tears in anterior cruciate ligament deficiency: stratifying the risk of surgical delay. Knee Surg Sports Traumatol Arthrosc 2009;17:30–4.
39. Yoo J, Ahn J, Lee S, et al. Increasing incidence of medial meniscal tears in non-operatively treated anterior cruciate ligament insufficiency patients documented by serial magnetic resonance imaging studies. Am J Sports Med 2009;37: 1478–83.
40. Fairbank T. Knee joint changes after meniscectomy. J Bone Joint Surg Am 1948; 30:664–70.
41. Jomha N, Borton D, Clingeleffer A, et al. Long term osteoarthritic changes in anterior cruciate ligament reconstructed knees. Clin Orthop Relat Res 1999; 358:188–93.
42. Brophy R, Zeltser D, Wright R, et al. Anterior cruciate ligament reconstruction and concomitant articular cartilage injury: incidence and treatment. Arthroscopy 2010;26:112–20.
43. van der Kraan P, van den Berg W. Chondrocyte hypertrophy and osteoarthritis: role in initiation and progression of cartilage degeneration? Osteoarthritis Cartilage 2012;20:223–32.
44. Oiestad B, Engebretsen L, Storheim K, et al. Knee osteoarthritis after anterior cruciate ligament injury. Am J Sports Med 2009;37:1434–43.
45. Meunier A, Odensten M, Good L. Long-term results after primary repair or non-surgical treatment of anterior cruciate ligament rupture: a randomized study with a 15-year follow-up. Scand J Med Sci Sports 2007;17:230–7.
46. Lebel B, Hulet C, Galaud B, et al. Arthroscopic reconstruction of the anterior cruciate ligament using bone-patellar tendon-bone autograft: a minimum 10 year follow-up. Am J Sports Med 2008;36:1275–82.
47. Neuman P, Englund M, Kostogiannis I, et al. Prevalence of tibiofemoral osteoarthritis 15 years after nonoperative treatment of anterior cruciate ligament injury: a prospective cohort study. Am J Sports Med 2008;36:1717–25.
48. Keays S, Newcombe P, Bullock-Saxton J, et al. Factors involved in the development of osteoarthritis after anterior cruciate ligament surgery. Am J Sports Med 2010;38:455–63.
49. Lohmander L, Roos H, Dahlberg L, et al. Temporal patterns of stromelysin-1, tissue inhibitor, and proteoglycan fragments in human knee joint fluid after injury to the cruciate ligament or meniscus. J Orthop Res 1994;12:21–8.

50. Sward P, Frobell R, Englund M, et al. Cartilage and bone markers and inflammatory cytokines are increased in synovial fluid in the acute phase of knee injury (hemarthrosis)–a cross-sectional analysis. Osteoarthritis Cartilage 2012;20:1302–8.
51. Wong J, Khan T, Jayadev C, et al. Anterior cruciate ligament rupture and osteoarthritis progression. Open Orthop J 2012;6:295–300.
52. Fetto J, Marshall J. The natural history and diagnosis of anterior cruciate ligament insufficiency. Clin Orthop 1980;147:29–38.
53. Andriacchi T, Dyrby C. Interactions between kinematics and loading during walking for the normal and ACL deficient knee. J Biomech 2005;38:293–8.
54. Tashman S, Kolowich P, Collon D, et al. Dynamic function of the ACL-reconstructed knee during running. Clin Orthop Relat Res 2007;454:66–73.
55. Chaudhari A, Briant P, Bevill S, et al. Knee kinematics, cartilage morphology, and osteoarthritis after ACL injury. Med Sci Sports Exerc 2008;40:215–22.
56. Ahmed A, Burke D. In-vitro measurement of static pressure distribution in synovial joints–part I: tibial surface of the knee. J Biomech Eng 1983;105:216.
57. Lee D, Bader D. Compressive strains at physiological frequencies influence the metabolism of chondrocytes seeded in agarose. J Orthop Res 1997;15:181–8.
58. Elder S, Goldstein S, Kimura J, et al. Chondrocyte differentiation is modulated by frequency and duration of cyclic compressive loading. Ann Biomed Eng 2001;29:476–82.
59. Meisterling S, Schoderbek R, Andrews J. Anterior cruciate ligament reconstruction. Operat Tech Sports Med 2009;17:2–10.
60. Frank C, Douglas J. The science of reconstruction of the anterior cruciate ligament. J Bone Joint Surg Am 1997;79:1556–76.
61. Frobell R, Roos E, Roos H, et al. A randomized trial of treatment for acute anterior cruciate ligament tears. N Engl J Med 2010;363:331–42.
62. Macaulay A, Perfetti D, Levine W. Anterior cruciate ligament graft choices. Sports Health 2012;4:63–8.
63. Foster R, Wolfe B, Ryan S, et al. Does the graft source really matter in the outcome of patients undergoing anterior cruciate ligament reconstruction? An evaluation of autograft versus allograft reconstruction results: a systematic review. Am J Sports Med 2010;38:189–99.
64. Biau D, Tournoux C, Katsahian S, et al. ACL reconstruction: a meta-analysis of functional scores. Clin Orthop Relat Res 2007;458:180–7.
65. Biau D, Katsahian S, Kartus J. Patellar tendon versus hamstring tendon autografts for reconstructing the anterior cruciate ligament: a meta-analysis based on individual patient data. Am J Sports Med 2009;37:2470–8.
66. Li S, Chen Y, Lin Z, et al. A systematic review of randomized controlled clinical trials comparing hamstring autografts versus bone-patellar tendon-bone autografts for the reconstruction of the anterior cruciate ligament. Arch Orthop Trauma Surg 2012;132:1287–97.
67. Moksnes H, Risberg M. Performance-based functional evaluation of nonoperative and operative treatment after anterior cruciate ligament injury. Scand J Med Sci Sports 2009;19:345–55.
68. Meuffels D, Favejee M, Vissers M, et al. Ten year follow-up study comparing conservative versus operative treatment of anterior cruciate ligament ruptures. A matched-pair analysis of high level athletes. Br J Sports Med 2009;43:347–51.
69. Barenius B, Forssblad M, Engstrom B, et al. Functional recovery after anterior cruciate ligament reconstruction, a study of health-related quality of life based on the Swedish National Knee Ligament Register. Knee Surg Sports Traumatol Arthrosc 2012. [Epub ahead of print].

70. Barenius B, Nordlander M, Ponzer S, et al. Quality of life and clinical outcome after anterior cruciate ligament reconstruction using patellar tendon graft or quadrupled semitendinosus graft: an 8-year follow-up of a randomized controlled trial. Am J Sports Med 2010;38:1533–41.
71. Oiestad B, Holm I, Aune A, et al. Knee function and prevalence of knee osteoarthritis after anterior cruciate ligament reconstruction: a prospective study with 10 to 15 years of follow-up. Am J Sports Med 2010;38:2201–10.
72. Linko E, Harilainen A, Malmivaara A, et al. Surgical versus conservative interventions for anterior cruciate ligament ruptures in adults. Cochrane Database Syst Rev 2005;(2):CD001356.
73. Janssen K, Orchard J, Driscoll T, et al. High incidence and costs for anterior cruciate ligament reconstructions performed in Australia from 2003-2004 to 2007-2008: time for an anterior cruciate ligament register by Scandinavian model? Scand J Med Sci Sports 2011;22(4):495–501.
74. Bach B Jr, Boonos C. Anterior cruciate ligament reconstruction. AORN J 2001;74: 152–64.
75. Arden C, Webster K, Taylor N, et al. Return to sport following ACL reconstruction surgery: are our expectations for recovery too high? J Sci Med Sport 2010;13(1):5.
76. Arden C, Webster K, Taylor N, et al. Return to sport following anterior cruciate ligament reconstruction surgery: a systematic review and meta-analysis of the state of play. Br J Sports Med 2011;45:596–606.
77. Myer G, Ford K, Palumbo J, et al. Neuromuscular training improves performance and lower-extremity biomechanics in female athletes. J Strength Cond Res 2005; 19:51–60.
78. Neitzel J, Kernozek T, Davies G. Loading response following anterior cruciate ligament reconstruction during the parallel squat exercise. Clin Biomech 2002; 17:551–4.
79. Myer G, Schmitt L, Brent J, et al. Utilization of modified NFL combine testing to identify functional deficits in athletes following ACL reconstruction. J Orthop Sports Phys Ther 2011;41:377–87.
80. Brophy R, Wright R, Matava M. Cost analysis of converting from single-bundle to double-bundle anterior cruciate ligament reconstruction. Am J Sports Med 2009; 37:683–7.
81. Gottlob C, Baker C Jr, Pellissier J, et al. Cost effectiveness of anterior cruciate ligament reconstruction in young adults. Clin Orthop Relat Res 1999;367: 272–82.
82. Lubowitz J, Appleby D. Cost-effectiveness analysis of the most common orthopaedic surgery procedures: knee arthroscopy and knee anterior cruciate ligament reconstruction. Arthroscopy 2011;27:1317–22.
83. Farshad M, Gerber C, Meyer D, et al. Reconstruction versus conservative treatment after rupture of the anterior cruciate ligament: cost effectiveness analysis. BMC Health Serv Res 2011;11:317.
84. Gilchrist J, Mandelbaum B, Melancon H. A randomized controlled trial to prevent noncontact anterior cruciate ligament injury in female collegiate soccer players. Am J Sports Med 2008;36:1476–83.
85. Myklebust G, Engebretsen L, Braekken I, et al. Prevention of noncontact anterior cruciate ligament injuries in elite and adolescent female handball athletes. Instr Course Lect 2007;56:407–18.
86. Mandelbaum B, Silvers H, Watanabe D. Effectiveness of neuromuscular and proprioceptive training program in preventing anterior cruciate ligament injuries in female athletes: 2-year follow-up. Am J Sports Med 2005;33:1003–10.

87. Steffen K, Myklebust G, Olsen O, et al. Preventing injuries in female youth football–a cluster randomized controlled trial. Scand J Med Sci Sports 2008;18: 605–14.

88. Walden M, Atroshi I, Magnusson H, et al. Prevention of acute knee injuries in adolescent female football players: cluster randomised controlled trial. Br Med J 2012;344:e3042.

89. Gagnier J, Morgenstern H, Chess L. Interventions designed to prevent anterior cruciate ligament injuries in adolescents and adults: a systematic review and meta-analysis. Am J Sports Med 2012. [Epub ahead of print].

90. Hewett T, Ford K, Myer G. Anterior cruciate ligament injuries in female athletes, part 2: a meta-analysis of neuromuscular interventions aimed at injury prevention. Am J Sports Med 2006;34:490–8.

91. Grindstaff T, Hammill R, Tuzson A, et al. Neuromuscular control training programs and noncontact anterior cruciate ligament injury rates in female athletes: a numbers-needed-to-treat analysis. J Athl Train 2006;41:450–6.

92. Shea K, Grimm N, Jacobs J, et al. ACL and knee injury prevention programs for young athletes: do they work? In: Annual Meeting of the American Orthopaedic Society for Sports Medicine. Providence, July 15–18, 2010.

93. Howell J, Handoll H. Surgical treatment for meniscal injuries of the knee in adults. Cochrane Database Syst Rev 2000;(2):CD001353.

Chronic Disease Management
A Review of Current Performance Across Quality of Care Domains and Opportunities for Improving Osteoarthritis Care

Caroline A. Brand, MBBS, BA, MPH, FRACP[a,b,c,]*,
Ilana N. Ackerman, BPhysio(Hons), PhD[a,c],
Megan A. Bohensky, BA, MPH, PhD[a,c],
Kim L. Bennell, BAppSci(physio), PhD[d]

KEYWORDS

- Osteoarthritis • Knee • Hip • Hand • Quality of care • Models of care

KEY POINTS

- Key OA hip and knee guideline recommendations are for non-pharmacological interventions such as exercise and weight optimization, and for severe disease, joint replacement surgery.
- There is suboptimal management of OA across a number of quality of care domains, including; effectiveness, safety, access and support for patient self-management.
- There are limitations in current services associated with inadequate information systems, variable team-based care and suboptimal service linkages.
- There is a need for improved delivery of decision support for clinicians and patients to support shared decision-making and uptake of cost-effective interventions.
- There is a need for further research directed at harnessing social networks to support people at risk or with mild to moderate osteoarthritis.

Disclosure: C.A.B., I.A., M.B., none; K.B. receives royalties from ASICS Oceania Pty Ltd.
[a] Melbourne EpiCentre, Royal Melbourne Hospital, Melbourne Health, University of Melbourne, Level 7 East, Main Block, Grattan Street, Parkville, Victoria 3052, Australia; [b] Centre for Research Excellence in Patient Safety, Monash University, Commercial road, Melbourne 3004, Australia; [c] Department of Medicine, Melbourne EpiCentre, Royal Melbourne Hospital, The University of Melbourne, Level 7 East, Main Block, Grattan Street, Parkville, Victoria 3052, Australia; [d] Department of Physiotherapy, Centre for Health, Exercise and Sports Medicine, School of Health Sciences, University of Melbourne, Berkeley Street, Parkville, Victoria 3010, Australia
* Corresponding author. Melbourne EpiCentre, Royal Melbourne Hospital, Melbourne Health, University of Melbourne, Level 7 East, Main Block, Grattan Street, Parkville, Victoria 3052, Australia.
E-mail address: caroline.brand@mh.org.au

BACKGROUND

Osteoarthritis (OA) is the most common chronic joint disease. It is highly prevalent and a leading cause of disability worldwide.[1] As such, OA poses a substantial societal burden, predominantly because of growing health care costs and lost productivity. The increasing incidence and prevalence of chronic diseases such as OA are driving health care reform internationally, particularly health care redesign to provide service models that better support the needs of people with these conditions.[2]

In addition, as greater attention is focused toward resolving gaps in implementing evidence into practice and preventing underuse, overuse, and sometimes misuse of effective interventions, a previously narrow focus on clinical outcomes such as mortality has expanded to consider broader measurement of quality of care. The Institute of Medicine in the United States advocates for 6 pillars to improve care: safety, effectiveness, patient-centered care, timeliness, efficiency, and equity (**Table 1**).[2]

Table 1 Improving care for chronic conditions: the 6 pillars of improving health care	
Quality Outcome Domain	**Definitions and Principles of Care Redesign**
Safety	Patients should be safe from injury caused by the system
Effectiveness	Patients should receive care based on the best available scientific knowledge Health care providers and organizations should actively collaborate and communicate to ensure appropriate exchange of information and coordination of care
Patient-centered care	Care is customized and based on patients' needs and values The health system should make available to patients and their families information that allows them to make informed decisions when selecting a health plan, hospital, or clinical practice. This information should include descriptions of the system's performance on safety, evidence-based practice, and patient satisfaction Patients are given necessary information and the opportunity to exercise the degree of control they choose over the health care decisions that affect them Health care providers and patients should communicate effectively and share information The health system should make available to patients and their families information that allows them to make informed decisions when selecting a health plan, hospital, or clinical practice. This information should include descriptions of the system's performance on safety, evidence-based practice, and patient satisfaction
Timeliness and appropriateness	The system should anticipate patient needs, rather than reacting to events Care should be continuous Health care providers and institutions should actively collaborate and communicate to ensure appropriate exchange of information and coordination of care
Efficiency	The health system should not waste resources or patient time
Equity	Care should not vary in quality because of gender, ethnicity, geographic location, or socioeconomic status

Adapted from Institute Of Medicine. Crossing the quality chasm: a new health system for the 21st century. The National Academy of Sciences; 2000. Available at: http://www.nap.edu/openbook/03090728/html/l.html. Accessed February 21, 2003.

There is a useful existing commentary about the ways in which care for people with OA can be improved.[3–7] This article builds on these sources by exploring system, health care provider, and patient barriers and enablers to improving care for OA in relation to the Institute of Medicine's 6 pillars for improving chronic care health services.

CURRENT PERFORMANCE IN MANAGEMENT OF OA

Recommendations for OA care can be found in several jurisdictional evidence-based clinical practice guidelines,[8–12] the most recent of which are the American College of Rheumatology (ACR) 2012 updated guidelines for conservative management of hand, hip, and knee OA.[10] The degree to which current practice reflects these guidelines is uncertain because it is difficult to access data about longitudinal performance in the management of OA. The exception to this is joint arthroplasty, for which high-quality clinical registries are maintained to monitor joint prosthesis survival outcomes and limited patient outcomes, such as revision rates and mortality.

Data from previous studies indicate that up to one-third of people with chronic conditions in general do not receive recommended care.[13,14] Suboptimal care may be even higher for those with OA, with 1 study reporting an average indicator pass rate for primary care of only 57%.[15] For OA, there is reported suboptimal use of effective interventions,[15–20] inequity in access to arthroplasty,[21–23] inappropriate use of arthroscopy,[24–26] unmet need for pain assessment and management, and potentially preventable safety issues associated with use of pharmacologic therapies for people with OA.[27] Variation in provision of evidence-based care also occurs. A recent patient survey using questions based on the Arthritis Foundation Quality Indicators for OA[20] found that provision of advice about nonpharmacologic care was not only suboptimal but that this differed according to sex, age, disability, and educational levels.[19]

Unlike previous clinical practice guidelines, the ACR has taken a case-based scenario approach to their recently updated OA recommendations, on the basis that studies to date have not tested sequential management strategies, and case scenarios allow clinicians to better provide an individualized management approach. Thus there are 6 cases and scenarios comprising mild to severe symptomatic OA as well as gastrointestinal and cardiovascular comorbidity scenarios. The guideline summary focuses on the initiation of therapy (**Tables 2** and **3**), although other case scenarios can be accessed through supplementary material online. Whether this guideline approach will be more effective than others is yet to be tested.

Effective, Safe, and Equitable Care for OA

Nonpharmacologic therapy

Clinical guidelines highlight the role of conservative nonpharmacologic treatments as the first-line approach to management of OA and emphasize their important role at all stages of disease. The bulk of research into nonpharmacologic treatments is focused on knee OA. Core nonpharmacologic treatments generally recommended by clinical guidelines for hip and knee OA include patient education, exercise, and, for those who are overweight or obese, weight loss.

In line with OA as a chronic disease, patient education is a key component of treatment and can take many forms in terms of content and mode of delivery. ACR guidelines conditionally recommend that people with hip or knee OA participate in formal self-management programs.[10] However, although OA self-management programs are available in many countries, health practitioners do not necessarily refer patients. A qualitative study found several barriers and enablers to general practitioner (GP) referral of people with OA to self-management programs in Australia.[28] These included

Table 2
Summary of initial conservative nonpharmacologic management options for OA hand, knee, and hip based on the ACR guidelines[a]

Treatment	OA Hand	OA Knee	OA Hip
Patient education/ self-management programs	√ For joint protection techniques	√	√
Exercise: aerobic, strengthening, aquatic	No recommendation	√√	√√
Weight loss if overweight/obese	Not applicable	√√	√√
Manual therapy	No recommendation	√ With exercise	√ With exercise
Acupuncture[b]	No recommendation	√	No recommendation
Transcutaneous electrical stimulation[b]	No recommendation	√	No recommendation
Thermal agents	√	√	√
Psychosocial interventions	No recommendation	√	√
Patellar taping	Not applicable	√ For medially directed No recommendation for laterally directed	Not applicable
Balance exercises	Not applicable	No recommendation	No recommendation
Tai Chi	Not applicable	√	No recommendation
Walking aids or assistive devices	√	√	√
Lateral wedge insoles	Not applicable	No recommendation √ If subtalar strapped	Not applicable
Medial wedge insoles	Not applicable	√	Not applicable
Braces/splints	√	No recommendation	Not applicable

√, Conditional recommendation; √√, strong recommendation.
[a] These recommendations are based on the scenario of an adult with symptomatic knee OA without cardiovascular comorbidities, current or past upper gastrointestinal (GI) problems, or chronic kidney disease presenting to the primary care provider for treatment. The patient complains of mild to severe pain in and/or around the knee(s) and of not having had an adequate response to either intermittent dosing of over-the-counter (OTC) acetaminophen or OTC nonsteroidal antiinflamatory drugs (NSAIDs) or OTC nutritional supplements.
[b] Only when the patient with knee OA has chronic moderate to severe pain and is a candidate for total joint arthroplasty but is unwilling or unable to have surgery.
Data from Hochberg MC, Altman RD, April KT, et al. American College of Rheumatology 2012 recommendations for the use of nonpharmacologic and pharmacologic therapies in osteoarthritis of the hand, hip, and knee. Arthritis Care Res 2012;64(4):455–74.

GP-related factors (knowledge about availability and types of services on offer, perceptions about patients' capacity to attend and motivation, beliefs about the benefit of referral), patient-related factors (awareness of the value and availability of services, patient-driven referrals), and program factors (design, content, location, cost, and waiting time). A range of barriers to participation in community-based arthritis self-management programs including travel difficulties and work commitments have also been reported by people with hip or knee OA.[29]

Table 3
Summary of initial pharmacologic management options for OA hand, knee, and hip based on the ACR guidelines[a]

Pharmaceutical Agent	OA Hand	OA Knee	OA Hip
Acetaminophen	No recommendation	√	√
Oral NSAIDs	√+	√	√
Topical NSAIDs	√	√	No recommendation
Tramadol	√	√	√
Intra-articular corticosteroid injections	x	√	√
Intra-articular hyaluronates	x	No recommendation	No recommendation
Opioid analgesia	x	No recommendation	No recommendation
Duloxetine	No recommendation	No recommendation	No recommendation
Glucosamine	No recommendation	x	x
Chrondroitin sulfate	No recommendation	x	x

√, conditional recommendation for the intervention; x, conditional recommendation that this intervention is not used; +, topical NSAIDs rather than oral NSAIDs are recommended in people more than 75 years old.

[a] These recommendations are based on the scenario of an adult with symptomatic knee OA without cardiovascular comorbidities, current or past upper GI problems, or chronic kidney disease presenting to the primary care provider for treatment. The patient complains of mild to severe pain in and/or around the knee(s) and of not having had an adequate response to either intermittent dosing of OTC acetaminophen or OTC NSAIDs or OTC nutritional supplements.

Data from Hochberg MC, Altman RD, April KT, et al. American College of Rheumatology 2012 recommendations for the use of nonpharmacologic and pharmacologic therapies in osteoarthritis of the hand, hip, and knee. Arthritis Care Res 2012;64(4):455–74.

For specific exercise prescription, an individualized approach is required. The ACR guidelines strongly recommend both aquatic and land-based exercises, and conditionally recommend tai chi, with the decision on choice of exercise approach based on patient preferences and functional ability.[10] Strengthening exercises for the lower limb muscles, particularly the quadriceps, and aerobic exercises such as walking are also recommended by several other guidelines.[8,11,30] Different exercise delivery modes (individual, group, home based) have all been found to be effective in improving pain and function.[31] However, 12 or more directly supervised exercise sessions seem to be more effective than fewer than 12.[31] Patient adherence is also a key factor in determining long-term outcome from exercise therapy in patients with OA.[32,33] Given that patient adherence to exercise declines over time, strategies to maximize adherence are needed.[34]

Despite strong evidence from randomized controlled trials (RCTs) showing the beneficial effects of exercise for people with OA[35] and numerous clinical guidelines advocating exercise, international surveys have found that exercise is underused by medical practitioners as a treatment of OA.[19,36,37] Furthermore, the attitudes and beliefs of health care professionals regarding exercise may be counterproductive to the patient behavioral changes needed to ensure ongoing exercise participation by the patient.[38] Provision of advice on exercise to patients with OA may also differ across age, sex, disability, and education levels.[19]

Clinical guidelines recommend weight loss for those with lower limb OA who are overweight or obese.[10,39] For knee OA, a meta-analysis of weight loss trials found that disability could be significantly improved when weight is reduced by more than 5%, or at a rate of greater than 0.24% reduction per week over a 20-week period.[40]

Ottawa Panel Guidelines, developed specifically for overweight or obese people with OA, recommend a combination of physical activity (aerobic exercise plus or minus strength training) and diet (caloric restriction).[41] The panel recommends weight loss before implementing weight-bearing exercise to maintain joint integrity. One RCT has shown that rheumatologist adoption of standardized goal-oriented patient visits can positively influence weight loss, exercise, and pain at 4 months follow-up, and improved physical activity, pain, and function at 1 year.[42]

A range of other conservative nonpharmacologic treatments are available for the management of OA, with varying recommendations from clinical guidelines based on limited or low-quality evidence to support their efficacy. Recent ACR recommendations for initial treatment are summarized in **Table 2**.[10]

Pharmacologic therapy

Research interest and evidence generated about pharmacologic management of OA has also focused largely on knee OA and, to a lesser extent, hip and hand OA. The pharmacologic armamentarium for OA, unlike that for rheumatoid arthritis (RA), remains directed primarily toward symptom management rather than structural modification and prevention of disease progression.

Overall, the recent ACR recommendations are largely in keeping with previous guidelines,[8,43] with some interesting differences. For instance, there is inclusion of a new psychoactive agent, duloxetine, a balanced serotonin and norepinephrine reuptake inhibitor (SNRI), for which there is RCT evidence of a benefit in reduction of pain and improvement of function over a 13-week trial period compared with placebo.[44] Although there was no statistical difference noted in harms, a greater proportion of the treated group experienced adverse events compared with placebo, and these results require testing in other settings and older OA populations.

In contrast with nonpharmacologic management, in which there is strong support for exercise, aquatic therapy, and weight loss for those who are overweight, all pharmacologic recommendations about initiation of therapy for hand, hip, and knee OA were of lower grade; that is, conditional recommendations (see **Table 3**). Recommendations for use of simple analgesia and nonsteroidal antiinflamatory drugs (NSAIDs) remain similar to those in the European League Against Rheumatism (EULAR)[43] and Osteoarthritis Research Society International (OARSI)[8] guidelines; however, there is now a recommendation that glucosamine and chondroitin sulfate should not be given, based on evidence from a meta-analysis[45] and a systematic review.[46] This is a contentious area because another recent meta-analysis supports use of chondroitin sulfate, based on a small but significant effect on cartilage loss for OA knee.[47]

In 2001 it was suggested that guidelines should be reviewed every 3 years[48]; however, given the rapidly changing evidence, a more responsive knowledge synthesis and dissemination process is required. For instance, the EULAR and OARSI guidelines supported use of hyaluronic acid, and the ACR guidelines provide no recommendation; however, a new systematic review reported only small and clinically irrelevant benefit from use of intra-articular hyaluronate therapy, suggesting that a stronger negative recommendation may now be appropriate.[49]

Safety of pharmacologic therapy

Understanding of safety in relation to OA care is largely based on information gathered in individual therapeutic intervention trials or meta-analyses and joint registry reported outcomes. NSAID gastrointestinal and cardiovascular risks and preventive strategies are well described,[50] and prescribing practices, associated with reduction in prescription of NSAIDs, have changed over the past 10 years.[51] However, an area of increasing interest is use of opioid medications. The ACR data indicate that, although there is strong evidence to support a benefit for pain (number needed to treat [NNT] = 5) and functional outcomes (NNT = 7), the number needed to harm with nausea (NNT = 5) and constipation (NNT = 4) is similar.[10] The rapid increase in use of opioids for management of nononcological chronic pain, including OA, in the last 10 years, particularly in developed countries, is of significant concern.[52,53] Data from Australia suggest that the peak age for prescribing opioids is 45 to 64 years, with high levels also noted for older people and 60% of prescriptions being for musculoskeletal problems.[54] A further study reported that in 2007 to 2008 the rate of hospital separations for poisoning associated with use of morphine, oxycodone, and codeine had increased from 0.05/1000 population to 0.11/1000. There is therefore an imperative to develop drug surveillance systems for monitoring long-term outcomes to inform guideline recommendations and clinical practice management of OA.

Surgery
Access and equity for hip and knee arthroplasty in OA There is good evidence that knee and hip arthroplasty are cost-effective interventions for the management of end-stage OA.[55,56] Although equitable access to arthroplasty for those who require it is a key goal in the management of severe OA, access to surgery is not always dictated by clinical need. Access can be limited by a range of health professional–related and health system–related factors such as delayed referral to an orthopedic surgeon, protracted waiting times for orthopedic consultation and surgery, inconsistent methods for prioritizing surgical waiting lists, and the availability of hospital resources. International studies have revealed great variation between settings in the severity of OA before surgery,[57,58] and this is likely to reflect the lack of concrete indications for arthroplasty and the lack of consensus regarding the appropriate timing of surgery. There is also substantial evidence of disparities in access to hip and knee arthroplasty in many countries, including those that have universal health care or parallel public and private health care systems. Disparities exist across demographic factors including race or ethnicity[59] and gender,[60] and socioeconomic factors such as level of education, income, and health care cover.[23] For example, a Canadian population-based study found that people with less education or lower income had the greatest unmet need for hip and knee arthroplasty,[61] and the likelihood of undergoing surgery has been shown to increase significantly with higher socioeconomic status in England and Canada.[62,63] In the United States, significantly lower rates of hip and knee arthroplasty have been reported for African American and Hispanic individuals.[64,65] Studies from Australia and the United Kingdom have found that people from lower socioeconomic backgrounds had greater symptom severity before arthroplasty[66] and poorer preoperative well-being,[67,68] suggesting delayed access to care.

Facilitating equitable access to arthroplasty is a complex task that requires an improved understanding of the barriers faced by people with OA. Frameworks that adopt a holistic approach to determining need for surgery could also be valuable.[69] Dieppe and colleagues[70] described a capacity to benefit algorithm. Incorporating both disease-related and treatment-related aspects, this algorithm brings together a range of factors for consideration by health professionals, including the personal impact of the condition, the likely benefit of arthroplasty, and individual preferences for treatment. This type of framework could assist in prioritizing access to arthroplasty for people with the greatest need and potential for improvement, given their individual circumstances. However, the conceptual framework for capacity to benefit could be expanded to incorporate system factors (**Fig. 1**). Although arthroplasty is cost-effective, there is evidence that total knee arthroplasty is more costly and less effective in low-volume centers

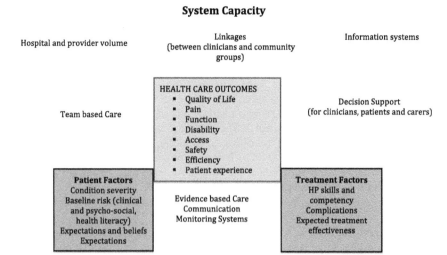

Fig. 1. Capacity to improve osteoarthritis health care outcomes. HP, health care provider.

compared with high-volume centers,[56] and a recent systematic review reports a clear and consistent relationship between higher provider (surgeon) or hospital volumes and improved patient outcomes.[71] At the clinical interface, use of patient decision aids, which been shown to improve knowledge, improves treatment expectation and reduces decisional conflict,[72] and could assist patients with decision making about arthroplasty.[73]

Appropriate use of arthroscopy in OA In contrast with arthroplasty, there is a lack of evidence for use of arthroscopy in OA, uncomplicated by major mechanical derangement. The use of lavage and arthroscopic debridement for the treatment of knee OA has been common since the 1970s for patients whose joint disease is not severe enough to require arthroplasty. Most of the early studies evaluating knee arthroscopy for treatment of OA showed a benefit in the most patients, but these studies were small, uncontrolled, and did not use validated outcomes measures.[74–77]

In 2002, Moseley and colleagues[78] randomly assigned 180 military veterans with knee OA to receive an arthroscopic debridement, arthroscopic lavage, or placebo surgery. During the 2-year follow-up period, no significant benefit was evident for patients who received arthroscopy, compared with those who received placebo surgery. Although this study was criticized for several methodological concerns,[79,80] subsequent studies support lack of benefit for patients without symptoms of mechanical derangement and bone fragments.[81] Despite this evidence, studies in the United Kingdom, Canada, and Australia have shown that rates of knee arthroscopies among patients with OA have not decreased since 2002.[24,26]

Guidelines are available to support decision making for surgical intervention for OA,[39,82] and the reasons for failure to take up this evidence are unclear. The UK and Canadian data, including data to 2004, may have been too early to capture change; however, the Australian study reviewed data up to 2009. Patients may preferentially seek surgical intervention before trying more conservative approaches, and younger patients may seek less invasive surgical options to delay arthroplasty. In addition, clinical decision making involves balancing research evidence with clinical experience.[83] A health care provider whose experience with using a procedure conflicts with research evidence may judge the former more highly (availability bias).

Overall, although there is good evidence that clinical practice guidelines positively influence delivery of the process of care,[84] the reported benefits for patient health outcomes are less well established, and sometimes conflicting.[85–88] The reasons for variable uptake are many, but evidence suggests that effective decision support systems need to:

- Be automatically provided as part of work flow
- Provide recommendations rather than assessments
- Be provided at the point (time and location) of decision making
- Be computer based[84]

Further, there needs to be assessment of the practicality of implementation, and potential adaptation of recommendations to different settings, while retaining fidelity of recommendation key principles.[89,90] Other methods of delivering guideline recommendations also need to be researched. For instance, use of social media, for which there are high levels of physician acceptance, although, again, effectiveness is likely to depend on perceived ease of use and usefulness.[91]

Changes in funding models could also influence treatment patterns. For instance, since 2004, the US Medicare system no longer reimburses providers for knee arthroscopies used to treat OA in the public system. However, because most knee arthroscopies occur in private settings, this policy may not gain traction and influence practice. It may also result in perverse changes in coding behaviors. Kim and colleagues[25] suggest that surgeons in the United States are now listing the diagnostic codes for patients with OA as having meniscal tears for the purposes of insurance authorization. As for arthroplasty, the usefulness of decision aids should be investigated for decision making about arthoscopy intervention in OA.

Efficiency and OA Care

An efficient health care system uses resources to get the best value for the money spent.[92] It is important to patients, managers, and funding providers that services are provided efficiently, although how efficiency is perceived and measured may differ between stakeholders. For example, patients may value timely, responsive care; managers may prioritize patient flow or throughput; and funding providers may prefer cost per quality-adjusted life year (QALY). The literature provides information about OA health care efficiency in various ways, but primarily through economic evaluations undertaken within the context of clinical trials and the use of economic modeling methods.

Aside from arthroplasty, there is more limited information about the cost-effectiveness of other interventions for OA. A 2012 meta-analysis located only 11 RCTs or quasi-RCTs of conservative nonpharmacologic interventions (exercise programs, acupuncture, rehabilitation, and lifestyle interventions) for hip and knee OA reporting health care costs, of which most had high risk of bias for the cost and/ or treatment effects of the study.[93] All studies reported cost savings where exercise programs were evaluated; however, there were conflicting results for rehabilitation programs, and none of the studies evaluating lifestyle programs (including education and self-management strategies) were cost-effective when QALYs were the measure of benefit. Although a single acupuncture trial showed cost-effectiveness, the investigators indicated that this study was associated with high risk of bias, lack of a sensitivity analysis, and was limited to a 3-month time frame.[93] In an Australian study, priority-setting models were used to compare the relative cost-effectiveness of different OA interventions.[94] The study confirmed total hip and knee arthroplasty as being the most cost-effective interventions for OA management. Exercise in different settings was also cost-effective, although less so for home-based programs. Cost-effectiveness for weight loss and patient education interventions could not be modeled because of lack of RCT data and/or inconsistencies in reported study outcomes.

Andrews and colleagues[95] have also used economic modeling methods to estimate the cost of providing optimal care for OA and RA based on measurement of years lived with disability. The health gain for OA was based on shifting from NSAIDs to simple analgesics, increasing the level of exercise activity among those with mild to moderate OA and provision of arthroplasty to all those with severe disease. In contrast with RA, for which optimal therapy entailed a 7% cost increase for an 85% health gain, the benefit for OA was less impressive, with a 40% increase in funds required to gain a 40% increase in health improvement.

Overall, costing studies have been limited by their frequent reliance on extrapolation from multiple data sources and questionable external validity, because data sources and funding models may not be comparable between settings. The lack of robust data about cost-effectiveness for interventions other than arthroplasty is also concerning. If there is to be advocacy for new models of OA care, for instance team-based services, there will need to be robust evaluation, including cost analyses, to support changes in policy and funding models. Although large-scale studies, based on routine, less resource intensive collection of administrative data may contribute to future costing studies, there are well-documented data quality issues associated with administrative data sources.[96] There is a need for data linkage between longitudinal administrative systems providing service use data and robust clinical data systems that provide adequate information about patient risk and their current OA condition, as well as a need for more research pertaining to direct and indirect costs for patients with OA. This research should include the cost of preventive care as well as treatment of established disease. Pinto and colleagues[93] made several useful recommendations to improve economic analyses, including the need for more uniform reporting of outcomes, regular use of health-related quality-of-life data, and use of comparators with known cost-effectiveness or usual care controls for at least 1 year.

Patient-centered Care

There is no single definition of patient-centered care.[97] However, the Institute of Medicine definition that has been informed by Sackett and colleagues'[98] description of evidence-based Medicine is "providing care that is respectful of and responsive to individual patient preferences, needs, and values and ensuring that patient values guide all clinical decisions," which captures several attributes of patient-centered care.[2] To meet this definition, the health system needs to be oriented toward patient-centered care and must have the capacity to provide it.

Current evidence suggests this is not yet the case,[99] and that patient experience of care (measured using a survey validated for OA that captures key elements of chronic-care service experience) is lower for OA than for other chronic conditions.[100] Factors contributing to suboptimal OA care delivery and uptake and potential solutions lie at all levels of the health system, even in developed countries.[101] Qualitative research in OA contributes to understanding service level barriers such as:

- Knowledge-based factors (lack of decision support for health care providers and patients)
- Service-based factors (service inflexibility and suboptimal responsiveness to perceived need, inadequate support for patient self-management of their

condition, lack of communication between health care providers, and inadequate coordination of care, particularly between primary and higher levels of care sectors[102]

These barriers are in keeping with those reported for other chronic conditions.[2]

Several chronic disease management models have emerged to improve chronic care and these have been shown to be effective for some conditions.[103] The various models differ according to the primary purpose for which they are designed; for instance, primary care models that focus on people managing with OA in the community,[104,105] and specialist care models designed to ensure that optimal conservative therapy has been undertaken before facilitating timely access to arthroplasty for those who can most benefit.[106,107] However, most chronic disease models include similar key components (**Table 4**), including use of clinical information systems and decision support, service delivery redesign (eg, team-based care), a focus on linkages across community health care provider and patient groups and between different levels of health care, and a focus on patient self-management support.[2,104,105] An important extension of the primary care model over time has been to focus more strongly on preventive care (see **Table 4**).[108–110]

In contrast with other chronic conditions, there is a lack of supportive evidence of effectiveness for OA chronic care models and, to date, the OA primary care models have largely focused on patient self-management components.[111] Single component models can be effective[103] and there is evidence that patient arthritis self-management programs are associated with modest benefits for improved psychological health status, self-efficacy, and some health behaviors lasting for up to 12 months.[112] Although small trial-based benefits could potentially translate to much larger population benefits, there is currently a lack of supportive cost-effectiveness data for education and self-management in isolation from exercise.[93]

Newer team-based OA service models, in which expanded roles have been designed for nurses and allied health professionals, are emerging. There have been mixed outcomes reported for nurse-led models that focus on education and self-management, with 1 RCT reporting positive improvements in patient knowledge and satisfaction and lack of inferiority for other health outcomes, compared with consultation with a junior doctor in a hospital clinic.[113] In contrast, there was no demonstrable benefit for 2 community-based nurse RCT studies.[114,115] A pilot RCT for a physiotherapist-delivered exercise program and pain coping skills training provided benefit compared with exercise alone,[116] and a more definitive RCT study is now being undertaken.[117]

Although it is important to explore expanded clinician roles and the way in which team-based care can contribute to improved OA outcomes, the size of the existing unmet need and future need in designing service delivery systems must be considered. Given the shortage of all health care providers, increasing burden of OA, and data from economic modeling studies,[95] it is unlikely that models reliant on sustained input from medical or other health care providers will be cost-effective for those with mild to moderate OA or those at risk of developing OA. The community will require innovative, low-cost methods of disseminating and supporting primary and secondary preventive strategies targeted toward lifestyle behavior change; for instance, the use of social media.[118] Five social processes have been reported to affect health behaviors and outcomes: social influence, social engagement and attachment, social recommendations, social contagion, and social support. Such methods have been reported to show benefit; for instance, for regular prompting to support self-monitoring behaviors.[119] These options have yet to be explored adequately for their usefulness in providing

Table 4
Chronic care models: key components for providing clinical management for established OA and preventive care for those at risk

OA Chronic Care Model Components	Clinical Management	Preventive Management
Organization of care	Chronic illness is a key goal of practices and organization Leaders are committed and actively engaged in supporting change and developing strategies for health care providers and patients to take up evidence-based interventions to improve care	Leaders are actively engaged in advocating for social, economic, and environmental improvements to improve care and in supporting patients to address lifestyle behavioral risk factors
Delivery system design Designing service components to meet the needs of patients with chronic conditions and to support health care providers in their roles Who is on the team and how they interact with patients	Developing teams (within and external to an individual health care provider practice or organizational setting) and defining roles of team members for delivering different aspects of care (eg, goal setting, referrals, medication management, education, support for self-management, coordination of care Structuring planned visits, follow-up, and acute-access systems	Developing teams to screen, advise, and coordinate preventive services within and external to the individual practice or organizational setting Consider group visits, proactive mailings, telephone counseling, and emerging electronic social media strategies/options
Clinical information systems Capturing and using critical information for clinical care	Capture populations with OA, development of individually tailored care plans and reminder systems, ability to support recall and provide feedback on performance and patient safety outcomes	Capture populations at risk of OA, provides status summaries on preventive services, prompt planned visits for review and preventive services

Component		
Decision support systems What is the best care and how it can be provided every time Integration of evidence-based recommendations about condition management at the point of care delivery for health care providers and patients	Delivers up-to-date information about effective nonpharmacologic and pharmacologic interventions and medication interactions for health care providers Delivers decision aids for patients to support shared decision making about therapeutic interventions	Delivers up-to-date information for health care providers and patients about effective preventive strategies to maintain a healthy lifestyle and reduce the risk of OA and other chronic conditions
Self-management support A focus on the central role of patients as self-managers of their condition and associated risk factors	How clinicians help people live with their conditions Develop a collaborative model for health care provider/patient interaction to define problems, set priorities and goals, and identify and manage barriers to achieving those goals Deliver care in a culturally competent manner	Focus on a supportive model that helps patients recognize their need for preventive services and take action to access them Focus on support for sustained behavior change
Community Resources and policies that influence care delivery	Creation of effective linkages between health care providers and different health care sectors; for example, allied health care providers, specialists, and hospitals where care is provided for people with severe conditions Linkages with community and patient organizations to support patient self-management of their conditions	Focus on linkages to community organizations and consumer groups for support in preventive care and lifestyle behavior change

Adapted from Refs.[105,109,110]

meaningful support for OA self-management. Special attention needs to be paid to designing OA models to meet the needs of those with low levels of health literacy.[108]

SUMMARY

This article presents an overview of many issues currently facing patients, health care providers, funding providers, and policy makers who are working to improve OA health outcomes. In doing so, it suggests that a broad approach that considers individual and system quality of care outcomes is a useful way to identify future research and improvement opportunities.

A key system barrier is the current lack of clinical information systems that support identification and monitoring of OA populations, and evaluation of newer service models and health outcomes performance. The National Joint Registries have provided an example of the power of robust outcome data, and, as novel therapies are being tested, including biological therapies, consideration for developing other OA intervention outcomes registries should also be considered.

Specialist and primary care services remain poorly integrated, and new service models should be focusing on these vertical linkages, as well as more effective horizontal linkages to patient groups.

At the clinical interface, it is still not known how best to support people with OA in shared decision making and in implementing and sustaining lifestyle behavior change. Although services have shifted toward a stronger biopsychosocial model, they need to go further, perhaps toward a model in which clinicians play a minor role for those at risk or with mild to moderate OA symptoms, if there are no other clinical comorbidities. As patients access more and more information from the Internet and social networking sites, evidence-based guidelines and decision aids will need to be accessible in appropriate lay formats and patients provided with appropriate guidance about the quality of the information they are accessing.

Many areas in OA management could be improved; however, in our view, in relation to the issues discussed in this article, there are some key priorities for research and advocacy. First, for mild to moderate OA and for those at risk of developing OA or OA progression, there must be a focus on translational research that targets behavior change, to identify service components and service delivery options that cost-effectively support and sustain lifestyle change, particularly for exercise and weight loss. Second, further research is needed to understand ways in which newer technologies and social learning networks can support clinicians and patients in shared decision making about OA therapeutic interventions such that those that are cost-effective and safe are prioritized. Third, there needs to be research and advocacy to improve use of information systems at the clinical practice level, to increase development of OA intervention outcomes registries, and to harness the maximal potential of existing data through data linkage.

REFERENCES

1. World Health Organization (WHO). The global burden of disease 2004 update. Geneva (Switzerland): WHO; 2008.
2. Institute of Medicine. Crossing the quality chasm: a new health system for the 21st century. The national Academy of Sciences; 2000. Available at: http://www.nap.edu/openbook.php?record_id=10027&page=1. Accessed November 11, 2012.
3. Hunter DJ. Quality of osteoarthritis care for community-dwelling older adults. Clin Geriatr Med 2010;26(3):401–17.

4. Hunter DJ, Neogi T, Hochberg MC. Quality of osteoarthritis management and the need for reform in the US. Arthritis Care Res 2011;63(1):31–8.

5. Dieppe P, Doherty M. Contextualizing osteoarthritis care and the reasons for the gap between evidence and practice. Clin Geriatr Med 2010;26(3):419–31.

6. Dieppe P. From protocols to principles, from guidelines to toolboxes: aids to good management of osteoarthritis. Rheumatology (Oxford) 2001;40:841–2.

7. Dieppe P. Osteoarthritis: time to shift the paradigm. BMJ 1999;318(7194): 1299–300.

8. Zhang W, Nuki G, Moskowitz RW, et al. OARSI recommendations for the management of hip and knee osteoarthritis: part III: changes in evidence following systematic cumulative update of research published through January 2009. Osteoarthritis Cartilage 2010;18(4):476–99.

9. Porcheret M, Jordan K, Croft P. Treatment of knee pain in older adults in primary care: development of an evidence-based model of care. Rheumatology 2007; 46(4):638–48.

10. Hochberg MC, Altman RD, April KT, et al. American College of Rheumatology 2012 recommendations for the use of nonpharmacologic and pharmacologic therapies in osteoarthritis of the hand, hip, and knee. Arthritis Care Res 2012; 64(4):455–74.

11. Conaghan PG, Dickson J, Grant RL. Care and management of osteoarthritis in adults: summary of NICE guidance. BMJ 2008;336(7642):502–3.

12. The Royal Australian College of General Practitioners (RACGP). Guideline for the non-surgical management of hip and knee osteoarthritis. South Melbourne (Victoria): RACGP; 2009.

13. Jencks S, Cuerdon T, Burwen D, et al. Quality of medical care delivered to Medi-care beneficiaries: a profile at state and national levels. JAMA 2000;284(13): 1670–6.

14. McGlynn EA, Asch SM, Adams J, et al. The quality of health care delivered to adults in the United States. N Engl J Med 2003;348(26):2635–45.

15. Ganz DA, Chang JT, Roth CP, et al. Quality of osteoarthritis care for community-dwelling older adults. Arthritis Rheum 2006;55(2):241–7.

16. Broadbent J, Maisey S, Holland R, et al. Recorded quality of primary care for osteoarthritis: an observational study. Br J Gen Pract 2008;58(557):839–43.

17. DeHaan M, Guzman J, Bayley M, et al. Knee osteoarthritis clinical practice guidelines – how are we doing? J Rheumatol 2007;34(10):2099–105.

18. Li LC, Maetzel A, Pencharz JN, et al. Use of mainstream nonpharmacologic treatment by patients with arthritis. Arthritis Rheum 2004;51(2):203–9.

19. Li LC, Sayre EC, Kopec JA, et al. Quality of nonpharmacological care in the community for people with knee and hip osteoarthritis. J Rheumatol 2011; 38(10):2230–7.

20. Pencharz JN, MacLean CH. Measuring quality in arthritis care: the Arthritis Foundation's Quality Indicator set for osteoarthritis. Arthritis Rheum 2004; 51(4):538–48.

21. Suarez-Almazor ME. Unraveling gender and ethnic variation in the utilization of elective procedures: the case of total joint replacement. Med Care 2002;40(6): 447–50.

22. Ellis H, Bucholz R. Disparity of care in total hip arthroplasty. Curr Opin Orthop 2007;18:2–7.

23. Ackerman IN, Busija L. Access to self-management education, conservative treatment and surgery for arthritis according to socioeconomic status. Best Prac Res Clin Rheumatol, in press.

24. Hawker G, Guan J, Judge A, et al. Knee arthroscopy in England and Ontario: patterns of use, changes over time, and relationship to total knee replacement. J Bone Joint Surg Am 2008;90(11):2337–45.

25. Kim S, Bosque J, Meehan JP, et al. Increase in outpatient knee arthroscopy in the United States: a comparison of National Surveys of Ambulatory Surgery, 1996 and 2006. J Bone Joint Surg Am 2011;93(11):994–1000.

26. Bohensky MA, Sundararajan V, Andrianopoulos N, et al. Trends in elective knee arthroscopies in a population-based cohort, 2000-2009. Med J Aust 2012; 197(7):399–403.

27. Chodosh J, Solomon DH, Roth CP, et al. The quality of medical care provided to vulnerable older patients with chronic pain. J Am Geriatr Soc 2004;52(5): 756–61.

28. Pitt VJ, O'Connor D, Green S. Referral of people with osteoarthritis to self-management programmes: barriers and enablers identified by general practitioners. Disabil Rehabil 2008;30(25):1938–46.

29. Ackerman IN, Buchbinder R, Osborne RH. Factors limiting participation in arthritis self-management programs: an exploration of barriers and patient preferences within a randomised controlled trial. Rheumatology 2012. [Epub ahead of print].

30. Peter WF, Jansen MJ, Hurkmans EJ, et al. Physiotherapy in hip and knee osteoarthritis: development of a practice guideline concerning initial assessment, treatment and evaluation. Acta Reumatol Port 2011;36(3):268–81.

31. Fransen M, McConnell S. Land-based exercise for osteoarthritis of the knee: a metaanalysis of randomized controlled trials. J Rheumatol 2009;36(6): 1109–17.

32. Mazieres B, Thevenon A, Coudeyre E, et al. Adherence to, and results of, physical therapy programs in patients with hip or knee osteoarthritis. Development of French clinical practice guidelines. Joint Bone Spine 2008;75(5):589–96.

33. Pisters MF, Veenhof C, Schellevis FG, et al. Exercise adherence improving long-term patient outcome in patients with osteoarthritis of the hip and/or knee. Arthritis Care Res 2010;62(8):1087–94.

34. Jordan JL, Holden MA, Mason EE, et al. Interventions to improve adherence to exercise for chronic musculoskeletal pain in adults. Cochrane Database Syst Rev 2010;(1):CD005956.

35. Fransen M, McConnell S. Exercise for osteoarthritis of the knee. Cochrane Database Syst Rev 2008;(4):CD004376.

36. Cottrell E, Roddy E, Foster NE. The attitudes, beliefs and behaviours of GPs regarding exercise for chronic knee pain: a systematic review. BMC Fam Pract 2010;11:4.

37. Chevalier X, Marre JP, de Butler J, et al. Questionnaire survey of management and prescription of general practitioners in knee osteoarthritis: a comparison with 2000 EULAR recommendations. Clin Exp Rheumatol 2004;22(2):205–12.

38. Holden MA, Nicholls EE, Young J, et al. UK-based physical therapists' attitudes and beliefs regarding exercise and knee osteoarthritis: findings from a mixed-methods study. Arthritis Rheum 2009;61(11):1511–21.

39. Zhang W, Moskowitz RW, Nuki G, et al. OARSI recommendations for the management of hip and knee osteoarthritis, Part II: OARSI evidence-based, expert consensus guidelines. Osteoarthritis Cartilage 2008;16(2):137–62.

40. Christensen R, Bartels EM, Astrup A, et al. Effect of weight reduction in obese patients diagnosed with knee osteoarthritis: a systematic review and meta-analysis. Ann Rheum Dis 2007;66(4):433–9.

41. Brosseau L, Wells GA, Tugwell P, et al. Ottawa Panel evidence-based clinical practice guidelines for the management of osteoarthritis in adults who are obese or overweight. Phys Ther 2011;91(6):843–61.
42. Ravaud P, Flipo RM, Boutron I, et al. ARTIST (osteoarthritis intervention standardized) study of standardised consultation versus usual care for patients with osteoarthritis of the knee in primary care in France: pragmatic randomised controlled trial. BMJ 2009;338:b421.
43. Jordan KM, Arden NK, Doherty M, et al. EULAR Recommendations 2003: an evidence based approach to the management of knee osteoarthritis: report of a Task Force of the Standing Committee for International Clinical Studies Including Therapeutic Trials (ESCISIT). Ann Rheum Dis 2003;62(12):1145–55.
44. Chappell AS, Ossanna MJ, Liu-Seifert H, et al. Duloxetine, a centrally acting analgesic, in the treatment of patients with osteoarthritis knee pain: a 13-week, randomized, placebo-controlled trial. Pain 2009;146(3):253–60.
45. Wandel S, Juni P, Tendal B, et al. Effects of glucosamine, chondroitin, or placebo in patients with osteoarthritis of hip or knee: network meta-analysis. BMJ 2010; 341:c4675.
46. Reichenbach S, Sterchi R, Scherer M, et al. Meta-analysis: chondroitin for osteoarthritis of the knee or hip. Ann Intern Med 2007;146(8):580–90.
47. Hochberg MC. Structure-modifying effects of chondroitin sulfate in knee osteoarthritis: an updated meta-analysis of randomized placebo-controlled trials of 2-year duration. Osteoarthritis Cartilage 2010;18(Suppl 1):S28–31.
48. Shekelle PG, Woolf SH, Eccles M, et al. Clinical guidelines: developing guidelines. BMJ 1999;318(7183):593–6.
49. Rutjes AW, Juni P, da Costa BR, et al. Viscosupplementation for osteoarthritis of the knee: a systematic review and meta-analysis. Ann Intern Med 2012;157(3): 180–91.
50. Patrignani P, Tacconelli S, Bruno A, et al. Managing the adverse effects of nonsteroidal anti-inflammatory drugs. Expert Rev Clin Pharmacol 2011;4(5):605–21.
51. Britt H, Miller GC, Charles J, et al. A decade of Australian general practice activity 2001–02 to 2010–11. Sydney (Australia): Sydney University Press; 2011.
52. Hall WD, Farrell MP. Minimising the misuse of oxycodone and other pharmaceutical opioids in Australia. Med J Aust 2011;195(5):248–9.
53. Roxburgh A, Bruno R, Larance B, et al. Prescription of opioid analgesics and related harms in Australia. Med J Aust 2011;195(5):280–4.
54. Harrison CM, Charles J, Henderson J, et al. Opioid prescribing in Australian general practice. Med J Aust 2012;196(6):380–1.
55. Rissanen P, Aro S, Sintonen H, et al. Costs and cost-effectiveness in hip and knee replacements. A prospective study. Int J Technol Assess Health Care 1997;13(4):575–88.
56. Losina E, Walensky RP, Kessler, et al. Cost-effectiveness of total knee arthroplasty in the United States: patient risk and hospital volume. Arch Intern Med 2009;169(12):1113–21 [discussion: 21–2].
57. Ackerman IN, Dieppe PA, March LM, et al. Variation in age and physical status prior to total knee and hip replacement surgery: a comparison of centers in Australia and Europe. Arthritis Rheum 2009;61(2):166–73.
58. Dieppe P, Judge A, Williams S, et al. Variations in the pre-operative status of patients coming to primary hip replacement for osteoarthritis in European orthopaedic centres. BMC Musculoskelet Disord 2009;10:19.
59. Irgit K, Nelson CL. Defining racial and ethnic disparities in THA and TKA. Clin Orthop Relat Res 2011;469(7):1817–23.

60. Novicoff WM, Saleh KJ. Examining sex and gender disparities in total joint arthroplasty. Clin Orthop Relat Res 2011;469(7):1824–8.
61. Hawker GA, Wright JG, Glazier RH, et al. The effect of education and income on need and willingness to undergo total joint arthroplasty. Arthritis Rheum 2002; 46(12):3331–9.
62. Judge A, Welton NJ, Sandhu J, et al. Equity in access to total joint replacement of the hip and knee in England: cross sectional study. BMJ 2010;341:c4092.
63. Rahman MM, Kopec JA, Sayre EC, et al. Effect of sociodemographic factors on surgical consultations and hip or knee replacements among patients with osteoarthritis in British Columbia, Canada. J Rheumatol 2011;38(3):503–9.
64. Steel N, Melzer D, Gardener E, et al. Need for and receipt of hip and knee replacement–a national population survey. Rheumatology 2006;45(11):1437–41.
65. Skinner J, Weinstein JN, Sporer SM, et al. Racial, ethnic, and geographic disparities in rates of knee arthroplasty among Medicare patients. N Engl J Med 2003; 349(14):1350–9.
66. Clement ND, MacDonald D, Howie CR, et al. The outcome of primary total hip and knee arthroplasty in patients aged 80 years or more. J Bone Joint Surg Br 2011;93(9):1265–70.
67. Ackerman IN, Graves SE, Wicks, et al. Severely compromised quality of life in women and those of lower socioeconomic status waiting for joint replacement surgery. Arthritis Rheum 2005;53(5):653–8.
68. Jenkins PJ, Perry PR, Yew Ng C, et al. Deprivation influences the functional outcome from total hip arthroplasty. Surgeon 2009;7(6):351–6.
69. Pollard B, Johnston M, Dieppe P. Exploring the relationships between International Classification of Functioning, Disability and Health (ICF) constructs of Impairment, Activity Limitation and Participation Restriction in people with osteoarthritis prior to joint replacement. BMC Musculoskelet Disord 2011; 12:97.
70. Dieppe P, Lim K, Lohmander S. Who should have knee joint replacement surgery for osteoarthritis? Int J Rheum Dis 2011;14(2):175–80.
71. Critchley RJ, Baker PN, Deehan DJ. Does surgical volume affect outcome after primary and revision knee arthroplasty? A systematic review of the literature. Knee 2012;19(5):513–8.
72. Stacey D, Bennett CL, Barry MJ, et al. Decision aids to help people who are facing health treatment or screening decisions. Cochrane Database Syst Rev 2011;(10):CD001431. http://dx.doi.org/10.1002/14651858.CD001431.pub3.
73. Arterburn D, Wellman R, Westbrook E, et al. Introducing decision AIDS at group health was linked to sharply lower hip and knee surgery rates and costs. Health Aff (Millwood) 2012;31(9):2094–104.
74. Sprague NF 3rd. Arthroscopic debridement for degenerative knee joint disease. Clin Orthop Relat Res 1981;(160):118–23.
75. Ogilvie-Harris DJ, Fitsialos DP. Arthroscopic management of the degenerative knee. Arthroscopy 1991;7(2):151–7.
76. Gross DE, Brenner SL, Esformes I, et al. Arthroscopic treatment of degenerative joint disease of the knee. Orthopedics 1991;14(12):1317–21.
77. Baumgaertner MR, Cannon WD Jr, Vittori, et al. Arthroscopic debridement of the arthritic knee. Clin Orthop Relat Res 1990;(253):197–202.
78. Moseley JB, O'Malley K, Petersen NJ, et al. A controlled trial of arthroscopic surgery for osteoarthritis of the knee. N Engl J Med 2002;347(2):81–8.
79. Chambers K, Schulzer M, Sobolev B. A controlled trial of arthroscopic surgery for osteoarthritis of the knee. Arthroscopy 2002;18(7):683–7.

80. Johnson LL. A controlled trial of arthroscopic surgery for osteoarthritis of the knee. Arthroscopy 2002;18(7):683–7.
81. Kirkley A, Birmingham TB, Litchfield RB, et al. A randomized trial of arthroscopic surgery for osteoarthritis of the knee. N Engl J Med 2008;359(11):1097–107.
82. American Academy of Orthopaedic Surgeons(AAOS). Clinical practice guideline on the treatment of osteoarthritis of the knee (non-arthroplasty). Rosemont (IL): AAOS; 2008.
83. Meakins JL. Evidence-based surgery. Surg Clin North Am 2006;86(1):1–16, vii.
84. Kawamoto K, Houlihan CA, Balas EA, et al. Improving clinical practice using clinical decision support systems: a systematic review of trials to identify features critical to success. BMJ 2005;330(7494):765.
85. Lugtenberg M, Zegers-van Schaick JM, Westert GP, et al. Why don't physicians adhere to guideline recommendations in practice? An analysis of barriers among Dutch general practitioners. Implement Sci 2009;4:54.
86. Grimshaw JM, Russell IT. Effect of clinical guidelines on medical practice: a systematic review of rigorous evaluations. Lancet 1993;342(8883):1317–22.
87. Woolf SH, Grol R, Hutchinson A, et al. Clinical guidelines: potential benefits, limitations, and harms of clinical guidelines. BMJ 1999;318(7182):527–30.
88. Garg AX, Adhikari NK, McDonald H, et al. Effects of computerized clinical decision support systems on practitioner performance and patient outcomes: a systematic review. JAMA 2005;293(10):1223–38.
89. Misso ML, Pitt VJ, Jones KM, et al. Quality and consistency of clinical practice guidelines for diagnosis and management of osteoarthritis of the hip and knee: a descriptive overview of published guidelines. Med J Aust 2008;189(7): 394–9.
90. Shiffman RN, Dixon J, Brandt C, et al. The GuideLine Implementability Appraisal (GLIA): development of an instrument to identify obstacles to guideline implementation. BMC Med Inform Decis Mak 2005;5:23.
91. McGowan BS, Wasko M, Vartabedian BS, et al. Understanding the factors that influence the adoption and meaningful use of social media by physicians to share medical information. J Med Internet Res 2012;14(5):e117.
92. Palmer S, Torgerson DJ. Economic notes: definitions of efficiency. BMJ 1999; 318(7191):1136.
93. Pinto D, Robertson MC, Hansen P, et al. Cost-effectiveness of nonpharmacologic, nonsurgical interventions for hip and/or knee osteoarthritis: systematic review. Value Health 2012;15(1):1–12.
94. Segal L, Day S, Chapman A, et al. Can we reduce disease burden from osteoarthritis? An evidence-based priority-setting model. Med J Aust 2004;180(5): S11–7.
95. Andrews G, Simonella L, Lapsley H, et al. Evidence-based medicine is affordable: the cost-effectiveness of current compared with optimal treatment in rheumatoid and osteoarthritis. J Rheumatol 2006;33(4):671–80.
96. Iezzoni LI. Assessing quality using administrative data. Ann Intern Med 1997; 127(8 Pt 2):666–74.
97. Wagner EH, Bennett SM, Austin BT, et al. Finding common ground: patient-centeredness and evidence-based chronic illness care. J Altern Complement Med 2005;11(Suppl 1):S7–15.
98. Sackett DL, Rosenberg WM, Gray JA, et al. Evidence based medicine: what it is and what it isn't. BMJ 1996;312(7023):71–2.
99. Audet AM, Davis K, Schoenbaum SC. Adoption of patient-centered care practices by physicians: results from a national survey. Arch Intern Med 2006;166(7):754–9.

100. Rosemann T, Laux G, Szecsenyi J, et al. The chronic care model: congruency and predictors among primary care patients with osteoarthritis. Qual Saf Health Care 2008;17(6):442–6.
101. Brand C, Hunter D, Hinman R, et al. Improving care for people with osteoarthritis of the hip and knee: how has national policy for osteoarthritis been translated into service models in Australia? Int J Rheum Dis 2011;14(2):181–90.
102. Brand C, Cox S. Systems for implementing best practice for a chronic disease: management of osteoarthritis of the hip and knee. Intern Med J 2006;36(3):170–9.
103. Tsai AC, Morton SC, Mangione CM, et al. A meta-analysis of interventions to improve care for chronic illnesses. Am J Manag Care 2005;11(8):478–88.
104. Bodenheimer T, Wagner EH, Grumbach K. Improving primary care for patients with chronic illness: the chronic care model, part 2. JAMA 2002;288(15):1909–14.
105. Wagner EH, Austin BT, Von Korff M. Organizing care for patients with chronic illness. Milbank Q 1996;74(4):511–44.
106. Brand CA, Amatya B, Gordon B, et al. Redesigning care for chronic conditions: improving hospital-based ambulatory care for people with osteoarthritis of the hip and knee. Intern Med J 2010;40(6):427–36.
107. Victorian Government Department of Health. Orthopedic waiting list project: summary report. Melbourne (Victoria): Victorian Government Department of Health; 2006.
108. Taggart J, Williams A, Dennis S, et al. A systematic review of interventions in primary care to improve health literacy for chronic disease behavioral risk factors. BMC Fam Pract 2012;13:49.
109. Glasgow RE, Orleans CT, Wagner EH. Does the chronic care model serve also as a template for improving prevention? Milbank Q 2001;79(4):579–612, iv–v.
110. Barr VJ, Robinson S, Marin-Link B, et al. The expanded Chronic Care Model: an integration of concepts and strategies from population health promotion and the Chronic Care Model. Hosp Q 2003;7(1):73–82.
111. Zwar N, Harris M, Griffiths R, et al. A systematic review of chronic disease management. Sydney (Australia): Research Centre for Primary Health Care and Equity, School of Public Health and Community Medicine; 2006.
112. Centers for Disease Control and Prevention (CDC). Sorting through the evidence for the arthritis self-management program and the chronic disease self-management program. Atlanta (GA): Centers for Disease Control and Prevention; 2011.
113. Hill J, Lewis M, Bird H. Do OA patients gain additional benefit from care from a clinical nurse specialist?–a randomized clinical trial. Rheumatology 2009; 48(6):658–64.
114. Victor CR, Triggs E, Ross F, et al. Lack of benefit of a primary care-based nurse-led education programme for people with osteoarthritis of the knee. Clin Rheumatol 2005;24(4):358–64.
115. Wetzels R, van Weel C, Grol R, et al. Family practice nurses supporting self-management in older patients with mild osteoarthritis: a randomized trial. BMC Fam Pract 2008;9:7.
116. Hunt MA, Keefe FJ, Bryant C, et al. A physiotherapist-delivered, combined exercise and pain coping skills training intervention for individuals with knee osteoarthritis: a pilot study. Knee 2012. [Epub ahead of print].
117. Bennell KL, Ahamed Y, Bryant C, et al. A physiotherapist-delivered integrated exercise and pain coping skills training intervention for individuals with knee osteoarthritis: a randomised controlled trial protocol. BMC Musculoskelet Disord 2012;13(1):129.

118. Lau AY, Siek KA, Fernandez-Luque L, et al. The role of social media for patients and consumer health. Contribution of the IMIA consumer health informatics working group. Yearb Med Inform 2011;6(1):131–8.
119. Greaney ML, Sprunck-Harrild K, Bennett GG, et al. Use of email and telephone prompts to increase self-monitoring in a Web-based intervention: randomized controlled trial. J Med Internet Res 2012;14(4):e96.

Update on the Role of Muscle in the Genesis and Management of Knee Osteoarthritis

Kim L. Bennell, BAppSci(physio), PhD[a],*, Tim V. Wrigley, BSc, MSc[a],
Michael A. Hunt, PT, PhD[b], Boon-Whatt Lim, MSc, PhD[c],
Rana S. Hinman, BPhysio, PhD[a]

KEYWORDS

- Muscle • Knee • Osteoarthritis • Proprioception • Strength • Rehabilitation
- Exercise

KEY POINTS

- Deficits in muscle function, including muscle strength, activation, and proprioception, are found in people with knee osteoarthritis.
- Stronger quadriceps muscle may reduce the risk of knee osteoarthritis onset but the role of muscle strength in influencing disease progression is conflicting.
- Exercise can improve deficits in muscle function.
- Improvement in muscle function, especially strength, is associated with reduced pain and improved function in people with knee osteoarthritis.

INTRODUCTION

The muscles of the lower limb, particularly the quadriceps, play an important role in the genesis and management of knee osteoarthritis (OA). At the knee, muscles function to produce movement but also to absorb limb loading and provide dynamic joint stability. Muscle weakness has been identified as a potential risk factor for disease development due to increased joint loading. In addition, the presence of OA has a negative impact on the integrity of the structure and function of muscles, potentially further affecting the disease process.

Research has provided a rationale for the use of muscle rehabilitation as part of the overall treatment regimen for knee OA to reduce symptoms, increase function, and possibly protect against disease onset or progression. A detailed understanding of

[a] Department of Physiotherapy, Centre for Health, Exercise and Sports Medicine, Faculty of Medicine, Dentistry and Health Sciences, The University of Melbourne, 200 Berkeley Street, Parkville, Victoria 3010, Australia; [b] Department of Physical Therapy, University of British Columbia, Vancouver, Canada; [c] School of Sports, Health and Leisure, Republic Polytechnic, Singapore
* Corresponding author.
E-mail address: k.bennell@unimelb.edu.au

Rheum Dis Clin N Am 39 (2013) 145–176
http://dx.doi.org/10.1016/j.rdc.2012.11.003
0889-857X/13/$ – see front matter Crown Copyright © 2013 Published by Elsevier Inc. All rights reserved.

the role of muscles in knee OA can, therefore, aid in the implementation of effective rehabilitation strategies and form the basis of primary prevention strategies against disease development.

This review, updated from 1 published in 2008,[1] outlines the influence of muscle activity on knee joint loading, describes the deficits in muscle function observed in people with knee OA, and summarizes available evidence pertaining to the role of muscle in the development and progression of knee OA. The review also focuses on whether muscle deficits can be modified in knee OA and whether improvements in muscle function lead to improved symptoms and joint structure. The review concludes with a discussion of exercise prescription for muscle rehabilitation in knee OA.

INFLUENCE OF MUSCLE ACTIVITY ON KNEE JOINT LOADING

Because knee OA is believed to be due to joint loading acting within the context of systemic and local susceptibility, it is important to understand the influence of muscle activity on knee joint load. To achieve equilibrium of motion and joint stability, all external forces acting on a joint must be counteracted by internal forces equal in magnitude, but opposite in direction. External knee joint loading experienced during human movement is primarily derived from the ground reaction forces and inertial properties of the lower limb, resulting in a total tibiofemoral joint force approaching 3 times body weight.[2,3] The individual contributions of internal structures such as muscles, ligaments, subchondral bone, and cartilage varies, and is highly influenced by the anatomic arrangement of each structure and their capacity to absorb load.

Of particular interest to the pathogenesis of knee OA is the ability to counteract the external adduction moment applied about the knee as this moment is suggested to influence disease initiation,[4] disease severity,[5] and disease progression.[6,7] Part of the reason why so much work has been done with this measure is that it is easy to obtain via three-dimensional gait analysis. Measures that may better reflect true medial compartment load are under development but have yet to be related to OA disease in the same way as the external adduction moment has been. There may be circumstances in which other moments (such as the sagittal flexor-extensor moment) need to be take into account as well,[8] but the extent to which this might be routinely important is somewhat unclear.

The external adduction moment, present throughout much of the stance phase of gait, results from the ground reaction force passing medial to the knee joint center of rotation.[9] It affects the load distribution between the medial and lateral tibiofemoral joint compartments and it has been used as a proxy for medial tibiofemoral joint load,[10,11] where most knee OA occurs. The external adduction moment not only compresses the tibiofemoral joint medially but distracts the joint laterally.[11] Thus, contributions from lateral and medial structures are required to maintain joint stability internally. Dynamic stability of the knee depends on the load-sharing characteristics of many passive soft tissues and active muscle forces.[11] Although in vivo data quantifying the relative contributions of knee joint structures in generating internal forces do not exist, many biomechanical modeling studies provide estimations of these forces.

Schipplein and Andriacchi[11] were among the first to evaluate passive soft tissue and active muscle contributions to dynamic knee stability during walking. They found that activation of the quadriceps muscles in isolation was insufficient to balance the external adduction moment and that cocontraction from the hamstrings and/or tension in lateral soft tissues was required to produce an internal abduction moment to maintain dynamic equilibrium in the frontal plane. This requirement for active muscle contributions to internal abduction moment generation has been supported by subsequent studies examining isometric loading.[12,13] Buchanan and Lloyd[13] reported individual activation patterns of many lower-limb muscles during static loads in the frontal plane. Muscles active during the production of internal abduction forces included sartorius, gracilis, quadriceps (primarily rectus femoris), long head of biceps femoris, and lateral gastrocnemius. Shelburne and colleagues[2] showed in a biomechanical modeling study that, although these muscles are capable of producing internal abduction moments isometrically, much of the contribution to the total abduction moment during normal gait came from the quadriceps (early stance) and gastrocnemius (late stance). These muscles were able to generate a sufficient internal abduction moment to counteract the external adduction moment, despite small frontal plane muscle moment arms. Recent work in healthy young individuals has suggested that muscles that do not span the knee can also contribute to compressive tibiofemoral joint forces along with those muscles that do span the joint (**Fig. 1**).[14] This general principle has been known for some time but has yet to be studied specifically in knees with OA.

These findings indicate that for a given external load, muscles are capable of generating enough force to produce most of the internal balancing load. However, there is still a requirement of other soft tissue structures such as ligaments to sustain load. Muscle force generation is of particular interest to clinicians given that it can be consciously controlled by the individual and improved with training. Improving the load-bearing capacities of lower-limb muscles through strength training and muscle rehabilitation programs may protect against soft tissue damage resulting from excessive load.

It is unclear, however, if the increase in the total joint reaction force occurring with muscle contraction may actually accelerate the degeneration of articular cartilage, rather than prevent it. Although muscle activity, particularly cocontraction of the quadriceps and hamstrings, may balance the external adduction moment and improve the dynamic stability of the knee joint during walking by limiting lateral condylar liftoff and shearing in the transverse plane, axial compression due to the muscles' line of pull

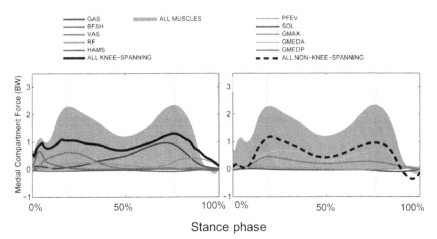

Fig. 1. Contributions of selected knee-spanning and non–knee-spanning muscles to the medial knee compartment force (compressive forces are positive). The first vertical gray line represents contralateral toe off and the second gray line represent contralateral heel strike. BFSH, biceps femoris; GAS, gastrocnemius; GEMEDA, anterior portion of gluteus medius; GMAX, gluteus maximus; GMEDP, posterior portion of gluteus medius; HAMS, medial hamstrings; PFEV, plantar flexor evertor; RF, rectus femoris; SOL, soleus; VAS, vastii. (*From* Sritharan P, Lin YC, Pandy MG. Muscles that do not cross the knee contribute to the knee adduction moment and tibiofemoral compartment loading during gait. J Orthop Res 2012;30(10):1586–95; with permission.)

may place the cartilage in an environment of excessive and prolonged load. Alterations in muscle activation in association with OA are discussed in the following section but it is apparent that further research into the effects of muscle cocontraction on the health of articular cartilage in the tibiofemoral joint is needed.

Muscle activation patterns influence not only the overall magnitude of the knee joint load but also the rate of loading. Coordinated timing of appropriate muscles during the weight-acceptance phase of gait ensures proper attenuation of axial compressive or impact loads suggested to be associated with the onset of knee OA.[15,16] Specifically, it is thought that adequate eccentric loading of the quadriceps during this phase of the gait cycle allows for a safe and controlled descent of the center of mass and protection against high impact loads. Mikesky and colleagues[17] reported a significant increase in the rate of loading during gait in a group of sedentary women compared with those who actively participated in strength training. However, faster walking speed seems to be more important in the generation of higher impact forces in OA than quadriceps muscle strength.[18] Consistent with what is known about the deleterious effects of high impact loading on cartilage degeneration from animal studies[19] and previous reports of the association between rate of loading and presence of knee pain,[20] it has been suggested that impact forces and loading rate may contribute to the development and/or progression of knee OA. However, no longitudinal studies have investigated this, and cross-sectional studies so far have not found a difference in impact forces between patients with OA and healthy controls.[21]

The hip muscles responsible for stabilizing the pelvis on the weight-bearing lower limbs during walking may also play a role in knee OA by altering knee loads. People with insufficient stance limb hip abductor strength to control the pelvis can exhibit a contralateral pelvic drop, the Trendelenburg sign.[22] This drop theoretically shifts the body's center of mass away from the stance limb toward the swing limb, thereby increasing the distance between the ground reaction force vector and the knee joint center of rotation, and hence increasing the knee adduction moment. It also increases the external hip adduction moment which, given such a patient's weak hip abductors, is not sustainable. Therefore, patients often adopt compensatory trunk lean back to the affected side, reducing the load on both the knee and the hip muscles.

Lower hip adduction moments consistent with these patterns have been found in studies using gait analysis in patients with more severe and progressive knee OA,[23,24] as has increased trunk lean to the affected side.[25,26] The hip adductor muscles may also assist in resisting the knee adduction moment particularly in a varus malaligned knee. By virtue of their attachment to the distal medial femoral condyle, the adductors theoretically could eccentrically restrain the tendency of the femur to move into further varus during the stance phase of gait.[27]

DEFICITS IN MUSCLE FUNCTION IN KNEE OA

Given the role of muscles in influencing knee joint load and knee stability, an understanding of deficits in muscle function associated with knee OA is important. Most studies of muscle function in knee OA have concerned muscle strength. However, other aspects of muscle function are also affected by the OA disease process, including activation patterns and proprioceptive acuity. Understanding how muscle function is impaired can assist clinicians in prescribing more effective rehabilitation programs.

Strength

Muscle weakness is a well-accepted impairment in knee OA (see Bennell and colleagues[28] for an in-depth review). However, assessment of strength is not straightforward and has not always been well conducted in OA studies. Clinical methods may not be as sophisticated as research methods, but should follow similar principles. The ability to generate muscle force is a function of muscle cross-sectional area and the ability to recruit and fire descending alpha motor neurons to muscle fibers at sufficient frequencies.[29,30] That force then acts in conjunction with the muscle's moment arm to generate a torque or moment about a particular joint.[29,30]

Ideally, strength should be measured to reflect this muscle-generated torque. Torque is thus measured as the product of the force (in Newtons) exerted at the point of attachment of a force-measuring transducer to the limb, and the distance (in meters) of that attachment from the axis of rotation of the joint in question; thus strength is reported in units of Newton meters (N m). Strength varies with body size (which affects muscle size and the moment arm length), in patients with OA as in athletes.[31,32] In some studies on OA, the investigators have failed to normalize the torque measurements for differences in body size (most logically body mass in kilograms).

Results of studies that have correctly measured strength as torque, and normalized for body mass differences (ie, N m/kg) show that patients with knee OA are 20% to 40% weaker in relative quadriceps strength than healthy controls.[33–39] Although other lower-limb muscles in knee OA have received less attention, strength of the hip muscles also seems to be reduced with 1 study reporting strength deficits ranging from 16% (hip extensors) to 27% (hip external rotators) compared with controls.[40]

There are several contributors to muscle weakness in individuals with knee OA. Pain, anxiety, motivation, effusion, muscle atrophy, and aberrant joint mechanics can all contribute to a loss of measurable strength. Some of the weakness in relation to body size seen in OA is likely caused by the obesity that is also commonly present, as the proportion of total body mass made up of force-generating muscle is by definition reduced. Primary deficits in muscle strength may be associated with muscle fiber atrophy (ie, loss of muscle cross-sectional area), reduced ability to activate muscle fibers, or both.

There are few studies investigating muscle atrophy in OA. Ikeda and colleagues[41] found that quadriceps cross-sectional area was significantly reduced by an average of 12% in women with incident radiological OA without symptoms, compared with women matched for age and body mass with no signs of OA. In later stage disease, more obvious signs of actual muscle fiber atrophy have been reported.[42,43] In patients before knee replacement, Pettersen and colleagues[44] found quadriceps lean muscle cross-sectional area to be 12% lower in the affected limb compared with the contralateral lateral side. Thus, it seems likely that at least some of any strength loss in OA is caused by loss of muscle cross-sectional area.

When muscle atrophy cannot explain the full extent of muscle weakness, inhibition in the ability to activate muscle is implicated. Detection of inhibition is primarily a research tool, whereby an electrical stimulus over the muscle is applied during a maximal contraction to determine whether the patient's voluntary activation is less than maximal. Overall, there is a large variation in the results of studies assessing the extent of maximal voluntary muscle activation typically possible in OA. For example, 1 study[45] found that patients before high tibial osteotomy had an average quadriceps activation of 71% (ie, 29% inhibited), with a range of 41% to 86%. Pettersen and colleagues[44] found that inhibition explained most of the strength variance in end-stage knee OA. Despite some variation in research findings, the literature overall does show that patients with OA commonly exhibit impaired activation compared with healthy controls, as was the conclusion of a recent meta-analysis of published studies.[46] This analysis also concluded that there was some evidence for activation deficits in the unaffected opposite limb.

The causes of muscle inhibition in knee OA are likely to be multifactorial. Pain is commonly presumed to be a major source of inhibition in the ability to voluntarily activate muscle surrounding arthritic joints.[47] Pain relief via local anesthetic injection resulted in an 11% to 12% increase in percentage activation of the quadriceps in people with knee OA,[48] confirming that at least some of the reduced voluntary activation observed in knee OA is caused by the presence of pain inhibition. Joint effusion on its own has also been found to be a potent inhibitor of maximal muscle activation in non-OA studies, even at low levels that might otherwise not be deemed clinically important (see Wrigley[49] for review of classic work in this area). Effusion is often associated with OA and associated pain.[50] Experimentally induced knee joint effusion has previously been found to generate pathologic gait changes.[51] Recently, Rutherford and colleagues[52] found that 17 medial patients with OA who presented with clinical knee joint effusions (bulge test) actually showed increased quadriceps activation and hamstring duration during gait compared with 18 patients without effusion. The patients also demonstrated greater stance flexion and a reduced external knee extensor moment. There were no differences in walking speed or pain between the groups. This supports the notion that effusions should be addressed in patients with OA, as they may be a barrier to rehabilitation and function.

Knowledge of the sources of muscle weakness in a patient is important, as it will determine how restoration of muscle strength might be approached therapeutically. If the deficit is primarily due to atrophy, then a pure muscle-strengthening approach should be taken. Alternatively, if the deficit is primarily in the ability to activate an essentially normal muscle, then attention might be directed toward removing the inhibitory sources that prevent sufficient activation (such as pain and effusion), and retraining the patient to activate their muscles fully.

Muscle Activation Patterns

In recent years, there has been increasing interest in the patterns of muscle activation associated with knee OA. As muscles are often the major contributors to joint loading,[53] their inefficient activation during walking and other functional tasks could be implicated in disease progression. It seems that some patients with OA are able to activate their knee muscles in a way that is most efficient for dealing with the commonly increased joint loading, especially of the medial compartment during gait, while satisfying the other requirements for weight support and propulsion. However, other patients adopt a less efficient strategy that involves activating many muscles in a less specific fashion that may increase overall joint loading.

Several cross-sectional studies have noted differences in muscle activation patterns comparing people with knee OA of varying disease severity to age-matched controls.[54–61] Using surface electromyography (EMG), Hubley-Kozey and colleagues[56] found that patients with moderate OA biased the activation of quadriceps and hamstrings toward the lateral components of these muscle groups in early stance, compared with healthy controls. Schmitt and Rudolph[57] found that patients with mild to severe medial tibiofemoral joint OA showed increased activation of lateral hamstrings and gastrocnemius before foot contact and increased cocontraction of the lateral quadriceps and gastrocnemius as well as medial quadriceps and hamstrings during weight acceptance.

Astephen and colleagues[58] found that patients with severe tibiofemoral OA could be distinguished from healthy controls by increased medial and lateral hamstring activity during stance; they were also different from those with moderate OA in terms of higher medial gastrocnemius activity in swing and early stance phases, but lower activity during late stance. In patients with a range of OA severity, Childs and colleagues[59] found that muscles were activated for longer durations in the period just before and during stance compared with healthy age-matched and gender-matched controls. Heiden and colleagues[60] found that cocontraction biased more toward lateral knee muscles increased with higher external knee adduction moments; this suggests that this pattern of muscle activation is directly linked to resisting associated increases in medial compartment loading. Thus, it seems that, as the disease progresses, a less specific and efficient activation of a greater number of knee muscles may become more apparent.

All the alterations in activation patterns in knee OA described in the literature are not necessarily consistent, and part of the variability may relate to methodological issues particularly in EMG measurement and analysis.[28] Nevertheless, it seems that muscle activation patterns do differ in people with knee OA and may be influenced by the stage of OA disease and aspects of the disease process. For example, a recent study found that, in people with knee OA, those with a joint effusion had greater overall quadriceps activation and prolonged hamstring activation during midstance compared with those without a joint effusion.[52] Whether these differences reflect the increasing difficulty in activating muscles efficiently for ambulation in the face of pain, effusion, and deteriorating joint mechanics, and/or are involved in disease progression itself, needs to be clarified. There is also little evidence that such patterns can be altered; nor is it clear what would constitute a desirable alteration.

Proprioception

Knee joint proprioception is important for the coordinated activity of surrounding muscles to protect against excessive movements, stabilize during static postures, and coordinate movement.[62] Proprioceptive afferent information from mechanoreceptors, particularly in muscles but also in ligaments, capsule, menisci, and skin, contributes at the spinal level to arthrokinetic and muscular reflexes, which play a large part in dynamic joint stability.[63] The information is also conveyed to supraspinal centers where it is integral to motor learning and the ongoing programming of complex movements. Abnormal proprioception could predispose to musculoskeletal lesions by altering the control of movement leading to abnormal stresses on tissues.[64] Alternatively, a pathologic condition, effusion, and pain may impair proprioceptive information,[65–67] possibly further compounding functional deficits.

Proprioception is typically measured in OA studies as conscious perception of joint position sense using accuracy of reproduction or threshold of movement detection tests. However, proprioception during normal function rarely requires conscious perception. Furthermore, just because a patient perceives proprioceptive information (consciously or unconsciously) does not mean that it is efficiently used by the nervous system to modulate movement.[28] Measurements of knee position sense and knee motion sense are not well correlated and as such seem to indicate different aspects of knee proprioception and probably stimulate different receptors.[62]

Most studies have found deficits in knee joint proprioception in patients with knee OA compared with similarly aged asymptomatic individuals.[68–72] A recent study also showed consistent differences in knee proprioception between groups with and without knee OA across all knee movement directions (varus, valgus, flexion, and extension) suggesting a global, rather than a direction-specific, reduction in sensation in patients with knee OA.[73] In addition to impaired proprioception at the affected knee joint, there is also evidence of proprioceptive deficits at other nonaffected sites including the contralateral knee[74] and the elbow.[75] This has led to suggestions that OA may be associated with a generalized defect in proprioception. The topic of proprioception in knee OA has recently been reviewed by Knoop and colleagues.[62]

EVIDENCE FOR A RELATIONSHIP BETWEEN MUSCLE FUNCTION AND OA ONSET AND PROGRESSION

As previously described, muscles influence knee joint loading, and impairments in muscle function have been observed in people with knee OA. This section (summary in **Table 1**) discusses the longitudinal cohort studies and randomized controlled trials (RCTs) that link impaired muscle function to the development and progression of knee OA. These studies have focused primarily on muscle strength with a limited number investigating proprioception. The RCTs that investigate the effects of strengthening exercise (as distinct from strength per se) on structural outcomes are discussed in a following section.

Disease Onset

There is some evidence to suggest that quadriceps weakness precedes the onset of knee OA and hence could increase the risk of disease development, particularly in women. The first longitudinal study to investigate this issue more than a decade ago demonstrated 15% to 18% lower baseline isokinetic quadriceps strength (adjusted for body and muscle mass) in women who went on to develop incident radiographic knee OA than in women who did not develop OA.[76] This was not seen in men nor was there a relationship between hamstring strength and OA onset in either sex. Although the study had some methodological issues, including lack of adjusting for potential covariates, these results were subsequently confirmed in a larger longitudinal cohort study involving 3081 adults.[77] In this study, higher isokinetic quadriceps strength (relative to body mass) was associated with a 55% to 64% reduced risk of developing knee or hip OA (self-reported) in women with similar, albeit nonsignificant, results in men (~25% less risk). Support for a link between quadriceps strength and disease onset also comes from a study on a group of 94 people aged 35 to 54 years with chronic knee pain but normal radiographs at baseline, in which the maximal number of one-legged rises, a functional measure that can indicate quadriceps strength, predicted radiographic knee OA 5 years later.[78]

More recent data from the large Multicenter Osteoarthritis Study (MOST) published in several papers have provided further insights into the relationship between muscle strength and OA development.[79–82] In 1 study, absolute isokinetic knee extensor and flexor strength was adjusted for age, body mass index, hip bone density, surgical history, pain, and physical activity score in multivariate models, and related to the onset of symptomatic and radiographic OA 30 months later.[80] Compared with the

---

Table 1
Summary of findings of the relationship between muscle function and knee OA onset and progression

Disease Onset	Disease Progression
Quadriceps muscle weakness may increase risk of symptomatic knee OA particularly in women	Conflicting evidence but higher strength may be related to slower progression in women and at the patellofemoral joint
Hamstring muscle weakness does not seem to be related	Strengthening exercise for the quadriceps and hip muscles does not alter knee adduction moment
Knee joint proprioception does not seem to be related to either radiographic or symptomatic onset	Weaker quadriceps, hamstrings, and hip abductor muscles as well as poorer knee joint proprioception are related to greater functional decline

lowest tertile, the highest tertile of adjusted isokinetic knee extensor strength pro-tected against development of incident symptomatic tibiofemoral or patellofemoral OA in both sexes. However, neither adjusted knee extensor strength nor the hamstring to quadriceps ratio was predictive of incident radiographic tibiofemoral OA. This suggests that, in this cohort at least, quadriceps muscle weakness may play a greater role in OA symptom development than structural changes per se. These results were confirmed using knee extensor specific strength (knee extensor torque divided by total thigh muscle mass).[82] This study also found that absolute total thigh muscle mass, as measured by dual energy x-ray absorptiometry, was not related to OA incidence.[82] This might be interpreted as implicating other sources of weakness than reduced contractile material (such as the inhibition discussed earlier). However, it would be interesting to further explore adjustment for the expected effects of body size on a volumetric quantity such as absolute muscle mass.

People who have sustained a knee joint injury, particularly a tear of the anterior cruciate ligament (ACL) or meniscus, are at an increased risk of developing knee OA compared with those with uninjured knees.[83,84] Whether subsequent muscle weakness further predisposes these individuals to developing knee OA has only been investigated in 1 longitudinal study to date.[85] In this study, concentric quadriceps muscle function measured using isokinetic dynamometry (60°/s, 5-repetition total work divided by body mass) at 6, 12, and 24 months following patellar tendon ACL reconstruction was not associated with the development of radiographic or symptom-atic radiographic knee OA 10 to 15 years later. Further research is needed to deter-mine the role of muscle function in influencing knee joint health in this patient population.

The link between knee proprioception and OA disease onset has been investigated in 2 recent large longitudinal studies using data from MOST.[81,86] Active knee joint position sense measured without weight bearing at baseline was not significantly associated with incident radiographic or symptomatic knee OA[81] or with the new onset of frequent knee pain[86] over a 30-month follow-up. Although it was hypothe-sized that sensorimotor factors may interact to mediate OA risk, the combination of high absolute isokinetic knee extensor strength and better knee joint position sense did not protect against development of knee OA.[81] These findings suggest that propri-oception, at least as assessed by knee joint position sense, does not predict the onset of either radiographic or symptomatic knee OA.

Disease Progression

Although it seems that quadriceps muscle strength is related to OA disease onset, the longitudinal evidence to suggest that stronger muscles can protect against OA progression in those with established disease is conflicting. Most studies used isoki-netic dynamometry to assess concentric quadriceps strength (albeit at various speeds) and different methods and grading systems to assess disease progression.

The earliest study, published in 1999, found that the mean absolute quadriceps strength of women with progressive OA (defined as worsening of the Kellgren and Lawrence grade over 2.5 years) was about 9% lower than those with radiographically stable OA.[87] However, this strength difference between the groups was not statisti-cally significant, which could be due to the small number of participants (17 out of 82) exhibiting radiographic progression. Strength relative to body mass did not differ between progressors and nonprogressors. The use of nonstandardized conventional radiographs for evaluating progression could also reduce the potential of this study to detect structural progression. Nevertheless, in support of this nonsignificant finding, a larger more recent study involving 265 individuals and using the supposedly more sensitive technique of magnetic resonance imaging (MRI) to assess tibiofemoral carti-lage loss over 30 months also failed to find an effect of relative isokinetic quadriceps strength on disease progression.[88] Conversely, a study using data from MOST showed that women in the lowest tertile of relative isokinetic quadriceps strength (normalized for height and weight) had an increased risk of tibiofemoral joint space narrowing over 30 months (odds ratio 1.69, 95% confidence interval 1.26, 2.28) compared with women in the highest strength tertile.[89] These results suggest that in women, but not men, quadriceps weakness may be a risk factor for structural deteri-oration in those who already have knee OA. A differential gender result also concurs with previous findings for incident symptomatic knee OA in MOST. Segal and Glass[90] postulated that this gender difference may relate to the strength capacity of women being closer to a threshold for risk, whereas greater absolute strength in men provides greater reserve such that a loss of strength is insufficient to lead to greater risk of progression.

Muscle strength may have differential effects depending on the joint involved. Greater isokinetic quadriceps strength (60°/s) relative to body mass has been found to protect against cartilage degeneration in the lateral aspect of the patellofemoral joint.[88] The findings were supported by another study showing a similar trend in women but not men, although that study used absolute isokinetic strength (60°/s) not strength relative to body size (eg, body mass).[89] Quadriceps weakness could alter patellar tracking and walking biomechanics, which could lead to disproportionate compressive forces across the patellofemoral joint.

It has been proposed that the local mechanical environment may also influence the relationship between strength and disease progression. A study by Sharma and colleagues[91] found that greater absolute quadriceps peak torque (at 120°/s) at base-line increased the risk of tibiofemoral joint disease progression in individuals with malaligned knees (defined as >5° deviation from the mechanical axis) or high-laxity knees (defined as >6.75° varus valgus deviation), but not in those who had neutral alignment or low-laxity knees. The investigators suggested that the inability of mala-ligned knees to evenly distribute muscle forces could result in focal stress, and the increase in muscle contraction to stabilize lax knees could lead to higher joint reaction forces. The inferred clinical implication of these results, espoused in an editorial that accompanied this study, was that quadriceps strengthening, the cornerstone of exer-cise therapy in OA, might actually be detrimental in those people with knee OA and malalignment or laxity.[92] However, a more recent study in 265 elderly individuals[88] has not supported the results of Sharma and colleagues.[91] In this study, there was no relationship between the relative isokinetic quadriceps strength (60°/s) at baseline and loss of medial tibiofemoral joint cartilage using MRI in those with or without knee malalignment.[88] As longitudinal studies assess relationships and cannot directly assess causality, clinical trials are needed to definitively investigate the effects of strengthening exercise on structural outcomes at different joint compartments, in different sexes, and in the presence of different mechanical factors.

Although the quadriceps muscle has been the major focus, there has also been interest in the role of the hip abductors. It has been suggested that stronger hip abduc-tors may be associated with a reduced risk of knee OA progression in the ipsilateral knee. In an 18-month study of 57 patients with mild to moderate unilateral knee OA, every additional unit of normalized internal hip abductor moment during gait was asso-ciated with a 43% reduction in the risk of ipsilateral medial knee OA progression.[23] Although hip abductor strength was not measured, the investigators suggested that the internal hip abduction moment might be primarily related to abductor muscle strength. Mundermann and colleagues[24] reported higher peak internal hip abduction moments during gait in individuals with mild to moderate knee OA compared with those with severe OA, further suggesting a protective effect of hip abduction strength against knee OA progression.

Some studies have used the external knee adduction moment during gait to examine the indirect effects of muscle strengthening on OA disease progression,[93–98] by virtue of the moment's association with both medial compartment loading[10,99] and structural disease progression.[6,7] Of the 6 studies, only 2 found an effect of exercise in reducing the knee adduction moment; both were uncontrolled pilot studies.[97,98] In 1 study, an 8-week, supervised, lower-limb strength and neuromuscular control exercises program including functional strengthening was evaluated in 13 patients with early knee OA.[98] The investigators found that the peak knee adduction moment during gait was not significantly altered at completion of the exercise program but there was a 14% reduction in the adduction moment measured during a one-leg rise. However, the clinical relevance of small changes in loading only during a one-leg rise task is unknown. The other study of 6 patients found that a 4-week strengthening program involving the hip and other lower-limb muscles led to an average 9% reduction in the peak knee adduction moment during walking even though strength gains were not found.[97]

In contrast to these pilot studies, several larger RCTs[93–96,98] and an uncontrolled study of 40 people[96] have failed to find changes in the knee adduction moment with strengthening programs targeting the quadriceps and hip muscles, despite strength gains and symptomatic improvements. In 1 study, 107 participants were stratified according to knee malalignment (more varus or more neutral) and randomized into either a 12-week, supervised, home-based, quadriceps strengthening group or a control group with no intervention. Quadriceps strengthening did not significantly alter the adduction moment in people with more malaligned or more neutral knees.[94] In another recent RCT, a 12-week hip muscle-strengthening program did not affect the knee adduction moment in 89 people with medial knee OA.[93] These results were further confirmed by a study involving 54 women randomized into a 6-month high-intensity progressive resistance training program or sham exercise.[95] In summary, the evidence currently suggests that muscle-strengthening exercise does not alter the knee adduction moment in people with knee OA.

Limited longitudinal data do not support a link between proprioception and progression of knee OA in those with established disease.[86] From MOST, active joint position sense was not associated with radiographic worsening over 30 months in 2440 people with mild disease.[86] It is not known whether proprioceptive deficits become more important risk factors in later stage disease when greater impairments in the sensorimotor system are found.

Although the role of muscle function on structural disease development and progression has received most of the attention in the literature, its effects on functional progression are less well known. Sharma and colleagues[100] conducted a 3-year longitudinal cohort study investigating factors contributing to poor physical functioning in 257 patients with knee OA. They found that in addition to factors such as age, reduced absolute quadriceps and hamstrings strength and poor proprioceptive acuity (measured as joint position sense) increased the likelihood of poor physical functioning as measured by the time to perform 5 repetitions of rising and sitting in a chair. Similarly, in a cohort of more than 2000 individuals, those with worse proprioceptive acuity (measured as active non–weight-bearing joint position sense) at baseline had slightly greater worsening of WOMAC (Western Ontario and McMaster Universities) pain scores (0.47 on a 20-point scale) and physical function scores (by 1.5 points on a 0- to 68-point scale) compared with those with the best proprioceptive acuity (for pain $P = .05$; for physical function $P = .02$) over 30 months.[86] Lastly, a longitudinal cohort study found that reductions in hip abductor strength were related to poorer functional outcomes more than 3 years in people with knee OA.[101] Taken together, these findings suggest that impaired muscle function is related to greater pain and declines in physical in those with knee OA.

CAN MUSCLE DEFICITS BE MODIFIED IN KNEE OA?

Given that numerous deficits in muscle function are associated with knee OA, it is important for health professionals to understand which deficits may be amenable to change with intervention (**Table 2**). An appreciation of which treatment strategies are most effective at improving muscle function will allow clinicians to tailor treatment to the nature of the presenting muscle deficit for each individual with knee OA.

Muscle Strength

Extensive research indicates that muscle strength can be improved with an appropriately targeted strengthening program.[102] A large systematic review assessed the effectiveness of isolated resistance training in people with knee OA.[103] Fourteen RCTs were identified that measured parameters of muscle strength and compared the effects of isolated resistance training to a non-exercising control group. In general, muscle strength improved significantly with resistance training (mean improvement of 17.4%, range 10.5% decrease to 49.5% increase), with 9 out of 14 studies reporting significant strength gains. Relative effect sizes for strength outcomes ranged from -0.04 to 1.52, with an average of 0.38, indicating small to moderate effects of resistance training in this patient group. Whereas/although the most research has targeted strength training to the quadriceps muscle, strength gains have also been observed with targeted training for the hamstrings and hip musculature.[93,104–107] Strength gains are apparent with both supervised clinic-based programs and home exercise regimes,[103,108–110] although it is presently not clear which mode of delivery is superior for achieving strength gains as this has not been directly evaluated. The magnitude of strength gain achieved with resistance training varies according to the intensity of training (resistance applied as well as frequency), patient adherence and the specificity of training, which probably explains the variation in strength change observed

Table 2
Summary of interventions that have been investigated in the literature and may potentially affect deficits in muscle function

Muscle Deficit	Interventions
Weakness	Strengthening exercise EMG biofeedback
Atrophy	Strengthening exercise
Muscle inhibition	Exercise generally including quadriceps strengthening Transcutaneous electrical nerve stimulation Cryotherapy
Altered activation patterns	Unloading knee brace Stochastic resonance electrical stimulation with knee sleeve
Proprioceptive deficits	Proprioceptive exercise Whole-body vibration Knee bandaging Knee bracing

in the systematic review by Lange and colleagues.[103,108–110] More research is needed to establish dose-response relationships with respect to resistance training for people with knee OA.

There has been interest in whether modalities such as EMG biofeedback or whole-body vibration platforms can assist in augmenting strength gains achieved with exercise in people with knee OA. A recent systematic review to determine the magnitude of the treatment effect for EMG biofeedback on quadriceps strength compared with that of placebo and traditional exercise interventions in both healthy and pathologic populations found the strongest effect in knee OA populations.[111] However, more definitive evidence is needed to confirm the benefits. With regards to vibration, there is limited research in knee OA with conflicting results. Segal and colleagues[112] recently found that in women with risk factors for knee OA, the addition of vibration to a twice-weekly lower-limb exercise program did not result in significantly greater improvements in lower-limb strength or power than did performance of the exercise program without vibration. In another small RCT, knee muscle strength gains were significantly increased compared with control.[113] A recent systematic review on whole-body vibration programs in older populations in general concluded that the effects do not seem to be greater than those achieved with conventional exercise alone.[114]

Muscle Atrophy and Activation

Increases in muscle strength with resistance training are probably only partly explained by muscle hypertrophy, and research is required to investigate the relative contributions of neural adaptation and muscle hypertrophy to the strength increases observed.

One study evaluated the effects of isokinetic training on the cross-sectional area of the quadriceps and hamstrings in people with bilateral knee OA.[115] Significant within-group increases in cross-sectional area were observed for both muscle groups with both a concentric and a combined concentric-eccentric training program.

Some studies have demonstrated improvements in voluntary activation of the quadriceps following an exercise regime, usually including quadriceps strengthening exercise.[110,116] Mean within-group increases in activation ranging from 5 to 14% have been reported. Other treatment modalities that have been shown to influence motor neuron pool excitability in healthy subjects with experimentally effused knee joints include transcutaneous electrical nerve stimulation (TENS) and cryotherapy.[117] Pietrosimone and colleagues[118] randomly allocated participants with knee OA to receive either 45 minutes of TENS, 20 minutes of focal knee joint cooling with ice bags or control intervention (sitting quietly for 20 minutes) and evaluated the effect of treatment on the quadriceps central activation ratio. Application of TENS resulted in a significantly higher percent change in activation ratio scores compared with control at 20 min, 30 min, and 45 min. Focal knee joint cooling resulted in significantly higher percent change activation ratio scores compared with the control group at 20 min only. No significant differences in percent change for the central activation ratio were found between the TENS and the focal knee joint cooling group. The same investigators also showed that the addition of TENS to an exercise program increases quadriceps activation beyond that observed with exercise alone.[119] These studies provide evidence that modalities such as TENS and cryotherapy may be useful for increasing muscle activation in people with knee OA, at least in the quadriceps.

Scopaz and colleagues[120] evaluated whether pre-treatment magnitude of quadriceps activation predicted the change in quadriceps strength with exercise therapy in knee OA. The investigators hypothesized that people with lower magnitudes of muscle activation would have smaller gains in strength following exercise, when compared with those with higher magnitudes activation. Although correlations demonstrated that baseline quadriceps activation was positively associated with absolute isometric quadriceps strength at both baseline and 2-month follow-up, the level of relative quadriceps activation at baseline did not predict post-exercise absolute quadriceps strength when data were controlled for baseline absolute strength and type of exercise therapy. This data would suggest that factors other than baseline voluntary quadriceps activation may be more important in determining response to strengthening exercise. However, Pietrosimone and Saliba[121] did recently show that changes in voluntary activation predicted 47% of the change in quadriceps strength in a group of patients with OA undergoing 4 weeks of supervised resistance training. Thus improvement in voluntary activation was linked to improvement in strength. This would suggest that deficits in activation could be investigated and targeted as part of OA rehabilitation.

Although impairments in muscle activation *patterns* during gait are associated with knee OA (see earlier), there currently seem to be no studies evaluating whether exercise can change this specific impairment in people with OA, probably because it is not clear what constitutes an optimal or desirable muscle activation pattern in these people. However a recent study has shown that application of a new therapy, stochastic resonance electrical stimulation combined with a neoprene knee sleeve, significantly decreased the ratio of vastus lateralis to lateral hamstring activity during walking.[122] Similarly, a study in people with medial knee OA found that a valgus producing knee brace significantly reduced the cocontraction of both the vastus lateralis-lateral hamstrings and vastus medialis-medial hamstrings.[123] Thus, it is possible to alter muscle activation patterns but whether this translates into clinical or structural benefits is not yet known.

Proprioception

Although many treatment strategies are postulated to improve proprioception, relatively few intervention studies in knee OA evaluate proprioception in their assessment of treatment efficacy. There is some evidence that impairment in proprioceptive acuity associated with knee OA may be enhanced with exercise training more so with exercise that specifically targets the proprioceptive system. One novel program involves a computer game, where seated participants control movement of a snake on the computer screen by stepping on 4 foot pedals in multiple directions at increasing speeds.[124–126] In addition to training the proprioceptive system, task performance involves some resistance applied to the foot. This program has been evaluated alongside strength training and a no-exercise control in RCTs conducted by the same group of investigators,[124–126] although it is not clear if the data reported in each paper were collected from 3 separate cohorts of people with knee OA or a single group. Within-group analyses demonstrated significant improvements in absolute error in knee angle repositioning from baseline to follow-up in the proprioceptive training group in all 3 studies (changes approximating 2–3° in magnitude). No change was evident within the no exercise control group[127] or within the group undergoing seated concentric & eccentric quadriceps training.[125] Another RCT, which evaluated the additive effect of a sensorimotor training program using sling suspension to routine physical therapy,[128] found that the program resulted in improved knee repositioning compared with physical therapy without the sensorimotor component (mean change 1.9° ± 1.7). In contrast, another randomized study demonstrated that the addition of kinesthesia and balance exercises to a routine strengthening program did not offer any additional improvement in proprioceptive acuity than a strengthening program alone.[129]

The effects of whole-body vibration on proprioceptive function have been investigated in knee OA. An RCT compared whole-body vibration on a stable platform to whole-body vibration on a balance board to a non-treated control group.[113] Movement detection threshold was significantly improved in the vibrating balance board group compared with controls and there was a tendency for the vibrating stable platform group to perform better than the controls. It is not clear from this study whether improvement in proprioception was caused by/because of the whole-body vibration or simply an effect of the training on the balance board.

There is some evidence to suggest that knee bandaging or bracing can improve proprioception in knee OA,[69,130] but findings are inconsistent across the literature.[131] Neither taping,[132] stimulating massage,[133] magnetic knee wraps[134] nor stochastic resonance electric stimulation[135] seem to have an effect/affect on proprioception in people with knee OA. Thus it seems that some but not all treatments show promise for enhancing proprioceptive acuity in knee OA. However reported mean changes are generally quite small and it is unclear if such changes are clinically relevant or indeed, merely within the realm of measurement error.

DO IMPROVEMENTS IN MUSCLE FUNCTION LEAD TO IMPROVED SYMPTOMS AND JOINT STRUCTURE IN KNEE OA?

There is ample evidence demonstrating that muscle-strengthening exercises result in improvements in pain, physical function and quality of life in people with knee OA.[102,136] Again, the most research has focused on quadriceps strengthening programs. A systematic review of exercise that pooled data from the strengthening studies noted small to moderate effect sizes for both pain (pooled effect size 0.32, range 0.23–0.42) and physical function (pooled effect size 0.32, range 0.23–0.41) following quadriceps strengthening.[136] These findings are supported by the most recent systematic review of strengthening exercise for knee OA, conducted by Lange and colleagues.[103] Although the investigators did not pool data across trials, they reported that 56% (10 out of 18) of studies found significant decreases in pain with strengthening exercise and physical disability significantly improved in 79% (11 out of 14) of studies.

Whereas/although the improvements observed in pain and physical function following strengthening programs are often attributed to improvements in muscle strength, studies generally do not correlate changes in muscle function with clinical improvements following intervention. Indeed, most clinical trials of exercise do not include measures of muscle function in their test battery. The systematic review by Lange and colleagues[103] found only 2 studies that evaluated such relationships. They reported positive associations between increased muscle strength and walking self-efficacy,[108] reduced pain,[137] improved function[108,137] and total WOMAC score.[137] Thus, although the evidence is limited, it is likely that increases in muscle strength are at least partially responsible for improvements in pain or function with exercise.

Improvements in clinical state with strengthening exercise are generally not maintained once the patient stops exercising. This was clearly demonstrated in a study by van Baar and colleagues,[138] who evaluated the long-term effectiveness of a multifaceted exercise program that included muscle strengthening in hip and knee OA. Participants were evaluated 6 months after completion of the 3-month exercise program. Although exercise was associated with reductions in pain and observed disability at 3 months,[106] these improvements had disappeared 6 months later.[138] This may partially be due to the gradual loss of improvement in muscle function once exercise has ceased (**Fig. 2**). Thus, for ongoing improvements in pain and function, and to maintain increases in muscle strength, long-term involvement in exercise is necessary.

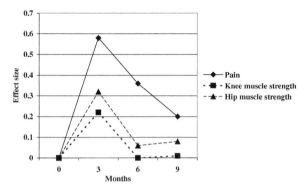

Fig. 2. Decline in effect size of muscle strength with exercise over time, as reported by van Baar and colleagues,[138] and its correlation with change in pain.

Compared with effects on symptoms, there are few RCTs evaluating whether improvements in muscle function have any discernable effect on joint structure in knee OA.[104,139,140] All these studies used radiographs to measure changes in joint structure and only 1 included a measure of joint structure as the primary outcome.[140] In this 30-month clinical trial, 105 people with knee OA were randomized to a strength-training group, with an emphasis on the quadriceps and hamstrings, or to a control range-of-motion exercise group.[140] The exercise programs were performed 3 times per week with supervision progressively withdrawn over the course of the study. The results showed a nonsignificant trend for a greater percentage of people in the control group (28%) to show an increase in grade of joint space narrowing on radiographs compared with the strength-training group (18%, $P = .09$) (**Fig. 3**). It is likely that this trial was underpowered to detect statistically significant differences in structural outcomes across groups, which may explain the nonsignificant findings of this study. Although the data suggest that it may be possible to slow structural joint deterioration over time with exercise, these results need to be interpreted cautiously given the low adherence to exercises, the high drop out rate, and the fact that the

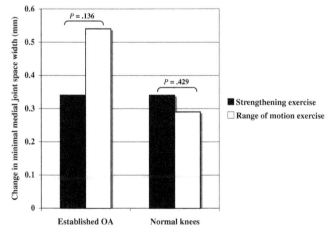

Fig. 3. Change in joint space width over 30 months with exercise as reported by Mikesky and colleagues,[140] relative to baseline disease state and according to treatment group.

strengthening groups actually lost, rather than gained, lower-extremity muscle strength over the 30-month trial. Trends in data from this study suggest that lower-limb strength training may play a role in slowing deterioration over time in established knee OA, but further large-scale studies using more sensitive imaging techniques (such as MRI) are needed.

Two other studies that included disease progression as a secondary outcome failed to find a significant effect of 18 months of exercise that included strength training in knee OA.[104,139] In 1 study, the exercise program comprised quadriceps, hamstrings, and calf strength training as well as moderate intensity walking 3 days per week[139]; the other study involved only strength training.[104] It has been proposed that the intensities or loads (% repetition maximum) used in OA exercise studies are well below those recommended for strength training in older individuals[141] and that long-duration, high-intensity strength training may be needed for structural effects. Given that knee malalignment increases the risk of structural progression over time,[142] exercise studies should also account for the severity of malalignment in data analysis so that the independent effects of exercise on disease progression can be elucidated. Further longer-term studies are needed before conclusions can be made on whether strengthening exercise can modify structural disease.

EXERCISE PRESCRIPTION FOR MUSCLE REHABILITATION

Muscle rehabilitation is an important component in the clinical management of knee OA and advocated for all patients with OA by clinical guidelines,[143] including the most recent (2012) from the American College of Rheumatology.[144] Given the muscle dysfunction (weakness, reduced proprioception) common in those with knee OA, restoration or improvement of muscle function is a key objective in the treatment of these individuals. Furthermore, because muscle dysfunction may have negative consequences on the loading environment within the knee joint, it is essential to include muscle rehabilitation exercises within the overall clinical management of knee OA to produce beneficial long-term outcomes. This section discusses practical aspects related to exercise prescription for patients and reviews current evidence about the best mode of delivery, type of exercise, and dosage (**Box 1**).

Mode of Delivery

Exercise may be delivered via individual treatments, supervised group classes, or performed at home; each has its own advantages and disadvantages. Advantages of

---

Box 1
Summary of exercise prescription for muscle rehabilitation in knee OA

- Refer to health professional for appropriate exercise prescription
- Supervised group or individual treatments are superior to independent home exercise for pain reduction
- Supplement home exercise with initial group exercise
- Exercise handouts or audiovisual material alone are ineffective
- Target quadriceps, hamstrings, and hip abductors for strengthening
- Minimize compressive joint forces
- Utilize a combined program of strengthening, flexibility, and functional exercises
- Use strategies to maximize long-term patient adherence to exercise

group-based exercise programs include the social aspects of group therapy and the ability to minimize the resources and costs to deliver the intervention. Disadvantages include difficulty in tailoring exercise to individual patients and the need to coordinate the schedules of multiple patients. Home exercise entails little financial outlay and provides the patient with greater flexibility regarding timing of the exercise session. However, there is a lack of supervision and often a lack of suitable equipment.

A recent Cochrane review compared the effect sizes of different exercise delivery modes in knee OA.[145] Results indicated that home-based exercise programs produced smaller effects on pain and physical function than individual supervised treatments or group-based interventions. However, these differences were not statistically significant. One potential explanation for the lack of statistical difference was that some of the home-based exercise programs also included visits from health care professionals. The review found that the magnitude of the treatment effect was significantly related to the number of supervised visits with a health care professional; 12 or more supervised sessions gave superior outcomes compared with less than 12 sessions. Thus, although home-based exercises may be the most feasible for some individuals with knee OA, it seems that supplementing home exercises with an initial class-based program supervised by a physiotherapist can lead to greater improvements in pain and locomotor function with home exercises in the longer term.[146] Economic analyses demonstrate that the additional cost of the group exercise classes can be offset by reductions in resource use elsewhere in the health care system.[147] Thus, exercise class supplementation represents a cost-effective method of maximizing the benefits of a home exercise program.

These findings indicate that some form of supervision from a qualified health care professional is needed to optimize outcomes. A minimalist approach whereby patients are simply given a pamphlet or audiovisual material outlining a standardized exercise program has not been found to be beneficial. In a large study, this exercise approach delivered by rheumatologists yielded similar clinical outcomes to usual care after 6 months.[148] Numerous factors likely contributed to the ineffectiveness of exercise in this study. Patients were poorly adherent and an unsupervised standardized exercise program and dosage was used, which may have been ineffective for such a heterogeneous patient group. Although a videotape demonstration of the exercises was provided, it would seem that technology is no substitute for personal demonstration and tuition in correct exercise technique. It is possible that many patients were performing the exercises incorrectly, further reducing their effectiveness.

Type of Program

Quadriceps strengthening has formed the cornerstone of traditional OA exercise therapy. Previous research into muscle dysfunction in people with knee OA has focused primarily on the quadriceps. Muscle-strengthening exercises may be performed in a variety of modes including isometric, isotonic, or isokinetic; the latter 2 may be concentric and/or eccentric. They may also be performed in an open kinetic or closed kinetic chain manner. Open kinetic chain exercises at the knee are non–weight bearing whereas closed kinetic chain exercises are typically weight bearing involving multiple joints and are believed to be more functional. However, the important issue for OA is keeping compressive joint forces as low as possible while still achieving an adequate muscle-strengthening stimulus. Thus, the advantages of functional closed kinetic chain exercises must be weighed against the potential disadvantages of increased joint loading. A meta-analysis published in 2009 identified 32 trials of exercise interventions for people with knee OA using a variety of modes including quadriceps strengthening, lower-limb muscle strengthening, combined strengthening and aerobic exercise, and other (unspecified exercises focusing on lower-limb muscle strengthening or aerobic conditioning).[149] Although the simple quadriceps strengthening programs produced only marginal significance for both pain and function and the other programs provided no significant benefit for physical function, the results of this meta-analysis found no significant differences in pain or function outcomes based on the type of exercise. Thus, clinicians can prescribe the type of exercise that best suits the individual patient. It is also likely that the effectiveness of joint-specific strengthening is maximized when combined with general strength, flexibility, and functional exercises.

Factors that may influence the type of exercise prescribed include the magnitude of joint pain and muscle weakness, disease severity, as well as the coexistence of symptoms arising from the patellofemoral joint. Given that patellofemoral involvement is generally prevalent in combination with tibiofemoral OA,[150] strengthening may need to be performed in positions that minimize patellofemoral contact forces and knee loading, which could include exercises that are performed in lesser degrees of knee flexion or in non–weight-bearing situations. Regardless of the compartmental involvement, aquatic exercise may be a useful way to strengthen muscles while minimizing joint loading particularly in the obese or in those with more advanced disease or with greater abnormalities in the local mechanical environment. A clinical trial comparing 18 weeks of aquatic exercise or land-based exercise in 64 people with knee OA found similar improvements in pain and function.[151] This suggests that aquatic exercise is a suitable and effective alternative to land-based exercise that should be considered when prescribing exercise.

Muscle rehabilitation for knee OA has largely focused on strengthening exercises given the desire to improve overall muscle force production. However, given the known impairments in muscle activation patterns in those with knee OA (see earlier section), investigation into the role of exercises that target muscle timing and function rather than purely strength (termed neuromuscular retraining exercises) has received increased interest in recent years. Neuromuscular retraining exercises may be important in people with knee OA who report instability, the symptom of buckling, slipping or giving way of the knee during functional activities.[152] Preliminary evidence for the role of neuromuscular retraining for people with knee OA has been largely surmised from treatment of other patient populations such as those with ACL injury or after meniscal surgery. A large prospective cohort study (n = 100) following individuals for 15 years after an ACL tear and subsequent neuromuscular retraining and activity modification showed similar strength and functional performance as the uninjured limb.[153] However, research into the clinical effects of neuromuscular retraining exercises in people with knee OA is limited and most research has been limited by single case studies or pilot studies. A recent RCT of 183 people with knee OA examined the addition of neuromuscular retraining exercises (including agility and perturbation exercises) to a standard strengthening exercise program.[154] The study found that the additional exercises did not improve pain and function any more than the standard exercise program alone. Further research in this area should focus on the identification of potential subgroups that would benefit most from neuromuscular retraining exercises as well as the longer-term effects on knee joint loading and disease progression.

Dosage

The frequency, duration, and intensity of the exercise program may affect clinical outcomes but these have not been well studied in people with knee OA. Although a definitive dose-based response to exercise has been reported in people with OA as well as many other populations, there may be issues with maintaining good adherence to programs with long durations. Most exercise guidelines would suggest a physiologic response can be attained with as little as 3 exercise sessions per week, and research into the effectiveness of exercise programs in individuals with knee OA have shown improvements after 8-week or 12-week programs.[155–157]

Although the notion of more is better is evident when determining the number of exercise sessions, the optimal intensity of resistance for a muscle-strengthening program for OA is unclear. High-intensity training (high resistance/load) might be expected to result in greater strength gains than low-intensity training and has been shown to be feasible in those with moderate to severe knee OA.[158] However, increased resistance during high-intensity exercise could potentially overload the joint and exacerbate symptoms such as pain, inflammation, and swelling. A study published in 2008 compared the effects of 8 weeks of high-intensity and low-intensity closed kinetic chain knee-strengthening exercise performed 3 times weekly in 102 people with knee OA.[159] High-intensity training was defined as 3 sets of 8 repetitions with an exercise weight set initially at 60% of 1 repetition maximum; low-intensity training was defined as 10 sets of 15 repetitions with an initial exercise weight of 10% of 1 repetition maximum. The results showed that both strengthening programs were beneficial for pain, function, walking time, and muscle strength. However, although not significantly different, the effect sizes were larger for high-resistance strength training. Similar findings have been reported recently by Foroughi and colleagues[95] who conducted an RCT on 54 women examining changes in biomechanical and clinical outcomes following a 6-month high-intensity (80% of 1 repetition maximum) muscle-strengthening intervention compared with a sham exercise program (similar exercises but with minimal resistance and no progression). Although muscle strength changes were significantly greater in the high-intensity group, no group differences were found in any measure of knee pain or function. Thus, it seems that with the exception of improved muscle strength, high-intensity resistance exercises do not provide greater clinical and biomechanical benefits than lower-resistance exercise interventions for people with knee OA. General guidelines for strength-training parameters in people with OA as developed by the American Geriatrics Society[160] and in older adults from the American College of Sports Medicine[161] are shown in **Table 3**. The choice of strength-training parameters depends on the patient's pain levels, tolerance, and functional level.

Enhancing Uptake of Exercise and Patient Adherence

Despite evidence of the benefits of exercise in OA and clinical guidelines recommending exercise,[143,144] it is clear that adherence to an exercise program is a major determinant of the longer-term benefits of exercise.[162] Thus, the challenge remains to increase the proportion of patients with knee OA who are exercising and to maintain active participation in their exercise program. Although there are many factors affecting the uptake of exercise in the OA population, 2 are of particular importance: (1) recommendation of exercise to patients by medical practitioners and appropriate referral to exercise professionals and (2) adherence of patients to prescribed exercise programs.

Exercise is under used by medical practitioners as a treatment strategy for OA.[163] For example, a recent Canadian survey evaluated the quality of care for people with OA.[164] The investigators found that only 25% of the people surveyed who required advice to exercise had actually seen a physiotherapist or attended a land-based or pool-based exercise program or had used fitness facilities over the past year. Furthermore, in a survey of 3000 French general practitioners, less than 15% reported that they would prescribe exercise for knee OA as a first-line therapeutic approach.[165]

Table 3			
General guidelines for strength-training parameters developed by the American Geriatrics Society for people with OA and by the American College of Sports Medicine for healthy older adults. Dosage can be modified taking into account the individual's ability and pain levels			
Exercise Type	Intensity	Volume	Frequency
American Geriatrics Society Recommendations for OA			
Isometric	Low-moderate: 40%–60% MVC	1–10 submaximal contractions/ muscle group; hold 1–6 s	Daily
Isotonic	Low: 40% 1 RM Moderate: 40%–60% 1 RM High: >60% 1 RM	10–15 repetitions 8–10 repetitions 6–8 repetitions	2–3/wk
American College of Sports Medicine Recommendations for older adults			
Isotonic	60%–80% of 1 RM	8–12 repetitions, 1–3 sets	2–3/wk

Abbreviations: 1 RM, 1 repetition maximum; MVC, maximum voluntary contraction.

Data from American Geriatrics Society Panel on Exercise and Osteoarthritis. Exercise prescription for older adults with osteoarthritis pain: consensus practice recommendations. J Am Geriatr Soc 2001;49:808–23; and American College of Sports Medicine. American College of Sports Medicine position stand. Progression models in resistance training for healthy adults. Med Sci Sports Exerc 2009:41(3);687–708.

A survey of patients with OA in Canada revealed that only one-third had been advised to use exercise for their condition,[166] however, 73% reported that they had tried exercise in the past. Given the large number of patients who chose to try exercise independently, it is possible that many failed to consult a professional regarding the most appropriate exercise. Given the known benefits of having therapist supervision during an exercise program (see earlier), it is imperative to identify ways to improve patient access to qualified health care professionals as well as inform clinicians of the benefits of exercise across the disease spectrum.

Patient adherence is a key factor in determining outcome from exercise therapy in patients with knee OA.[162,167] Although patient adherence to exercise is often good when commencing an exercise program, it typically declines over the longer term. Several factors can contribute to adherence rates for exercise programs in individuals with knee OA. Adherence is improved when patients receive attention from health professionals rather than a primarily home-based exercise program.[147] Psychosocial attributes of the individual also influence adherence. Better adherence with therapy has been found to be related to the perception of more severe knee symptoms, belief in the effectiveness of the intervention, and understanding of the pathogenesis of knee OA (those who are less adherent tend to believe that OA is part of the natural aging process or that it is simply a wear and tear disease).[168] Self-efficacy, or one's belief in one's own ability to perform tasks, is also associated with higher adherence and better outcome.[169]

Many strategies have been suggested to improve patient adherence when prescribing exercise interventions for those with knee OA.[170] Tailoring the exercise program to the unique requirements of the patient as well as ensuring availability of resources can be effective. Other methods suggested to improve adherence include monitoring via telephone contact[171] or self-reported diary,[172–174] graphic feedback on exercise goals and progress,[175] or lifestyle retraining.[172] Although monitoring from a health care professional is the preferred method of contact, patients can rely on their own social support network when an appropriate health care professional is unavailable.[172,176,177] In addition, self-monitoring via positive feedback loops based

---

Box 2
Strategies that may assist in improving adherence to exercise in people with OA

- Patient-centered and individually tailored exercise programs with respect to exercise capacity, pain levels, goals, and interests rather than standardized nonspecific programs
- Supervised exercise sessions rather than unsupervised where possible
- Supplement a home-based-program with group exercise
- Long-term monitoring/review by a health professional (phone, mail, or visits)
- Patient education regarding the importance and benefits of exercise
- Inclusion of spouse/family in the exercise program
- Self-monitoring by means of an exercise diary or pedometer
- Support from family and friends to incorporate exercise into lifestyle
- Intermittent booster or refresher exercise sessions with a health professional
- Ensure access to appropriate exercise resources and facilities

---

on level of physical function and attainment of goals may be useful for some patients. **Box 2** provides a summary of ways to improve adherence to exercise in people with knee OA.

Recently, integrated treatment combining both exercise and self-management strategies has been advocated for OA as a means of improving patient adherence as well as targeting physical and psychological factors associated with OA.[178] Traditionally, these interventions are usually delivered separately, and theoretically, the benefits of each strategy individually may be additive. In addition, although self-management programs for OA typically emphasize the importance of exercise for OA, most programs do not have an active exercise component. A recent cluster randomized trial evaluated the efficacy of an integrated rehabilitation program that included an individualized progressive exercise regime, education, and self-management strategies to alter behavior and dispel inappropriate health beliefs.[179] In this study involving 418 people with chronic knee pain, self-reported physical functioning was evaluated immediately after the 6-week intervention, as well as 6, 18, and 30 months later. Results showed that participants undergoing integrated rehabilitation (delivered by a physiotherapist either individually or in groups) had better functioning than those receiving only usual primary care after the intervention. Although improvements in function declined over time, the integrated program still resulted in better function and was more cost-effective than usual care at 30 months. Other strategies of combining exercise and psychological treatment such as pain coping skills training have been examined and show positive benefits of combined training either by a single practitioner or via discipline-specific health care professionals.[180,181] These approaches have the added advantage of directly addressing personal barriers to exercise adherence through practical examples unique to the individual embedded within the treatment program. More research in this area is needed to identify ways of optimizing the delivery of these combined treatments.

SUMMARY

Lower-limb muscles, particularly the quadriceps, influence knee joint load, a major contributor to knee OA. Impairments in muscle function including weakness, altered activation patterns, and proprioceptive deficits are commonly found in association with knee OA. Furthermore, there is some evidence that muscle weakness may predispose to the onset and potentially the progression of knee OA. Exercise is a key component of conservative management of knee OA and has been found to be effective in symptom reduction. Whether exercise influences disease development and progression requires further research.

REFERENCES

1. Bennell KL, Hunt MA, Wrigley TV, et al. Role of muscle in the genesis and management of knee osteoarthritis. Rheum Dis Clin North Am 2008;34(3):731–54.
2. Shelburne KB, Torry MR, Pandy MG. Contributions of muscles, ligaments, and the ground-reaction force to tibiofemoral joint loading during normal gait. J Orthop Res 2006;24(10):1983–90.
3. Taylor WR, Heller MO, Bergmann G, et al. Tibio-femoral loading during human gait and stair climbing. J Orthop Res 2004;22(3):625–32.
4. Amin S, Luepongsak N, McGibbon CA, et al. Knee adduction moment and development of chronic knee pain in elders. Arthritis Rheum 2004;51(3):371–6.
5. Sharma L, Hurwitz DE, Thonar EJ, et al. Knee adduction moment, serum hyaluronan level, and disease severity in medial tibiofemoral osteoarthritis. Arthritis Rheum 1998;41(7):1233–40.
6. Miyazaki T, Wada M, Kawahara H, et al. Dynamic load at baseline can predict radiographic disease progression in medial compartment knee osteoarthritis. Ann Rheum Dis 2002;61(7):617–22.
7. Bennell KL, Bowles KA, Wang Y, et al. Higher dynamic medial knee load predicts greater cartilage loss over 12 months in medial knee osteoarthritis. Ann Rheum Dis 2011;70(10):1770–4.
8. Walter JP, D'Lima DD, Colwell CW, et al. Decreased knee adduction moment does not guarantee decreased medial contact force during gait. J Orthop Res 2010;28(10):1348–54.
9. Hunt MA, Birmingham TB, Giffin JR, et al. Associations among knee adduction moment, frontal plane ground reaction force, and lever arm during walking in patients with knee osteoarthritis. J Biomech 2006;39(12):2213–20.
10. Zhao D, Banks SA, Mitchell KH, et al. Correlation between the knee adduction torque and medial contact force for a variety of gait patterns. J Orthop Res 2007;25(6):789–97.
11. Schipplein OD, Andriacchi TP. Interaction between active and passive knee stabilizers during level walking. J Orthop Res 1991;9:113–9.
12. Lloyd DG, Buchanan TS. A model of load sharing between muscles and soft tissues at the human knee during static tasks. J Biomech Eng 1996;118(3):367–76.
13. Buchanan TS, Lloyd DG. Muscle activation at the human knee during isometric flexion-extension and varus-valgus loads. J Orthop Res 1997;15(1):11–7.
14. Sritharan P, Lin YC, Pandy MG. Muscles that do not cross the knee contribute to the knee adduction moment and tibiofemoral compartment loading during gait. J Orthop Res 2012;30(10):1586–95.
15. Collins JJ, Whittle MW. Impulsive forces during walking and their clinical implications. Clin Biomech (Bristol, Avon) 1989;4:179–87.
16. Simon SR, Radin EL, Paul IL, et al. The response of joints to impact loading. II. In vivo behavior of subchondral bone. J Biomech 1972;5(3):267–72.
17. Mikesky AE, Meyer A, Thompson KL. Relationship between quadriceps strength and rate of loading during gait in women. J Orthop Res 2000;18(2):171–5.

18. Hunt MA, Hinman RS, Metcalf BR, et al. Quadriceps strength is not related to gait impact loading in knee osteoarthritis. Knee 2010;17(4):296–302.
19. Radin EL, Orr RB, Kelman JL, et al. Effect of prolonged walking on concrete on the knees of sheep. J Biomech 1982;15(7):487–92.
20. Radin EL, Yang KH, Riegger C, et al. Relationship between lower limb dynamics and knee joint pain. J Orthop Res 1991;9(3):398–405.
21. Henriksen M, Simonsen EB, Graven-Nielsen T, et al. Impulse-forces during walking are not increased in patients with knee osteoarthritis. Acta Orthop 2006;77(4):650–6.
22. Perry J. Gait analysis: normal and pathologic function. Thorofare (NJ): Slack; 1992.
23. Chang A, Hayes K, Dunlop D, et al. Hip abduction moment and protection against medial tibiofemoral osteoarthritis progression. Arthritis Rheum 2005; 52(11):3515–9.
24. Mundermann A, Dyrby CO, Andriacchi TP. Secondary gait changes in patients with medial compartment knee osteoarthritis: increased load at the ankle, knee, and hip during walking. Arthritis Rheum 2005;52(9):2835–44.
25. Hunt MA, Birmingham TB, Bryant D, et al. Lateral trunk lean explains variation in dynamic knee joint load in patients with medial compartment knee osteoarthritis. Osteoarthritis Cartilage 2008;16(5):591.
26. van der Esch M, Steultjens MP, Harlaar J, et al. Lateral trunk motion and knee pain in osteoarthritis of the knee: a cross-sectional study. BMC Musculoskelet Disord 2011;12:141.
27. Yamada H, Koshino T, Sakai N, et al. Hip adductor muscle strength in patients with varus deformed knee. Clin Orthop Relat Res 2001;(386):179–85.
28. Bennell K, Hinman RS, Wrigley TV, et al. Exercise and osteoarthritis: cause and effects. Compr Physiol 2011;1:1943–2008.
29. Lieber R. Skeletal muscle structure, function & plasticity: the physiological basis of rehabilitation. Philadelphia: Lippincott Williams & Wilkins; 2002.
30. Enoka R. Neuromechanics of human movement. Champaign (IL): Human Kinetics; 2002.
31. Wrigley TV, Strauss G. Strength assessment by isokinetic dynamometry. In: Gore C, editor. Physiological tests for elite athletes. Champaign (IL): Human Kinetics; 2000. p. 155–99.
32. Jaric S. Role of body size in the relation between muscle strength and movement performance. Exerc Sport Sci Rev 2003;31:8–12.
33. Slemenda C, Brandt KD, Heilman DK, et al. Quadriceps weakness and osteoarthritis of the knee. Ann Intern Med 1997;127(2):97–104.
34. Messier SP, Loeser RF, Hoover JL, et al. Osteoarthritis of the knee: effects on gait, strength, and flexibility. Arch Phys Med Rehabil 1992;73(1):29–36.
35. Jan MH, Lai JS, Tsauo JY, et al. Isokinetic study of muscle strength in osteoarthritic knees of females. J Formos Med Assoc 1990;9:873–9.
36. Cheing G, Hui-Chan C. The motor dysfunction of patients with knee osteoarthritis in a Chinese population. Arthritis Care Res 2001;45:62–8.
37. Diracoglu D, Baskent A, Yagci I, et al. Isokinetic strength measurements in early knee osteoarthritis. Acta Reumatol Port 2009;34(1):72–7.
38. Liikavainio T, Lyytinen T, Tyrvainen E, et al. Physical function and properties of quadriceps femoris muscle in men with knee osteoarthritis. Arch Phys Med Rehabil 2008;89(11):2185–94.
39. Palmieri-Smith RM, Thomas AC, Karvonen-Gutierrez C, et al. Isometric quadriceps strength in women with mild, moderate, and severe knee osteoarthritis. Am J Phys Med Rehabil 2010;89(7):541–8.

40. Hinman RS, Hunt MA, Creaby MW, et al. Hip muscle weakness in individuals with medial knee osteoarthritis. Arthritis Care Res 2010;62(8):1190–3.

41. Ikeda S, Tsumura H, Torisu T. Age-related quadriceps-dominant muscle atrophy and incident radiographic knee osteoarthritis. J Orthop Sci 2005;10:121–6.

42. Fink B, Egl M, Singer J, et al. Morphologic changes in the vastus medialis muscle in patients with osteoarthritis of the knee. Arthritis Rheum 2007;56:3626–33.

43. Glasberg MR, Glasberg JR, Jones RE. Muscle pathology in total knee replacement for severe osteoarthritis: a histochemical and morphometric study. Henry Ford Hosp Med J 1986;34:37–40.

44. Petterson SC, Barrance P, Buchanan T, et al. Mechanisms underlying quadriceps weakness in knee osteoarthritis. Med Sci Sports Exerc 2008;40(3):422–7.

45. Machner A, Pap G, Awiszus F. Evaluation of quadriceps strength and voluntary activation after unicompartmental arthroplasty for medial osteoarthritis of the knee. J Orthop Res 2002;20:108–11.

46. Pietrosimone BG, Hertel J, Ingersoll CD, et al. Voluntary quadriceps activation deficits in patients with tibiofemoral osteoarthritis: a meta-analysis. PM R 2011;3(2):153–62 [quiz: 162].

47. Moskowitz RW, Howell DS, Goldberg VM, et al. Osteoarthritis: diagnosis and medical/surgical management. Philadelphia: WB Saunders; 1992.

48. Hassan B, Doherty S, Mockett S, et al. Effect of pain reduction on postural sway, proprioception, and quadriceps strength in subjects with knee osteoarthritis. Ann Rheum Dis 2002;61(5):422–8.

49. Wrigley TV. Physiological responses to injury: muscle. In: Zuluaga M, Briggs C, Carlisle J, et al, editors. Sports physiotherapy: applied science & practice. Edinburgh (United Kingdom): Churchill Livingstone; 1995. p. 17–42.

50. Lo GH, McAlindon TE, Niu J, et al. Bone marrow lesions and joint effusion are strongly and independently associated with weight-bearing pain in knee osteoarthritis: data from the osteoarthritis initiative. Osteoarthritis Cartilage 2009; 17(12):1562–9.

51. Torry MR, Decker MJ, Viola RW, et al. Intra-articular knee joint effusion induces quadriceps avoidance gait patterns. Clin Biomech (Bristol, Avon) 2000;15(3): 147–59.

52. Rutherford DJ, Hubley-Kozey CL, Stanish WD. Knee effusion affects knee mechanics and muscle activity during gait in individuals with knee osteoarthritis. Osteoarthritis Cartilage 2012;20(9):974–81.

53. Winby CR, Lloyd DG, Besier TF, et al. Muscle and external load contribution to knee joint contact loads during normal gait. J Biomech 2009;42(14):2294–300.

54. Rutherford DJ, Hubley-Kozey CL, Stanish WD, et al. Neuromuscular alterations exist with knee osteoarthritis presence and severity despite walking velocity similarities. Clin Biomech (Bristol, Avon) 2011;26(4):377–83.

55. Rudolph KS, Schmitt LC, Lewek MD. Age-related changes in strength, joint laxity, and walking patterns: are they related to knee osteoarthritis? Phys Ther 2007;87(11):1422–32.

56. Hubley-Kozey CL, Deluzio KJ, Landry SC, et al. Neuromuscular alterations during walking in persons with moderate knee osteoarthritis. J Electromyogr Kinesiol 2006;16(4):365–78.

57. Schmitt LC, Rudolph KS. Influences on knee movement strategies during walking in persons with medial knee osteoarthritis. Arthritis Rheum 2007;57(6):1018–26.

58. Astephen JL, Deluzio KJ, Caldwell GE, et al. Gait and neuromuscular pattern changes are associated with differences in knee osteoarthritis severity levels. J Biomech 2008;41(4):868–76.

59. Childs JD, Sparto PJ, Fitzgerald GK, et al. Alterations in lower extremity movement and muscle activation patterns in individuals with knee osteoarthritis. Clin Biomech (Bristol, Avon) 2004;19(1):44–9.

60. Heiden TL, Lloyd DG, Ackland TR. Knee joint kinematics, kinetics and muscle co-contraction in knee osteoarthritis patient gait. Clin Biomech (Bristol, Avon) 2009;24(10):833–41.

61. Hortobagyi T, Westerkamp L, Beam S, et al. Altered hamstring-quadriceps muscle balance in patients with knee osteoarthritis. Clin Biomech (Bristol, Avon) 2005;20(1):97–104.

62. Knoop J, Steultjens MP, van der Leeden M, et al. Proprioception in knee osteoarthritis: a narrative review. Osteoarthritis Cartilage 2011;19(4):381–8.

63. Jerosch J, Prymka M. Proprioception and joint stability. Knee Surg Sports Traumatol Arthrosc 1996;4:171–9.

64. Sharma L, Pai YC. Impaired proprioception and osteoarthritis. Curr Opin Rheumatol 1997;9(3):253–8.

65. Cho YR, Hong BY, Lim SH, et al. Effects of joint effusion on proprioception in patients with knee osteoarthritis: a single-blind, randomized controlled clinical trial. Osteoarthritis Cartilage 2011;19(1):22–8.

66. Lephart SM, Pincivero DM, Giraldo JL, et al. The role of proprioception in the management and rehabilitation of athletic injuries. Am J Sports Med 1997;25: 130–7.

67. Fischer-Rasmussen T, Jensen P. Proprioceptive sensitivity and performance in anterior cruciate ligament-deficient knee joints. Scand J Med Sci Sports 2000; 10:85–9.

68. Barrack RL, Skinner HB, Cook SD, et al. Effect of articular disease and total knee arthroplasty on knee joint-position sense. J Neurophysiol 1983;50:684–7.

69. Barrett DS, Cobb AG, Bentley G. Joint proprioception in normal, osteoarthritic and replaced knees. J Bone Joint Surg Br 1991;73:53–6.

70. Hassan BS, Mockett S, Doherty M. Static postural sway, proprioception, and maximal voluntary quadriceps contraction in patients with knee osteoarthritis and normal control subjects. Ann Rheum Dis 2001;60:612–8.

71. Koralewicz LM, Engh GA. Comparison of proprioception in arthritic and age-matched normal knees. J Bone Joint Surg Am 2000;82:1582–8.

72. Pai YC, Rymer WZ, Chang RW, et al. Effect of age and osteoarthritis on knee proprioception. Arthritis Rheum 1997;40:2260–5.

73. Cammarata ML, Schnitzer TJ, Dhaher YY. Does knee osteoarthritis differentially modulate proprioceptive acuity in the frontal and sagittal planes of the knee? Arthritis Rheum 2011;63(9):2681–9.

74. Sharma L, Pai YC, Holtkamp K, et al. Is knee joint proprioception worse in the arthritic knee versus the unaffected knee in unilateral knee osteoarthritis? Arthritis Rheum 1997;40(8):1518–25.

75. Lund H, Juul-Kristensen B, Hansen K, et al. Movement detection impaired in patients with knee osteoarthritis compared to healthy controls: a cross-sectional case-control study. J Musculoskelet Neuronal Interact 2008;8(4): 391–400.

76. Slemenda C, Heilman DK, Brandt KD, et al. Reduced quadriceps strength relative to body weight: a risk factor for knee osteoarthritis in women? Arthritis Rheum 1998;41(11):1951–9.

77. Hootman JM, Fitzgerald SJ, Macera CA, et al. Lower extremity muscle strength and risk of self-reported hip or knee osteoarthritis. J Phys Activ Health 2004; 1(4):321–30.

78. Thorstensson CA, Petersson IF, Jacobsson LT, et al. Reduced functional performance in the lower extremity predicted radiographic knee osteoarthritis five years later. Ann Rheum Dis 2004;63(4):402–7.

79. Segal NA, Torner JC, Felson DT, et al. Knee extensor strength does not protect against incident knee symptoms at 30 months in the multicenter knee osteoarthritis (MOST) cohort. PM R 2009;1(5):459–65.

80. Segal NA, Torner JC, Felson D, et al. Effect of thigh strength on incident radiographic and symptomatic knee osteoarthritis in a longitudinal cohort. Arthritis Rheum 2009;61(9):1210–7.

81. Segal NA, Glass NA, Felson DT, et al. The effect of quadriceps strength and proprioception on risk for knee osteoarthritis. Med Sci Sports Exerc 2010; 42(11):2081–8.

82. Segal NA, Findlay C, Wang K, et al. The longitudinal relationship between thigh muscle mass and the development of knee osteoarthritis. Osteoarthritis Cartilage 2012;20(12):1534–40.

83. Oiestad BE, Engebretsen L, Storheim K, et al. Knee osteoarthritis after anterior cruciate ligament injury: a systematic review. Am J Sports Med 2009;37(7): 1434–43.

84. Lohmander LS, Englund PM, Dahl LL, et al. The long-term consequence of anterior cruciate ligament and meniscus injuries: osteoarthritis. Am J Sports Med 2007;35(10):1756–69.

85. Oiestad BE, Holm I, Gunderson R, et al. Quadriceps muscle weakness after anterior cruciate ligament reconstruction: a risk factor for knee osteoarthritis? Arthritis Care Res 2010;62(12):1706–14.

86. Felson DT, Gross KD, Nevitt MC, et al. The effects of impaired joint position sense on the development and progression of pain and structural damage in knee osteoarthritis. Arthritis Rheum 2009;61(8):1070–6.

87. Brandt KD, Heilman DK, Slemenda C, et al. Quadriceps strength in women with radiographically progressive osteoarthritis of the knee and those with stable radiographic changes. J Rheumatol 1999;26(11):2431–7.

88. Amin S, Baker K, Niu J, et al. Quadriceps strength and the risk of cartilage loss and symptom progression in knee osteoarthritis. Arthritis Rheum 2009;60(1):189–98.

89. Segal NA, Glass NA, Torner J, et al. Quadriceps weakness predicts risk for knee joint space narrowing in women in the MOST cohort. Osteoarthritis Cartilage 2010;18(6):769–75.

90. Segal NA, Glass NA. Is quadriceps muscle weakness a risk factor for incident or progressive knee osteoarthritis? Phys Sportsmed 2011;39(4):44–50.

91. Sharma L, Dunlop DD, Cahue S, et al. Quadriceps strength and osteoarthritis progression in malaligned and lax knees. Ann Intern Med 2003;138(8):613–9.

92. Brandt KD. Is a strong quadriceps muscle bad for a patient with knee osteoarthritis? Ann Intern Med 2003;138(8):678–9.

93. Bennell KL, Hunt MA, Wrigley TV, et al. Hip strengthening reduces symptoms but not knee load in people with medial knee osteoarthritis and varus malalignment: a randomised controlled trial. Osteoarthritis Cartilage 2010;18(5):621–8.

94. Lim BW, Hinman RS, Wrigley TV, et al. Does knee malalignment mediate the effects of quadriceps strengthening on knee adduction moment, pain, and function in medial knee osteoarthritis? A randomized controlled trial. Arthritis Rheum 2008;59(7):943–51.

95. Foroughi N, Smith RM, Lange AK, et al. Lower limb muscle strengthening does not change frontal plane moments in women with knee osteoarthritis: a randomized controlled trial. Clin Biomech (Bristol, Avon) 2011;26:167–74.

96. Sled EA, Khoja L, Deluzio KJ, et al. Effect of a home program of hip abductor exercises on knee joint loading, strength, function, and pain in people with knee osteoarthritis: a clinical trial. Phys Ther 2010;90(6):895–904.

97. Thorp LE, Wimmer MA, Foucher KC, et al. The biomechanical effects of focused muscle training on medial knee loads in OA of the knee: a pilot, proof of concept study. J Musculoskelet Neuronal Interact 2010;10(2):166–73.

98. Thorstensson CA, Henriksson M, von Porat A, et al. The effect of eight weeks of exercise on knee adduction moment in early knee osteoarthritis–a pilot study. Osteoarthritis Cartilage 2007;15(10):1163–70.

99. Erhart JC, Dyrby CO, D'Lima DD, et al. Changes in in vivo knee loading with a variable-stiffness intervention shoe correlate with changes in the knee adduction moment. J Orthop Res 2010;28(12):1548–53.

100. Sharma L, Cahue S, Song J, et al. Physical functioning over three years in knee osteoarthritis: role of psychosocial, local mechanical, and neuromuscular factors. Arthritis Rheum 2003;48(12):3359–70.

101. van Dijk GM, Veenhof C, Spreeuwenberg P, et al. Prognosis of limitations in activities in osteoarthritis of the hip or knee: a 3-year cohort study. Arch Phys Med Rehabil 2010;91(1):58–66.

102. Pelland L, Brosseau L, Wells G, et al. Efficacy of strengthening exercises for osteoarthritis (Part I): a meta-analysis. Phys Ther Rev 2004;9(2):77–108.

103. Lange AK, Vanwanseele B, Singh MA. Strength training for treatment of osteoarthritis of the knee: a systematic review. Arthritis Rheum 2008;59(10):1488–94.

104. Ettinger WH Jr, Burns R, Messier SP, et al. A randomized trial comparing aerobic exercise and resistance exercise with a health education program in older adults with knee osteoarthritis. The Fitness Arthritis and Seniors Trial (FAST). JAMA 1997;277(1):25–31.

105. Hinman R, Heywood S, Day A. Aquatic physical therapy for hip and knee osteoarthritis: results of a single-blind randomized controlled trial. Phys Ther 2007;87:32–43.

106. Van Baar ME, Dekker J, Oostendorp RA, et al. The effectiveness of exercise therapy in patients with osteoarthritis of the hip or knee: a randomized clinical trial. J Rheumatol 1998;25(12):2432–9.

107. Fisher NM, Gresham G, Pendergast DR. Effects of a quantitative progressive rehabilitation program applied unilaterally to the osteoarthritic knee. Arch Phys Med Rehabil 1993;74(12):1319–26.

108. Baker K, Nelson M, Felson D, et al. The efficacy of home-based progressive strength training in older adults with knee osteoarthritis: a randomized controlled trial. J Rheumatol 2001;28:1655–65.

109. Thomas KS, Muir KR, Doherty M, et al. Home based exercise programme for knee pain and knee osteoarthritis: randomised controlled trial. BMJ 2002;325(7367):752.

110. O'Reilly SC, Muir KR, Doherty M. Effectiveness of home exercise on pain and disability from osteoarthritis of the knee: a randomised controlled trial. Ann Rheum Dis 1999;58(1):15–9.

111. Lepley AS, Gribble PA, Pietrosimone BG. Effects of electromyographic biofeedback on quadriceps strength: a systematic review. J Strength Cond Res 2012;26(3):873–82.

112. Segal NA, Glass NA, Shakoor N, et al. Vibration platform training in women at risk for symptomatic knee osteoarthritis. PM R 2012. http://dx.doi.org/10.1016/j.pmrj.2012.07.011.

113. Trans T, Aaboe J, Henriksen M, et al. Effect of whole body vibration exercise on muscle strength and proprioception in females with knee osteoarthritis. Knee 2009;16(4):256–61.

114. Sitja-Rabert M, Rigau D, Fort Vanmeerghaeghe A, et al. Efficacy of whole body vibration exercise in older people: a systematic review. Disabil Rehabil 2012; 34(11):883–93.

115. Gur H, Cakun N, Akova B, et al. Concentric versus combined concentric-eccentric isokinetic training: effects on functional capacity and symptoms in patients with osteoarthrosis of the knee. Arch Phys Med Rehabil 2002;83: 308–16.

116. Hurley MV, Scott DL. Improvements in quadriceps sensorimotor function and disability of patients with knee osteoarthritis following a clinically practicable exercise regime. Br J Rheumatol 1998;37:1181–7.

117. Hopkins J, Ingersoll C, Edward J, et al. Cryotherapy and transcutaneous electric neuromuscular stimulation decrease arthrogenic muscle inhibition of the vastus medialis after knee joint effusion. J Athl Train 2002;37:25–31.

118. Pietrosimone BG, Hart JM, Saliba SA, et al. Immediate effects of transcutaneous electrical nerve stimulation and focal knee joint cooling on quadriceps activation. Med Sci Sports Exerc 2009;41(6):1175–81.

119. Pietrosimone BG, Saliba SA, Hart JM, et al. Effects of transcutaneous electrical nerve stimulation and therapeutic exercise on quadriceps activation in people with tibiofemoral osteoarthritis. J Orthop Sports Phys Ther 2011;41(1):4–12.

120. Scopaz K, Piva S, Gil A, et al. Effect of baseline quadriceps activation on changes in quadriceps strength after exercise therapy in subjects with knee osteoarthritis. Arthritis Care Res 2009;61(7):951–7.

121. Pietrosimone BG, Saliba SA. Changes in voluntary quadriceps activation predict changes in quadriceps strength after therapeutic exercise in patients with knee osteoarthritis. Knee 2012;19(6):939–43.

122. Collins A, Blackburn JT, Olcott C, et al. The impact of stochastic resonance electrical stimulation and knee sleeve on impulsive loading and muscle co-contraction during gait in knee osteoarthritis. Clin Biomech (Bristol, Avon) 2011;26(8):853–8.

123. Ramsey DK, Briem K, Axe MJ, et al. A mechanical theory for the effectiveness of bracing for medial compartment osteoarthritis of the knee. J Bone Joint Surg Am 2007;89(11):2398–407.

124. Jan M, Lin C, Lin Y, et al. Effects of weight-bearing versus nonweight-bearing exercise on function, walking speed, and position sense in participants with knee osteoarthritis: a randomized controlled trial. Arch Phys Med Rehabil 2009;90(6):897–904.

125. Lin D, Lin C, Lin Y, et al. Efficacy of 2 non–weight-bearing interventions, proprioception training versus strength training, for patients with knee osteoarthritis: a randomized clinical trial. J Orthop Sports Phys Ther 2009;39(6):450–7.

126. Lin D, Lin Y, Chai H, et al. Comparison of proprioceptive functions between computerized proprioception facilitation exercise and closed kinetic chain exercise in patients with knee osteoarthritis. Clin Rheumatol 2007;26(4):520–8.

127. Jan MH, Tang PF, Lin JJ, et al. Efficacy of a target-matching foot-stepping exercise on proprioception and function in patients with knee osteoarthritis. J Orthop Sports Phys Ther 2008;38(1):19–25.

128. Tsauo J, Cheng P, Yang R. The effects of sensorimotor training on knee proprioception and function for patients with knee osteoarthritis: a preliminary report. Clin Rehabil 2008;22(5):448–57.

129. Diracoglu D, Aydin R, Baskent A, et al. Effects of kinesthesia and balance exercises in knee osteoarthritis. J Clin Rheumatol 2005;11(6):303–10.
130. Birmingham T, Kramer J, Kirkley A, et al. Knee bracing for medial compartment osteoarthritis: effects on proprioception and postural control. Rheumatology (Oxford) 2001;40:285–9.
131. Hassan BS, Mockett S, Doherty M. Influence of elastic bandage on knee pain, proprioception, and postural sway in subjects with knee osteoarthritis. Ann Rheum Dis 2002;61(1):24–8.
132. Hinman R, Crossley K, McConnell J, et al. Does the application of tape influence quadriceps sensorimotor function in knee osteoarthritis? Rheumatology (Oxford) 2004;43:331–6.
133. Lund H, Henriksen M, Bartels EM, et al. Can stimulating massage improve joint repositioning error in patients with knee osteoarthritis? J Geriatr Phys Ther 2009; 32(3):111–6.
134. Chen CY, Fu TC, Hu CF, et al. Influence of magnetic knee wraps on joint proprioception in individuals with osteoarthritis: a randomized controlled pilot trial. Clin Rehabil 2011;25(3):228–37.
135. Collins AT, Blackburn JT, Olcott CW, et al. Stochastic resonance electrical stimulation to improve proprioception in knee osteoarthritis. Knee 2011;18(5): 317–22.
136. Roddy E, Zhang W, Doherty M. Aerobic walking or strengthening exercise for osteoarthritis of the knee? A systematic review. Ann Rheum Dis 2005;64:544–8.
137. Maurer BT, Stern AG, Kinossian B, et al. Osteoarthritis of the knee: isokinetic quadriceps exercise versus an educational intervention. Arch Phys Med Rehabil 1999;80(10):1293–9.
138. van Baar M, Dekker J, Oostendorp R, et al. Effectiveness of exercise in patients with osteoarthritis of the hip or knee: nine months follow up. Ann Rheum Dis 2001;60(12):1123–30.
139. Messier SP, Loeser RF, Miller GD, et al. Exercise and dietary weight loss in overweight and obese older adults with knee osteoarthritis: the arthritis, diet, and activity promotion trial. Arthritis Rheum 2004;50(5):1501–10.
140. Mikesky AE, Mazzuca SA, Brandt KD, et al. Effects of strength training on the incidence and progression of knee osteoarthritis. Arthritis Rheum 2006;55(5): 690–9.
141. Nelson ME, Rejeski WJ, Blair SN, et al. Physical activity and public health in older adults: recommendation from the American College of Sports Medicine and the American Heart Association. Med Sci Sports Exerc 2007;39(8):1435–45.
142. Tanamas S, Hanna FS, Cicuttini FM, et al. Does knee malalignment increase the risk of development and progression of knee osteoarthritis? A systematic review. Arthritis Rheum 2009;61(4):459–67.
143. Zhang W, Moskowitz RW, Nuki G, et al. OARSI recommendations for the management of hip and knee osteoarthritis. Part II: OARSI evidence-based, expert consensus guidelines. Osteoarthritis Cartilage 2008;16(2):137–62.
144. Hochberg MC, Altman RD, Toupin April K, et al. American College of Rheumatology 2012 recommendations for the use of nonpharmacologic and pharmacologic therapies in osteoarthritis of the hand, hip, and knee. Arthritis Care Res 2012;64(4):465–74.
145. Fransen M, McConnell S. Exercise for osteoarthritis of the knee. Cochrane Database Syst Rev 2008;(4):CD004376.
146. McCarthy C, Mills P, Pullen R, et al. Supplementation of a home-based exercise programme with a class-based programme for people with osteoarthritis of the

knees: a randomised controlled trial and health economic analysis. Health Technol Assess 2004;8(46):1–61.

147. McCarthy CJ, Mills PM, Pullen R, et al. Supplementing a home exercise programme with a class-based exercise programme is more effective than home exercise alone in the treatment of knee osteoarthritis. Rheumatology (Oxford) 2004;43(7):880–6.

148. Ravaud P, Giraudeau B, Logeart I, et al. Management of osteoarthritis (OA) with an unsupervised home based exercise programme and/or patient administered assessment tools. A cluster randomised controlled trial with a 2x2 factorial design. Ann Rheum Dis 2004;63(6):703–8.

149. Fransen M, McConnell S. Land-based exercise for osteoarthritis of the knee: a meta-analysis of randomized controlled trials. J Rheumatol 2009;36(6):1109–17.

150. Ledingham J, Regan M, Jones A, et al. Radiographic patterns and associations of osteoarthritis of the knee in patients referred to hospital. Ann Rheum Dis 1993; 52(7):520–6.

151. Silva LE, Valim V, Pessanha AP, et al. Hydrotherapy versus conventional land-based exercise for the management of patients with osteoarthritis of the knee: a randomized clinical trial. Phys Ther 2008;88(1):12–21.

152. Hurley MV. Muscle dysfunction and effective rehabilitation of knee osteoarthritis: what we know and what we need to find out. Arthritis Rheum 2003;49(3):444–52.

153. Ageberg E, Pettersson A, Friden T. 15-year follow-up of neuromuscular function in patients with unilateral nonreconstructed anterior cruciate ligament injury initially treated with rehabilitation and activity modification: a longitudinal prospective study. Am J Sports Med 2007;35(12):2109–17.

154. Fitzgerald GK, Piva SR, Gil AB, et al. Agility and perturbation training techniques in exercise therapy for reducing pain and improving function in people with knee osteoarthritis: a randomized clinical trial. Phys Ther 2011;91(4):452–69.

155. Rogind H, Bibow-Nielsen B, Jensen B, et al. The effects of a physical training program on patients with osteoarthritis of the knees. Arch Phys Med Rehabil 1998;79(11):1421–7.

156. Huang MH, Lin YS, Yang RC, et al. A comparison of various therapeutic exercises on the functional status of patients with knee osteoarthritis. Semin Arthritis Rheum 2003;32(6):398–406.

157. Suomi R, Collier D. Effects of arthritis exercise programs on functional fitness and perceived activities of daily living measures in older adults with arthritis. Arch Phys Med Rehabil 2003;84:1589–94.

158. King LK, Birmingham TB, Kean CO, et al. Resistance training for medial compartment knee osteoarthritis and malalignment. Med Sci Sports Exerc 2008;40(8):1376–84.

159. Jan M, Lin J, Liau J, et al. Investigation of clinical effects of high- and low-resistance training for patients with knee osteoarthritis: a randomized controlled trial. Phys Ther 2008;88:427–36.

160. American Geriatrics Society Panel on Exercise and Osteoarthritis. Exercise prescription for older adults with osteoarthritis pain: consensus practice recommendations. J Am Geriatr Soc 2001;49:808–23.

161. American College of Sports Medicine. American College of Sports Medicine position stand. Progression models in resistance training for healthy adults. Med Sci Sports Exerc 2009;41(3):687–708.

162. Pisters M, Veenhof C, Schellevis F, et al. Exercise adherence improves long-term patient outcome in patients with osteoarthritis of the hip and/or knee. Arthritis Care Res 2010;62(8):1087–94.

163. Cottrell E, Roddy E, Foster NE. The attitudes, beliefs and behaviours of GPs regarding exercise for chronic knee pain: a systematic review. BMC Fam Pract 2010;11:4.
164. Li LC, Sayre EC, Kopec JA, et al. Quality of nonpharmacological care in the community for people with knee and hip osteoarthritis. J Rheumatol 2011; 38(10):2230–7.
165. Chevalier X, Marre JP, de Butler J, et al. Questionnaire survey of management and prescription of general practitioners in knee osteoarthritis: a comparison with 2000 EULAR recommendations. Clin Exp Rheumatol 2004;22(2):205–12.
166. Li LC, Maetzel A, Pencharz JN, et al. Use of mainstream nonpharmacologic treatment by patients with arthritis. Arthritis Rheum 2004;51(2):203–9.
167. Mazieres B, Thevenon A, Coudeyre E, et al. Adherence to, and results of, physical therapy programs in patients with hip or knee osteoarthritis. Development of French clinical practice guidelines. Joint Bone Spine 2008;75(5):589–96.
168. Campbell R, Evans M, Tucker M, et al. Why don't patients do their exercises? Understanding non-compliance with physiotherapy in patients with osteoarthritis of the knee. J Epidemiol Community Health 2001;55:132–8.
169. Marks R, Allegrante JP. Chronic osteoarthritis and adherence to exercise: a review of the literature. J Aging Phys Act 2005;13(4):434–60.
170. Jordan JL, Holden MA, Mason EE, et al. Interventions to improve adherence to exercise for chronic musculoskeletal pain in adults. Cochrane Database Syst Rev 2010;(1):CD005956.
171. Castro CM, King AC, Brassington GS. Telephone versus mail interventions for maintenance of physical activity in older adults. Health Psychol 2001;20(6): 438–44.
172. Roddy E, Doherty M. Changing life-styles and osteoarthritis: what is the evidence? Best Pract Res Clin Rheumatol 2006;20(1):81–97.
173. King E, Rimer BK, Benincasa T, et al. Strategies to encourage mammography use among women in senior citizens' housing facilities. J Cancer Educ 1998; 13(2):108–15.
174. Noland MP. The effects of self-monitoring and reinforcement on exercise adherence. Res Q Exerc Sport 1989;60(3):216–24.
175. Duncan K, Pozehl B. Effects of an exercise adherence intervention on outcomes in patients with heart failure. Rehabil Nurs 2003;28(4):117–22.
176. Litt MD, Kleppinger A, Judge JO. Initiation and maintenance of exercise behavior in older women: predictors from the social learning model. J Behav Med 2002;25(1):83–97.
177. Oka RK, King AC, Young DR. Sources of social support as predictors of exercise adherence in women and men ages 50 to 65 years. Womens Health 1995;1(2):161–75.
178. Hurley MV, Walsh NE. Effectiveness and clinical applicability of integrated rehabilitation programs for knee osteoarthritis. Curr Opin Rheumatol 2009;21(2): 171–6.
179. Hurley MV, Walsh NE, Mitchell H, et al. Long-term outcomes and costs of an integrated rehabilitation program for chronic knee pain: a pragmatic, cluster randomized, controlled trial. Arthritis Care Res 2012;64(2):238–47.
180. Keefe FJ, Blumenthal J, Baucom D, et al. Effects of spouse-assisted coping skills training and exercise training in patients with osteoarthritic knee pain: a randomized controlled study. Pain 2004;110(3):539–49.
181. Keefe FJ, Somers TJ. Psychological approaches to understanding and treating arthritis pain. Nat Rev Rheumatol 2010;6(4):210–6.

Disease Modification
Promising Targets and Impediments to Success

Gloria L. Matthews, DVM, PhD, DACVS

KEYWORDS

- Osteoarthritis • Disease modification • Clinical trial • Joint

KEY POINTS

- Modifying the course of osteoarthritis is a significant unmet medical need, because the treatable population is enormous and current therapies are only palliative.
- The accepted definition of disease modification is expanding from its previous cartilage-centric focus as appreciation for the effect of the disease on other joint tissues has increased.
- Although anticatabolic strategies may still be of value, there is increasing interest in anabolic and biologic approaches to disease modification.
- Drug development hurdles in this area are significant and include challenges with sensitivity of current outcome measures, validation of surrogate endpoints such as imaging and biochemical biomarkers, establishment of a minimum clinically important difference with these biomarkers, and, to some extent, translatability of animal model data to the clinical setting.

INTRODUCTION

Because OA constitutes a substantial burden to afflicted individuals and the impact on the health care system, as well as overall loss of productivity, is large and growing, its successful treatment remains a significant and increasingly unmet need. Nearly 75% of patients want better treatment of their OA.[1] Current treatments of OA are palliative for symptoms with little demonstration of efficacy in modifying the structural changes induced by the disease or altering its clinical course. This overview intends to bring attention to a relatively recent evolution of the traditional definition of "disease modification," provide an overview of therapeutic strategies currently in late-stage development, and give special emphasis to challenges associated with therapeutic development in this area. This introduction to a shift in thinking about broader implications of the term "disease modification" is timely because the challenges to drug development in this area have resulted in the recent exodus of most pharmaceutical

Orthopaedic & Regenerative Medicine Research, Genzyme, A Sanofi Company, 49 New York Avenue, Framingham, MA 01701, USA
E-mail address: gloria.matthews@sanofi.com

Rheum Dis Clin N Am 39 (2013) 177–187
http://dx.doi.org/10.1016/j.rdc.2012.10.006
0889-857X/13/$ – see front matter © 2013 Elsevier Inc. All rights reserved.

companies from this area of focus, at a time when the unmet need is large and expanding annually in parallel with the growth of the mature adult population, many of whom are heavier and/or active longer in life and develop unacceptable activity-limiting OA earlier than has been the case in recent decades.

Thinking more broadly about what is considered modification of the disease to include both hard and soft tissues of the joint and neurovascular and adipose components may help reveal novel and targetable approaches to treating this debilitating disease and encourage the reinvestment of much needed resources in this area. This will of course need to be done in the context of regulatory agency acceptability to be successful, but a crucial first step in getting this process under way will be to reestablish the perceived validity of investing in OA research and development programs by producing sensible, credible, and readily translatable therapeutic targeting strategies, with a goal to improve the clinical and quality of life outcomes of affected patients, regardless of the type of tissue behavior modified in the process.

DEFINITION OF "DISEASE MODIFICATION"

Diarthrodial joints are a composite of cartilage, subchondral bone, synovial membrane, and extrasynovial tendons, ligaments, fascia, fat, and muscle. With the exception of cartilage, all of these tissues are supplied by local branches of larger peripheral blood vessel and nerves. The interior of the normal joint is bathed by a thin layer of synovial fluid, an ultrafiltrate of plasma enhanced by locally synthesized hyaluronic acid. Osteoarthritic joints exhibit a continuous cycle of whole organ metabolic and structural derangement including induction of catabolic cytokine cascades, impaired oxygenation, decreased local tissue pH, altered water balance, progressive cartilage loss, subchondral bone remodeling, osteophyte formation, local venous congestion, and mild to moderate synovial inflammation.[2]

The precise etiopathogenesis of OA is poorly understood, and the idea that the disease can be initiated or perpetuated by any or all of the multiple tissue types in the joint is not new. A great deal of attention has been paid in the literature to most of these affected joint tissues, particularly cartilage,[3] but also bone,[4–8] meniscal degeneration,[9] synovium,[10,11] and the intracapsular but extrasynovial infrapatellar fat pad.[12]

Despite recent recognition by various camps that bone and synovium are significant participants in OA disease manifestation and progression, the world of disease modification research and product development (see Approaches Currently Being Tested section) has largely been dominated by a cartilage-centric view. For several decades, cytokine-based cartilage culture models have been successfully used to model disease effects. Treatment of isolated chondrocytes and cartilage explants in culture with individual or combinations of cytokines such as interleukin (IL)-1 and tumor necrosis factor (TNF)α/oncostatin M combinations reliably drive up serine and cysteine proteinases, as well as the aggrecanases that degrade cartilage matrix and inhibit matrix production (proteoglycan, type II collagen) at the message level. This naturally spawned the notion that these pathways were central to OA pathophysiology and disease manifestation[13,14] and focused attention on the cartilage component of the disease. Historically, this led to a great deal of investment in anticytokine therapeutic strategies to help preserve cartilage, much of which has, unfortunately, been largely unrewarding. One good example of this is IL-1, the role of which has been recently reviewed in OA.[15] Although useful as a reliable short-term inducer of OA phenotype in cell and organ culture models, the clinical trial performance of IL-1 inhibitors as therapeutics has not been strong.[16,17]

Recent therapeutic development efforts (**Fig. 1**) have recognized the potential contribution of subchondral bone to the disease process and have begun to interrogate the value of targeting this tissue therapeutically. Risedronate, a bisphosphonate intended to maintain bone integrity to support the joint surface and thus help keep the cartilage surface healthy and intact, although unsuccessful as a disease-modifying agent or symptom modifier in a large clinical trial[18,19] (potentially caused in part to challenges with patient selection and unpredictable disease progression), nevertheless helped pave the way for other therapeutics with a similar strategic approach. It was recently reported that a single treatment of another bisphosphonate, zoledronic acid, resulted in significant pain reduction and decrease in pain and the size of disease progression–associated bone marrow lesions in patients with knee OA in a randomized placebo-controlled clinical study.[20] After these findings in the clinic, the effects of this agent were shown to be disease state specific in a surgical instability model of OA in rats.[21] Oral salmon calcitonin has also recently been in clinical development as a disease-modifying OA drug (DMOAD), seeking to reverse or slow the OA-induced disruption of the bone–cartilage unit. Although traditionally studied in the context of bone, there is mounting evidence that calcitonin has direct effects on both bone and cartilage.[22,23] Calcitonin can directly inhibit matrix metalloproteinases (MMPs) and block collagen degradation in $TNF\alpha$/oncostatin M–exposed cultured articular chondrocytes.[24] Enhancement of type II collagen and proteoglycan synthesis has been demonstrated in vitro in cultured human OA cartilage.[25] In vivo, calcitonin has demonstrated the ability to slow meniscectomy-induced damage in a rat ovariectomy model of postmenopausal OA,[26] as well as to confer some level of protection from cartilage degradation in an mouse model of OA.[27] A recently completed large (1169 enrolled subjects) multicenter double-blind, randomized, placebo-controlled 2-year phase III trial in Kellgren-Lawrence (K-L) grade 2–3 OA patients[28] demonstrated significant difference in cartilage volume loss by magnetic resonance (MR) imaging in favor of calcitonin, with significant analgesic effects seen compared with placebo control. No difference was seen, however, between treated and control subjects on radiographic joint space width change, still considered a critical endpoint by regulatory agencies.

Another approach that may have effects on both cartilage and bone is treatment with vitamin D, being the subject of trials that are now either complete or nearing completion, including a randomized, double-blind placebo-controlled study being conducted in Australia in subjects with low plasma vitamin D levels and OA for at least 6 months. The rationale for this treatment includes multiple facets, including direct chondrocyte effects and association of low vitamin D level with diminution in muscle strength, known to be associated with OA. Further, low vitamin D levels have been shown to negatively influence bone formation, metabolism, and mineral deposition, as well as osteoblast activity.[29]

Targeting other joint tissues, including synovial or neovascularization pathologies, is a path less well traveled. Certainly there is overlap between anticatabolic strategies intended to preserve cartilage and those that influence synovial production of degradative cytokines. Inducible nitric oxide synthase (iNOS) inhibition, a strategy recently interrogated in a phase III clinical trial, could be considered a good example of an agent likely to influence both synovial and cartilage nitric oxide production and to reduce pathologic effects in both tissues. iNOS is the enzyme responsible for cytokine-induced production of oxidatively toxic nitric oxide by chondrocytes under pathologic stress.[30] Experimentally, iNOS inhibition can reduce the size of cartilage lesions and osteophytes while reducing synovial production of IL-1β, MMPs, and prostaglandins, all potential drivers of structural damage and/or pain sensitization.[31–33] A large (1048

Technology	Rationale	Result	Company/Institution
Zoledronic acid	Support bone integrity	Decrease in subchondral bone marrow lesion size and pain	Menzies Research Institute
Inducible nitric oxide synthase inhibitor	Interrupt inflammatory cascade leading to cartilage degradation	K-L 2: inhibition of joint space narrowing at 48 weeks, not 96; no difference vs. placebo in total study population	Pfizer
Salmon calcitonin	Support cartilage matrix production and bone integrity	Decrease in cartilage volume loss by magnetic resonance imaging (MRI); no difference in joint space width; pain efficacy signal	Novartis, Nordic Biosciences
Fibroblast growth factor-18	Drive chondrocyte proliferation and maintain anabolic phenotype	Increase in lateral femorotibial cartilage volume by MRI, no difference in joint space width or pain	Merck KgaA
Vitamin D	Support healthy bone formation in Vitamin D deficient patients	Ongoing	University of Zurich; Menzies Research Institute
Mesenchymal stem cells, chondrocytes, bone marrow concentrate	Leverage paracrine effects on inflammatory and anabolic profile	Very small early phase trials underway	Stempeutics, Red de Terapia Celular, Royan Institute, Internat'l Stem Cell Services, others…

Fig. 1. Recent OA disease–modifying therapeutic strategies in development.

study completers of 1457 randomized subjects) 2-year multinational multicenter randomized double-blind trial was recently completed to evaluate the potential of iNOS to slow progression of radiographic joint space narrowing in the medial tibiofemoral joint compartment to a greater degree than placebo control.[34] In the overall analysis, joint space width was not significantly different between treated and placebo control groups, whereas in discrete subanalyses by OA radiographic severity, K-L grade 2 subjects demonstrated significantly lower rates of joint space narrowing during the first 48 weeks of treatment but K-L grade 3 subjects did not, which the investigators indicate suggests either that iNOS plays a more significant role in OA pathologic conditions earlier in the disease process or that late-stage disease has advanced biomechanically too far to be amenable to treatment with this inhibitor, or potentially both.

Other strategies that could prove useful include inhibition of such OA-related pathologic conditions as vascular leakage, neovascularization, neuronal cell death, osteophyte formation, and bone marrow lesion formation and growth. The potential value of these types of less-traditional approaches for either symptom or structure modification remains to be explored.

OTHER APPROACHES UNDER ACTIVE CONSIDERATION

A review[35] summarizing active clinical trials published in early 2010 shows a pipeline dominated by anticatabolic strategies, including inhibition of IL-1, TNFα, iNOS, MMPs, and aggrecanases. More recently, emphasis has been placed more on anabolic strategies, such as growth factors and cells as approaches to slow or stop joint degeneration in OA. A similar review of active late-stage clinical trials published in 2011[36] shows what may be considered a shifting landscape for active clinical trials from that published in early 2010. Anticatabolic strategies such as those targeting serine and cysteine proteinases, aggrecanases, interleukins, and members of the mitogen-activated protein kinase signaling pathway have for the most part been dropped from the therapeutic pipeline. Fibroblast growth factor-18 (FGF-18), a chondrogenic factor for chondrocytes and stem cells that can promote extracellular matrix synthesis,[37–39] has been the subject of a recent clinical proof-of-concept trial.[40] This factor has also been shown to have some catabolic activity in OA chondrocytes. Supporting this dual role is a microarray analysis of the effects of FGF-18 on IL-1–stimulated human articular chondrocytes in culture,[41] which demonstrated increased gene expression of cartilage protective factors aggrecan, bone morphogenetic protein-2, and COL2A1 with concomitant upregulation of catabolic factors such as the aggrecanases ADAMTS-4 and -5, IL-1β, IL-6, and MMP-13. It remains to be seen if this balance between anabolic and catabolic activities promotes anabolism with beneficial structural remodeling of newly formed repair tissue or results in either little effect or a disorganized or inconsistent response. Clinically, in a randomized, double-blind, placebo-controlled, multicenter study evaluating intra-articular injection of FGF-18 in patients with OA,[40] total cartilage volume was significantly increased in the treated group versus placebo, with most of the change seen in the lateral femorotibial compartment. Similar to other studies of this type, as described earlier for iNOS and salmon calcitonin, radiographic joint space width was not different between groups.

Osteogenic protein-1 (also known as bone morphogenetic protein-7), is a powerful bone and cartilage matrix anabolic factor expressed by adult human chondrocytes that may also demonstrate some level of IL-1 inhibitory activity. Similar to other members of the transforming growth factor-β superfamily, osteogenic protein -1 markedly drives up proteoglycan and collagen production by chondrocytes and may help to prevent chondrocytes from terminally differentiating and becoming hypertrophic as OA progresses.[42–44] This agent was in trial for pain-relieving effects and structural change, and although early clinical data seemed to hold promise, successful pain endpoints were not achieved in a larger later-stage trial.

Multiple small exploratory autologous and allogeneic cell therapy–based clinical trials with both pain and structure endpoints are currently registered (clinicaltrials. gov) evaluating efficacy of OA treatment. The mechanism of action of stem cells in a disease such as OA may be linked to the pluripotent differentiation capability of these cells providing additional stem cells and chondrocytes that are geared toward restoration of damaged tissues, but these cells are also factories for balanced levels of growth factors, cytokines, chemokines, and other factors that influence tissue repair, remodeling, and inflammation. This latter paracrine capacity is currently considered the primary mechanism of action of these therapies. Although this mechanistic complexity may make cell-based therapy a more biologically relevant treatment option, it will also hinder its regulatory and commercial acceptability. As for other biologic approaches, the therapeutic potential of these strategies remains to be proved.

CHALLENGES TO THERAPEUTIC DEVELOPMENT

Although a shift in therapeutic type being tested has been pointed out here, this change does not necessarily indicate that the therapeutic target selections were not valid. Although a given target may indeed not be appropriate, there are a wide variety of potential reasons clinical programs do not go forward, including significant development hurdles (discussed further in this section), change in business approach of the parent company sponsoring the development program (particularly common in the case of mergers and acquisitions), inability to move forward because of unforeseen and nonnegotiable intellectual property issues, and/or unanticipated safety issues that do not meet an acceptable risk/benefit threshold.

The biggest challenges facing DMOAD product development today are the slow and insidious progression of the disease, insensitive change-detection techniques available clinically, and correlation of detectable structure benefit change to a clinically meaningful change such as pain relief or enhanced function. These are addressed in more detail later. Other challenges stem from lack of validated therapeutic targets and the difficulty in achieving validation given the limited understanding of both disease etiopathogenesis and the translational power of preclinical models to predict clinical outcomes.[45,46]

Slow, Unpredictable Disease Progression

OA develops during decades and often starts to progress most rapidly at the end stage of the disease, a time when successful treatment of the pathologic conditions and slowing, stopping, or reversing structural damage may be nearly impossible. Even with careful standardization using a fixed-flexion view, rates of change of radiographic joint space during a 2-year period are reported to be a mere 0.18 mm,[46] which lies very close to the coefficient of variation of the imaging technique. Predicting patients who will progress measurably within a feasible clinical trial period of 1 to 2 years has been extremely problematic. Current research activities are under way to identify methods for selecting patients who will progress adequately during the trial period, and factors such as more advanced K-L grade (II or III), malalignment, bone marrow lesions, and meniscal injury[47] have been identified as potentially predicting progression. However, each of these conditions may also signal advanced disease and may significantly impair the ability of a therapeutic agent to be effective in that setting. Others have found generalized knee OA and hyaluronic acid levels to be predictive, whereas knee pain, radiologic severity at baseline, sex, quadriceps strength, knee injury, and regular athletic activity were unrelated to progression.[48]

Insensitivity of Change-Detection Techniques

The traditional and still only regulatory agency–accepted method of detecting OA progression is based on radiographic joint space narrowing. One challenge with this technique is difficulty standardizing views between patients and between visits from any individual patient. Another is the very small rate of change expected in a 2-year period,[46] which pushes the maximum amount of time sponsors are willing to carry out a clinical trial, as the costs and logistics become extensive and difficult to manage. A third challenge of radiographic joint space narrowing is that it is an indirect measure of cartilage integrity and thickness. Cartilage cannot be visualized by traditional radiography, and thus joint space narrowing can be a composite result over time of cartilage thinning, meniscal extrusion (common in patients with OA), and even bone shape changes through both normal age-related and pathologic remodeling. MR imaging techniques, which can more directly measure cartilage volume and thickness, have been developed with the hope of increasing sensitivity to small changes seen in cartilage of patients with OA. Although recent reports have indicated the sensitivity for change, detection is not substantially greater than properly positioned radiographic techniques[49,50] MR imaging, when used semiquantitatively, does give an added benefit of being able to assess synovitis and bone marrow lesions, 2 potentially important features in OA pathology and treatment.[51]

Establishing Clinically Relevant Change

The regulatory draft guidance document authored in 1999 by the US Food and Drug Administration, *Clinical Development Programs for Drugs, Devices, and Biologic Products Intended for the Treatment of Osteoarthritis (OA)*,[52] indicates, and subsequent public statements by agency representatives supports, that unless there is a profound effect of a DMOAD such that the disease is completely arrested or reversed (ie, cured), the candidate agent will need to demonstrate a clinically relevant benefit, such as pain relief, functional improvement, delay of total joint replacement, or a similar affect to be considered approvable. The challenge here is that pain and structural change are not well linked, and many of the current targets for DMOAD effects are unlikely to have pain relief or disability decreasing benefits, at least within a reasonable and acceptable trial period. Another challenge is that patient selection for a DMOAD trial may differ substantially from that optimal for demonstrating a clinically measurable patient benefit such as pain relief; thus, multiple additional trials could be necessary before approval. Combining a DMOAD with an analgesic drug is one strategy that could help overcome this challenge. However, this becomes a more ominous regulatory hurdle, because full factorial trials are frequently required, starting potentially as early as preclinical stages. These factors are challenges the industry continues to grapple with but will be essential to overcome for successful therapeutic development in this area.

SUMMARY

OA is a widespread debilitating disease that represents an enormous patient and public health burden. Currently, treatments are strictly palliative, and there is a great unmet need for novel therapeutics that can provide some level of disease modification. The traditional definition of "disease modification" has been accepted by most of the OA research community to have a cartilage-centric focus, but that definition is evolving to include the other affected tissues in this whole organ disease, including bone, synovium, vessels, nerves, and other joint-associated soft tissue structures such as menisci and the infrapatellar fat pad. This evolution is likely to be necessary to be successful in opening up new target potential for this field and rejuvenating investment interest in OA research and development from all sources, including government, industry, and foundation-based agencies.

Current DMOAD target focus has also shifted from primarily small molecule anticatabolic strategies to a more diverse mix of small molecules and biologics, tending to focus on the anabolic events in bone or cartilage, including bone-preserving agents and cells. Although this may mean the anticatabolic strategies were wrong, it is equally possible that other factors such as ominous development pathways, intellectual property issues, or loss of patience and interest on the part of developing entities are at the root of the dropout of at least some of these agents from the therapeutic development pipeline.

Although the path to successful DMOAD development is extremely challenging, passionate and dedicated research continues in this field, and this, combined with a broadening of the definition of disease modification, potentially opening the door to new target potential, gives reason to be optimistic.

REFERENCES

1. National Council on Aging. Harris interactive survey. 2005.
2. Wieland HA, Michaelis M, Kirschbaum BJ, et al. Osteoarthritis: an untreatable disease? Nat Rev Drug Discov 2005;4(4):331–44.
3. Goldring MB. Update on the biology of the chondrocyte and new approaches to treating cartilage diseases. Best Pract Res Clin Rheumatol 2006;20(5):1003–25.
4. Radin EL, Rose RM. Role of subchondral bone in the initiation and progression of cartilage damage. Clin Orthop Relat Res 1986;213:34–40.
5. Burr DB. Anatomy and physiology of the mineralized tissues: role in the pathogenesis of osteoarthrosis. Osteoarthritis Cartilage 2004;12(Suppl A):S20–30.
6. Spector TD. Bisphosphonates: potential therapeutic agents for disease modification in osteoarthritis. Aging Clin Exp Res 2003;15:413–8.
7. Bailey AJ, Mansell JP, Sims TJ, et al. Biochemical and mechanical properties of subchondral bone in osteoarthritis. Biorheology 2004;41:349–58.
8. Lories RJ, Luyten FP. The bone-cartilage unit in osteoarthritis. Nat Rev Rheumatol 2011;7(1):43–9.
9. Englund M, Guermazi A, Lohmander LS. The meniscus in knee osteoarthritis. Rheum Dis Clin North Am 2009;35(3):579–90.
10. Fell HB, Jubb RW. The effect of synovial tissue on the breakdown of articular cartilage in organ culture. Arthritis Rheum 1977;20(7):1359–71.
11. Aigner R, van der Kraan P, van den Berg W. Osteoarthritis and inflammation: Inflammatory changes in osteoarthritic synoviopathy. In: Buckwalter J, Lotz M, Stoltz J-F, editors. Osteoarthritis, inflammation and degradation: a continuum. Amsterdam: IOS Press; 2007. p. 219–35.
12. Clockaerts S, Batiaansen-Jenniskens YM, Runhaar J, et al. The infrapatellar fat pad should be considered as an active osteoarthritis joint tissue: a narrative review. Osteoarthritis Cartilage 2010;18(7):876–82.
13. Fernandes JC, Martel-Pelletier J, Pelletier JP. The role of cytokines in osteoarthritis pathophysiology. Biorheology 2002;39:237–46.
14. Kapoor M, Martel-Pelletier J, Lajeunesse D, et al. Role of proinflammatory cytokines in the pathophysiology of osteoarthritis. Nat Rev Rheumatol 2011;7(1):33–42.

15. Daheshia M, Yao JQ. The interleukin 1β pathway in the pathogenesis of osteoarthritis. J Rheumatol 2008;35(12):1–7.
16. Chevalier X, Girardeau B, Conrozier T, et al. Safety study of intraarticular injection of interleukin 1 receptor antagonist in patients with painful knee osteoarthritis: a multicenter study. J Rheumatol 2005;32:1317–23.
17. Chevalier X, Goupille P, Beaulieu AD, et al. Intraarticular injection of anakinra in osteoarthritis of the knee: a multicenter, randomized, double-blind, placebo-controlled study. Arthritis Rheum 2009;61:344–52.
18. Spector TD, Conaghan PG, Buckland-Wright JC, et al. Effect of risedronate on joint structure and symptoms of knee osteoarthritis: results of the BRISK randomized controlled trial. Arthritis Res Ther 2005;7:R625–33.
19. Bingham CO 3rd, Buckland-Wright JC, Garnero P, et al. Risedronate decreases biochemical markers of cartilage degradation but does not decrease symptoms or slow radiographic progression in patients with medial compartment osteoarthritis of the knee: results of the two-year multinational knee osteoarthritis structural arthritis study. Arthritis Rheum 2006;54(11):3494–507.
20. Laslett LL, Doré DA, Quinn SJ, et al. Zoledronic acid reduces knee pain and bone marrow lesions over 1 year: a randomised controlled trial. Ann Rheum Dis 2012; 71(8):1322–8.
21. Yu DG, Yu B, Mao YQ, et al. Efficacy of zoledronic acid in treatment of osteoarthritis is dependent on the disease progression stage in rat medial meniscal tear model. Acta Pharmacol Sin 2012;33(7):924–34.
22. Naot D, Cornish J. The role of peptides and receptors of the calcitonin family in the regulation of bone metabolism. Bone 2008;43(5):813–8.
23. Sondergaard BC, Madsen SH, Segovia-Silvestre T, et al. Investigation of the direct effects of salmon calcitonin on human osteoarthritic chondrocytes. BMC Musculoskelet Disord 2010;11:62.
24. Karsdal MA, Sondergaard BC, Arnold M, et al. Calcitonin affects both bone and cartilage: a dual action treatment for osteoarthritis? Ann N Y Acad Sci 2007;1117:181–95.
25. Sondergaard BC, Wulf H, Henriksen K, et al. Calcitonin directly attenuates collagen type II degradation by inhibition of matrix metalloproteinase expression and activity in articular chondrocytes. Osteoarthritis Cartilage 2006;14(8):759–68.
26. Nielsen RH, Bay-Jensen AC, Byrjalsen I, et al. Oral salmon calcitonin reduces cartilage and bone pathology in an osteoarthritis rat model with increased subchondral bone turnover. Osteoarthritis Cartilage 2011;19(4):466–73.
27. Sondergaard BC, Catala-Lehnen P, Huebner AK, et al. Mice over-expressing salmon calcitonin have strongly attenuated osteoarthritic histopathological changes after destabilization of the medial meniscus. Osteoarthritis Cartilage 2012;20(2): 136–43.
28. Karsdal MA, Alexandersen P, John MR, et al. Oral calcitonin demonstrated symptom-modifying efficacy and increased cartilage volume: results from a 2-year phase 3 trial in patients with osteoarthritis of the knee. Osteoarthritis Cartilage 2011;19(Suppl 1):S35.
29. Cao Y, Jones G, Cicuttini F, et al. Vitamin D supplementation in the management of knee osteoarthritis: study protocol for a randomized controlled trial. Trials 2012; 13(1):131.
30. Abramson SB, Amin AR, Clancy RM, et al. The role of nitric oxide in tissue destruction. Best Pract Res Clin Rheumatol 2001;15:831–45.
31. Pelletier JP, Jovanovic D, Fernandes JC, et al. Reduced progression of experimental osteoarthritis in vivo by selective inhibition of inducible nitric oxide synthase. Arthritis Rheum 1998;41:1275–86.

32. Pelletier JP, Jovanovic D, Fernandes JC, et al. Selective inhibition of iNOS in experimental OA is associated with reduction in tissue levels of catabolic factors. J Rheumatol 1999;26:2002–14.

33. Pelletier J-P, Jovanovic DV, Lascau-Coman V, et al. Selective inhibition of inducible nitric oxide synthase reduces progression of experimental osteoarthritis in vivo: possible link with the reduction in chondrocyte apoptosis and caspase 3 level. Arthritis Rheum 2000;43:1290–9.

34. Hellio le Graverand MP, Clemmer RS, Redifer P, et al. A 2-year randomised, double-blind, placebo-controlled, multicentre study of oral selective iNOS inhibitor, cindunistat (SD-6010), in patients with symptomatic osteoarthritis of the knee. Ann Rheum Dis 2012. [Epub ahead of print].

35. Berenbaum F. Targeted therapies in osteoarthritis: a systematic review of the trials on www.clinicaltrials.gov. Best Pract Res Clin Rheumatol 2010;24:107–19.

36. Matthews GL, Hunter DJ. Emerging drugs for osteoarthritis. Expert Opin Emerg Drugs 2011;16(3):479–91.

37. Ellsworth JL, Berry J, Bukowski T, et al. Fibroblast growth factor-18 is a trophic factor for mature chondrocytes and their progenitors. Osteoarthritis Cartilage 2002;10:308–20.

38. Davidson D, Blanc A, Filion D, et al. Fibroblast growth factor (FGF) 18 signals through FGF receptor 3 to promote chondrogenesis. J Biol Chem 2005;280: 20509–15.

39. Moore EE, Bendele AM, Thompson DL, et al. Fibroblast growth factor-18 stimulates chondrogenesis and cartilage repair in a rat model of injury-induced osteoarthritis. Osteoarthritis Cartilage 2005;13:623.

40. McPherson R, Flechsenhar K, Hellot S, et al. A randomized, double-blind, placebo-controlled, multicenter study of rhFGF18 administered intraarticularly using single or multiple ascending doses in patients with primary knee osteoarthritis (OA), not expected to require knee surgery within 1 year. Abstracts of the 2011 World Congress on Osteoarthritis. Osteoarthritis Cartilage 2011; 19(Suppl 1):S35.

41. Sandell LJ, Xing X, Franz C, et al. Exuberant expression of chemokine genes by adult human articular chondrocytes in response to IL-1beta. Osteoarthritis Cartilage 2008;16(12):1560–71.

42. Chubinskaya S, Merrihew C, Cs-Szabo G, et al. Human articular chondrocytes express osteogenic protein-I. J Histochem Cytochem 2000;48(2):239–50.

43. Huch K, Wilbrink B, Flechtenmacher J, et al. Effects of recombinant human osteogenic protein1 on the production of proteoglycan, prostaglandin E2, and interleukin-I receptor antagonist by human articular chondrocytes cultured in the presence of interleukin-1. Arthritis Rheum 1997;40:2157–61.

44. Koepp HE, Sampath KT, Kuettner KE, et al. Osteogenic protein-1 (OP-I) blocks cartilage damage caused by fibronectin fragments and promotes repair by enhancing proteoglycan synthesis. Inflamm Res 1999;47:1–6.

45. Le Graverand-Gastineau MP. Disease modifying osteoarthritis drugs: facing development challenges and choosing molecular targets. Curr Drug Targets 2010;11(5):528–35.

46. Botha-Scheepers S, Kloppenburg M, Kroon HM, et al. Fixed flexion knee radiography: the sensitivity to detect knee joint space narrowing in osteoarthritis. Osteoarthritis Cartilage 2007;15(3):350–3.

47. Hunter DJ. Risk stratification for knee osteoarthritis progression: a narrative review. Osteoarthritis Cartilage 2009;17(11):1402–7.

48. Belo JN, Berger MY, Reijman M, et al. Prognostic factors of progression of osteoarthritis of the knee: a systematic review of observational studies. Arthritis Rheum 2007;57(1):13–26.

49. Hellio Le Graverand MP, Buck RJ, Wyman BT, et al. Change in regional cartilage morphology and joint space width in osteoarthritis participants versus healthy controls – a multicenter study using 3.0 Tesla MRI and Lyon Schuss radiography. Ann Rheum Dis 2010;69:155–62.

50. Duryea J, Neumann G, Niu J, et al. Comparison of radiographic joint space width with magnetic resonance imaging cartilage morphometry: analysis of longitudinal data from the Osteoarthritis Initiative. Arthritis Care Res (Hoboken) 2010;62(7): 932–7.

51. Crema MD, Roemer FW, Guermazi A. Magnetic resonance imaging in knee osteoarthritis research: semiquantitative and compositional assessment. Magn Reson Imaging Clin N Am 2011;19(2):295–321.

52. US Department of Health and Human Services, Food and Drug Administration, Center for Drug Evaluation and Research (CDER), Center for Biologics Evaluation and Research (CBER), and Center for Devices and Radiological Health (CDRH). Guidance for Industry Clinical Development Programs for drugs, devices, and biological products intended for the treatment of osteoarthritis (OA). July 1999. Available at: www.fda.gov/downloads/Drugs/GuidanceComplianceRegulatory Information/Guidances/UCM071577.pdf. Accessed November 28, 2012.

Nonarthroplasty Hip Surgery for Early Osteoarthritis

Stephanie Y. Pun, MD[a],*, John M. O'Donnell, MBBS, FRACS[b],
Young-Jo Kim, MD, PhD[c]

KEYWORDS

- Hip osteoarthritis • Acetabular dysplasia • Femoroacetabular impingement
- Hip arthroscopy

KEY POINTS

- The most favorable mechanical environment for the hip is one that is free of both instability and impingement, creating a concentric articulation with optimum femoral head coverage by the acetabulum.
- Anatomic variations such as acetabular dysplasia with associated instability, and femoroacetabular impingement with abnormal constraint, will lead to abnormal joint mechanics, articular damage, and osteoarthritis.
- Surgical techniques such as periacetabular osteotomies, and femoral and acetabular osteoplasties enable correction of anatomic variations that cause mechanical damage to the hip joint, thereby potentially preventing or delaying development of osteoarthritis and subsequent need for joint replacement.

INTRODUCTION

Osteoarthritis (OA) is thought to be caused by a combination of intrinsic vulnerabilities of the joint, such as anatomic shape and alignment, and modulatory factors, such as body weight, injury, and activity level.[1] The current concept of the mechanical cause of hip OA is that anatomic variations create an unfavorable mechanical environment for the hip, leading to joint damage. OA is rarely considered purely idiopathic in this framework, and this observation is supported by previous studies. Aronson[2] noted that 43% of his population of OA hips had developmental dysplasia of the hip (DDH), 22% had Perthes disease, 11% had slipped capital femoral epiphysis (SCFE), and only 12% were classified as idiopathic. Even earlier, Murray,[3] Stulberg,[4] and Harris[5] recognized

[a] Young Adult and Adolescent Hip Unit, Harvard Medical School, Children's Hospital Boston, 300 Longwood Avenue, Hunnewell II, Boston, MA 02115, USA; [b] University of Melbourne, 21 Erin Street, Richmond, Melbourne, Victoria 3121, Australia; [c] Department of Orthopedic Surgery, Harvard Medical School, Children's Hospital Boston, 300 Longwood Avenue, Hunnewell II, Boston, MA 02115, USA
* Corresponding author.
E-mail address: stephanie.pun@childrens.harvard.edu

Rheum Dis Clin N Am 39 (2013) 189–202
http://dx.doi.org/10.1016/j.rdc.2012.11.004
0889-857X/13/$ – see front matter © 2013 Elsevier Inc. All rights reserved.

that prominence of the femoral head-neck junction, or the pistol grip deformity of the proximal femur, predisposed to OA.

Population-based studies on hip OA have shown some role for mild dysplasia as a significant risk factor.[6,7] Work by Ganz and colleagues[8–13] and others,[14] showed that subtle anatomic abnormalities of the hip, such as acetabular retroversion, acetabular overcoverage, and decreased head-neck offset of the femoral head-neck junction, are clinically significant anatomic variants that may lead to pain, intra-articular damage, and eventual OA in the young adult population. The limiting factor in treatment outcome in many mechanically compromised hips is the amount of cartilage damage that has occurred before treatment. Therefore, it is critical to understand and recognize the signs and symptoms of these painful hips in a timely fashion.

A useful paradigm for thinking about the mechanical function of the hip, as it relates to the development of OA, is that the most favorable mechanical environment of the hip is one that is free of both instability and impingement. Long-lasting and pain-free function of the hip joint requires a concentric articulation with optimum femoral head coverage by the acetabulum (**Fig. 1**A). Hip dysplasia represents an anatomic deformity in which the basic pathologic mechanical abnormality is instability. Lack of femoral head coverage (see **Fig. 1**B) in acetabular dysplasia can lead to hip instability and overloading of the articular cartilage, which can lead to joint damage.

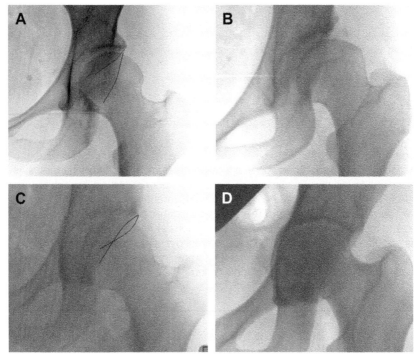

Fig. 1. Range of acetabular morphologies. (*A*) Normal hip joint should be concentric and spherical with the anterior and posterior acetabular edges (*outlined in black*) meeting at the lateral edge of the acetabulum. The weight-bearing surface, or sourcil, should be horizontal. (*B*) In the dysplastic hip, the sourcil is oblique and femoral head coverage by the acetabulum is insufficient. (*C*) In the retroverted acetabulum, the anterior lip of the acetabulum crosses the posterior lip over the femoral head. (*D*) Acetabular protrusio is characterized by femoral head medial to the ilioischial line and excessive acetabular coverage.

In contrast, femoroacetabular impingement represents an anatomic deformity at the other end of the mechanical spectrum, in which the primary mechanical disorder is abnormal constraint to normal hip motion. Overcoverage of the femoral head by the acetabulum anteriorly in acetabular retroversion (see **Fig. 1**C) or globally as in acetabular protrusio (see **Fig. 1**D) can lead to pincer-type impingement between the prominent acetabular rim and the femoral head-neck junction. A static form of impingement is seen in conditions such as Perthes disease, in which the articular surfaces are incongruent. A dynamic form of impingement is seen in subtler cases of aspherical femoral heads or prominent femoral head-neck junctions, in which the incongruency may only occur in certain positions of the hip.[8] The femoral CAM deformities can be subtle and only detected on lateral radiographs. Normal hips have a spherical femoral head on the anteroposterior (**Fig. 2**A) and lateral views (see **Fig. 2**B). If the femoral head-neck junction is too broad or aspherical (see **Fig. 2**C, D), this can lead to

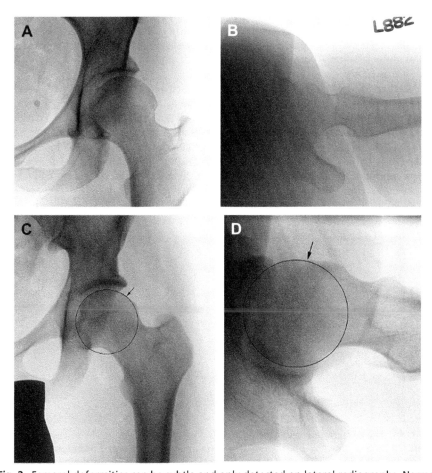

Fig. 2. Femoral deformities can be subtle and only detected on lateral radiographs. Normal hip should have a spherical head both on the anteroposterior (*A*) and lateral views (*B*). CAM-type impingement is caused by an aspherical femoral head, which is protrudes from the edges of a best-fit circle (*in black*) superimposed on femoral head. CAM deformity is subtly seen on the anterioposterior view (*C*) but best seen on the lateral view (*D*).

CAM-type impingement and pain. Therefore, all of these anatomic variations along this spectrum must be recognized to fully evaluate and treat the painful hip.

ANATOMIC ABNORMALITIES: DYSPLASIA AND INSTABILITY
Acetabular Dysplasia

Acetabular dysplasia is shallowness of the acetabulum and obliquity of the weight-bearing zone, leading to overloading of the acetabular cartilage, labral tears, and OA. It is often a component of DDH, which predominantly affects women. Patients with residual DDH as an adult may have been treated as an infant for either a dislocated or dysplastic hip with apparent success. However, many adults with symptomatic acetabular dysplasia have no history of clinical abnormality before adulthood.

Patients often present with anterior groin pain and sensations of instability during activities such as walking. Patients may also describe or demonstrate clicking or snapping of the hip with range of motion. Physical examination may show variable changes in range of motion. There may be a positive anterior impingement test with the hip in flexion and internal rotation, particularly if the labrum has been injured. Patients may also have a positive anterior apprehension test with the hip in extension and external rotation. There may be hip abductor weakness, an abductor lurch with ambulation, or a positive Trendelenburg sign.[15]

Acetabular dysplasia can range from the most severe form, which can result in a subluxated or dislocated hip, to subtle variants that may go unrecognized for a long period of time. The lateral acetabular deficiency is the most commonly recognized abnormality in acetabular dysplasia and is measured as the lateral center-edge angle (LCEA) (**Fig. 3**A). However, anterior deficiency as quantified by the anterior center-edge angle of Lequesne (ACEA), seen on the false profile view (see **Fig. 3**B), is also important to evaluate, because anterior deficiency is more severe than lateral deficiency in some hips.[16]

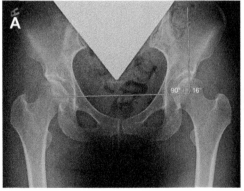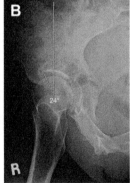

Fig. 3. (A) The center-edge angle of Wiberg is a measure of femoral head coverage. It is measured by first drawing a horizontal line connecting the centers of both femoral heads. The center-edge angle is subtended by a vertical line perpendicular to the horizontal line and a line connecting the center of the femoral head and the lateral edge of the weight-bearing dome of the acetabulum. (B) The anterior center-edge angle of Lequesne is measured on the false profile view of the hip. It is the angle subtended by a vertical line from the center of the femoral head and a line connecting the center of the femoral head and the anterior edge of the weight-bearing dome of the acetabulum.

Among the anatomic deformities of the hip that lead to OA, the natural history of acetabular dysplasia is the best understood. Wiberg[17] postulated that an LCEA less than 20° is abnormal. Murphy and colleagues[18] later showed that no hips with an LCEA less than 16° survived into the sixth decade of life without OA. Thus, symptomatic hips with an LCEA of less than 20° are generally considered for surgical intervention such as periacetabular osteotomy (PAO) to reorient the acetabulum and to provide more femoral head coverage.

Hip Instability and Borderline Dysplasia

A more recent focus of research has been the identification and treatment of hips that are not grossly dysplastic by traditional definitions but still behave in an unstable manner. Patients with hip instability may have underlying connective tissue disorders or generalized ligamentous laxity, and may describe a history of past events of subluxation or a sensation of instability during physical activities.[19–21] Hips with an LCEA between 20° and 25° are considered borderline dysplastic, especially if patients are symptomatic. If instability or borderline dysplasia is suspected, assessing the anterior coverage with a radiographic false profile view is important to rule out undercoverage of the femoral head anteriorly and instability in that anatomic plane. Arthroscopic studies have shown that, in instances of instability, the pattern of labral damage is typically more anterior and medial.[20]

The challenge in treating these patients is deciding whether a soft tissue procedure such as labral repair and capsular plication is sufficient, or whether the underlying structure of the acetabulum is sufficiently dysplastic that bony reorientation is necessary. Arthroscopic labral debridement,[22] labral repair,[23–26] and labral reconstructions,[27–29] with either thermal[30] or suture capsular plication[31] to address hip instability, have been described with success in short-term follow-up studies, but further studies on the long-term effects of such procedures are necessary.

ANATOMIC ABNORMALITIES: FEMOROACETABULAR IMPINGEMENT

Femoroacetabular impingement is a condition in which there is mechanical conflict between the femoral head-neck junction and the acetabular rim, causing intra-articular damage to the labrum and articular cartilage. This condition can either be caused by acetabular morphology, such as a deep or retroverted acetabulum causing overcoverage of the femoral head, or caused by femoral morphology, such as prominence or convexity of the femoral head-neck junction.

Coxa Profunda and Acetabular Protrusio

Although insufficient acetabular coverage leads to instability and mechanical overloading at the acetabular rim,[11] overcoverage may lead to a pincer-type impingement between the acetabular rim and the femoral head-neck junction. The acetabular overcoverage may be global and severe, as in acetabular protrusio (see **Fig. 1**D), or milder, as in coxa profunda.

Acetabular protrusio may be caused by conditions such as rheumatoid arthritis or Marfan[32] syndrome. However, most cases are idiopathic. The deep acetabulum leads to global limitation of hip motion and impingement of the femoral head-neck junction against the acetabular rim, resulting in labral degeneration/tear and pain. Patients may complain of anterior impingement as well as lateral and/or posterior impingement pain. It is generally considered that protrusio is present when the femoral head is medial to the ilioischial line.[32,33] However, the upper limits of normal femoral head coverage as measured on radiographs and the natural history of protrusio and coxa profunda are not well understood.

For deep acetabulums, safe acetabuloplasty or rim trimming through a surgical dislocation approach or arthroscopic approach have both been described. Although surgical dislocation may provide more global access to the acetabular rim, labral repair and reconstruction have been described with both approaches.

Acetabular Retroversion

Unlike acetabular protrusio and coxa profunda, which are global increases in femoral head coverage, acetabular retroversion creates isolated anterior overcoverage and anterior pincer impingement between the acetabular rim and the femoral head-neck junction, especially problematic in positions of hip flexion. Up to 33% of hips with acetabular dysplasia may also have acetabular retroversion, which must be recognized and taken into account when performing pelvic osteotomies for acetabular dysplasia.[34] In addition, acetabular retroversion is common in posttraumatic dysplasia,[35] Down syndrome,[36] SCFE,[37] and proximal femoral focal deficiency.[38] If mild, the anterior overcoverage may be addressed arthroscopically, but often the global malorientation of the acetabulum must be addressed with total acetabular reorientation, such as is achieved with a reverse PAO.[13]

CAM/Inclusion Femoroacetabular Impingement and Pistol Grip Deformity

Deformities on the femoral side can also lead to abnormal hip joint mechanics. The most commonly recognized femoral abnormality is the retrotilted femoral head or pistol grip deformity initially described by Murray.[3] This anatomic variant is thought to be a major cause of hip OA in men. Some of the pistol grip proximal femur is similar to that found in a mild SCFE and may be a developmental variant related to SCFE.[39] In severe SCFE, the prominent femoral metaphysis may be sufficiently large to cause a pincer-type impingement that crushes the acetabular labrum. In milder SCFE, the prominent metaphysis is small enough to enter the acetabulum, which may cause a greater mechanical problem for the articular cartilage than a more prominent metaphysis that is too large to enter the acetabulum; the intra-articular extent of the prominent neck causes increased loading within the joint, causing cartilage delamination[12] and OA. In addition to the pistol grip deformity, focal prominence in the head-neck junction may cause sufficient decrease in head-neck offset to cause a similar disorder.[40,41] Siebenrock and colleagues[42] showed that many CAM deformities are caused by an extension of the epiphysis onto the anterior femoral neck, which is distinct from an SCFE deformity. CAM morphology may be common in the community, with an incidence of around 30%.[43,44]

SURGICAL TREATMENT
Periacetabular Osteotomy

In North America, the predominant pelvic osteotomy performed for acetabular dysplasia is the Bernese periacetabular osteotomy.[16] This procedure preserves the pelvic ring but allows precise and full correction of even severe acetabular dysplasia. **Fig. 4** illustrates the type of correction that can be achieved with this procedure. The original procedure has been refined by Murphy and Millis[45] to protect the hip abductor muscles and hence lessen the morbidity and hasten the speed of recovery after surgery. Outcome studies have shown that this procedure is effective in relieving the early arthritic symptoms of acetabular dysplasia.

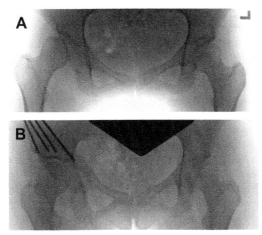

Fig. 4. Severe acetabular dysplasia is seen in the right hip (*A*) of this 19-year-old girl with hip pain. Bernese periacetabular osteotomy was performed (*B*) with improvement in hip mechanics and resolution of hip symptoms.

Murphy and colleagues[46] reported on 180 patients using the direct anterior approach. At 3-year follow-up of 88 patients, results were good and there was no abductor dysfunction. There was conversion of 2 hips to arthroplasty in the early results. Trumbe and colleagues[47] reported on 123 periacetabular osteotomies with an average increase in Harris hip score from 65 to 89 and a Merle d'Aubigné score from 13.6 to 16.3. The investigators performed approximately half of the osteotomies through an ilioinguinal approach and the others through a modified Smith-Petersen approach. More recently, Peters and colleagues[48] showed similar results with 83 periacetabular osteotomies that had an increase in Harris hip score from 54 to 87 at slightly less than 4 years of follow-up.

The short-term and long-term results predominantly depend on the amount of cartilage damage in the joint at time of surgery. The delayed gadolinium-enhanced magnetic resonance imaging (MRI) of cartilage (dGEMRIC) technique,[49] which measures the proteoglycan concentration in cartilage, can be used as a proxy to measure severity of cartilage damage and OA. Jessel and colleagues[50] showed that lower dGEMRIC indices representing more severe OA are associated with increasing age, presence of labral tear, and the severity of dysplasia. Trousdale and colleagues[51] showed that the amount of radiographic OA determines the longevity of a good result of joint-preserving surgery over time. If there is moderate to severe joint space narrowing, then the long-term outlook is guarded. The dGEMRIC technique has been used to select out poor candidates for pelvic osteotomy. The dGEMRIC index in the joint, as a surrogate marker of early OA, was the best predictor of early failure after osteotomy.[52] Using these techniques, it should be possible to reliably treat prearthritic/early arthritic joints by correcting the anatomic abnormality with a pelvic osteotomy.

The disease-modifying effect of a pelvic osteotomy for acetabular dysplasia remains an open question. Long-term follow-up studies are being pursued using biochemical imaging such as dGEMRIC to show slowing or reversal of articular cartilage damage with a pelvic osteotomy.

Safe Surgical Dislocation of the Hip

Dislocation of a native hip is traditionally thought of as a dangerous maneuver because of its association with avascular necrosis of the femoral head. Recent clarification of the vascular anatomy of the proximal femur[53,54] has allowed the development of a safe surgical dislocation technique for the hip.[55] Although there are several competing surgical techniques, such as hip arthroscopy and more traditional limited surgical exposure of the hip joint, complete safe surgical exposure of the hip joint affords many technical advantages in cases involving disorders inside and around the hip joint. Indications for the full surgical exposure of the hip joint through a dislocation technique are relative and are dictated by the risks and benefits of each individual case; they will evolve with advances in other surgical techniques.

In a series of 213 hips over 7 years, Ganz and colleagues[55] reported that a surgical dislocation of the hip can be performed safely without the development of avascular necrosis. More than 1000 hips were dislocated with the development of 1 osteonecrosis, which was thought to be caused by the trochanteric osteotomy extending into the femoral neck. There were 3 trochanteric nonunions and 1 transient sciatic nerve neuropraxia. Shore and colleagues[56] similarly showed that surgical dislocation is a safe and effective method of treating aspherical femoral head deformities in patients with healed Perthes disease. Given the many advantages that this approach provides, the complication rate seems acceptable and should decrease with surgical experience.

The surgical dislocation technique is useful in treating the femoral and acetabular abnormalities associated with femoroacetabular impingement (FAI). FAI causes chondral and labral lesions, which lead to OA of the hip (**Fig. 5**). Surgical dislocation of the

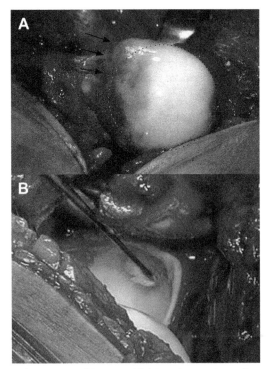

Fig. 5. The hip joint of a 20-year-old man with hip pain. At time of surgical dislocation of the hip, the femoral deformity (*A*) is noted. Plain radiographs did not show evidence of OA. The CAM-type impingement resulted in extensive articular cartilage delamination (*B*) that was seen at the time of surgery.

hip and acetabular and/or femoral osteoplasty treat the underlying bony disorder leading to impingement, which should relieve the patient's symptoms and prevent or delay further damage and degeneration of the hip. In a midterm analysis[57] (average 4.7 years' follow-up), the surgical results of 14 men and 5 women (19 hips) with a mean age of 36 years were analyzed. Using the Merle d'Aubigné score, 13 hips were rated excellent to good with a pain score improving from 2.9 to 5.1 points. Five hips with osteoarthrosis (Tönnis grade II) or severe cartilage destruction at surgery had subsequent total hip replacement. In hips without migration of the head into the acetabular cartilage defect on MRI, no additional cartilage narrowing occurred. In addition, preliminary analysis of 400 patients supports the finding that surgical dislocation with correction of FAI yields good results in patients with early degenerative changes not exceeding grade I osteoarthrosis. The North American experience has mirrored the Swiss experience, in which patients with minimal radiographic OA had good surgical outcomes after osteochondroplasty[58,59] for FAI.

Recent advances in understanding of the anatomy and function of the acetabular labrum has motivated the preservation of the labrum during surgery for FAI.[60–62] When the acetabular damage is mostly confined to the articular cartilage, the intact labrum can be detached, bony resection performed, and labrum reattached using bone anchors. The detached labrum seems to heal and may provide improved pain relief. The labrum may be repaired either through a surgical dislocation approach or hip arthroscopy.

Hip Arthroscopy

Hip arthroscopy has traditionally been used to diagnose and treat intra-articular disorders such as labral tears and ligamentum teres tears, and to remove intra-articular loose bodies such as synovial chondromatosis and posttraumatic osteochondral fragments. Arthroscopic techniques have been developed to resect both the overcovered acetabulum in pincer FAI (**Fig. 6**A, B) and the prominent bone along the femoral head-neck junction (see **Fig. 6**C, D) in CAM FAI. Newer techniques of labral reconstruction and capsular plication to decrease hip instability have been introduced more recently. Although resection of delaminated cartilage or repair of a torn labrum may provide symptomatic relief, it is essential to elucidate the reason for the soft tissue damage and to correct the underlying bony disorder, or else the risk of reinjury is high. Disorders such as dysplasia and FAI routinely cause labral tears and chondral injuries, and the underlying disorders must be addressed.[63]

Several studies have shown evidence of the clinical superiority of labral repair compared with resection. Schilders and colleagues[24] compared 96 patients (101 hips) with FAI and labral tears who had been treated arthroscopically with either labral repair or resection. At mean follow-up of 2 years, the labral repair group (group 1, 69 hips) had a mean Harris hip score (HHS) improvement that was 7.3 points greater ($P = .036$, 95% confidence interval 0.51–14.09) than in the labral resection group (group 2, 32 hips). Larson and colleagues[26] similarly showed in a case control study that, at a mean 3.5 years' follow-up, subjective outcomes were significantly improved ($P<.01$) for both groups compared with preoperative scores, but the HHS ($P = .001$), SF-12 ($P = .041$), and Visual Analog Scale (VAS) pain scores ($P = .004$) were all significantly better for the labral repair group compared with the labral resection group. As surgical techniques and familiarity with hip arthroscopy improve over time, the clinical outcomes will also likely improve.

Labral reconstruction may be considered in hips with a diminutive or degenerative labrum that precludes adequate repair. Both iliotibial band autograft[27] and ligamentum teres autograft[28] have been described in surgical techniques. In a recent study by Walker and colleagues,[29] 15 of 20 hips that underwent labral reconstruction

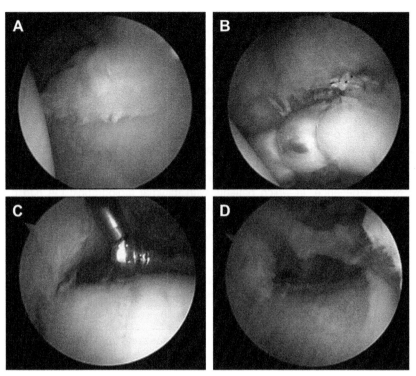

Fig. 6. Arthroscopic view of a degenerative labral tear with labral chondral separation (*A*). Arthroscopic techniques are available to repair the labrum (*B*). The cause of labral damage is often the CAM deformity on the femoral side (*C*). The anterior CAM deformity is easily resected arthroscopically (*D*).

showed subjective improvement in preoperative pain and function at minimum follow-up of 12 months. However, 3 hips in 3 patients were converted to total hip arthroplasty within 36 months of their labral reconstruction for continued preoperative pain. Longer-term follow-up studies are necessary to prove that labral reconstruction results in lasting clinical improvement and delay or prevention of OA.

Some success has also been achieved treating articular cartilage defects. Smaller defects (<2 cm^2) seem to respond well to microfracture, and larger defects have been treated with matrix autologous chondrocyte implantation and autologous matrix-induced chondrogenesis.

Capsular repair, plication, and capsulorrhaphy have been proposed as techniques to decrease iatrogenic instability of the hip after arthroscopy and to increase stability in hips with microinstability secondary to ligamentous laxity.[30,31] Although the concept of capsular repair and plication is supported by anatomic studies,[64] these surgical techniques need further study to support their clinical usefulness.

Ligamentum teres reconstruction has also been reported recently, using either synthetic ligament, semitendinosus tendon, or iliotibial band grafts.[65–67] Although results are only short term, initial marked improvement in stability has been noted.

SUMMARY

Understanding of the role of subtle anatomic abnormalities leading to mechanically induced OA is advancing quickly. These advances are primarily driven by progress in surgical technique and also by increasingly sophisticated imaging technology. To a large extent, it is possible to rectify anatomic abnormalities on the pelvic and femoral sides of the hip joint with an acceptable amount of risk and morbidity to the patient. Early results indicate that these procedures are able to relieve pain and restore function. The primary factor limiting successful outcome is the amount of cartilage damage at the time of surgery. Advanced MRI techniques are being used to help with patient selection as well as to help clinicians to understand the effect of these surgical interventions on the progression of OA in these hips. Although developments in surgical treatment have allowed the mechanical environment of the hip joint to be optimized, future biological therapies and pharmacologic disease-modifying therapies are also likely to play an important role in early treatment of hips with changes to the articular cartilage composition. In the future, when disease-modifying pharmacologic therapies or tissue-engineered cartilage therapies are available, all lessons learned in joint preservation surgery for the hip will be applicable and allow the need for prosthetic replacement in these young, active adults to be delayed.

REFERENCES

1. Felson DT. Risk factors for osteoarthritis: understanding joint vulnerability. Clin Orthop Relat Res 2004;S16–21.
2. Aronson J. Osteoarthritis of the young adult hip: etiology and treatment. Instr Course Lect 1986;35:119–28.
3. Murray RO. The aetiology of primary osteoarthritis of the hip. Br J Radiol 1965;38: 810–24.
4. Stulberg SD. Unrecognized childhood hip disease: a major cause of idiopathic osteoarthritis of the hip. In: Proceedings of the Third Open Scientific Meeting of the Hip Society. St Louis (MO): CV Mosby; 1975. p. 212–28.
5. Harris WH. Etiology of osteoarthritis of the hip. Clin Orthop Relat Res 1986; 20–33.
6. Lane NE, Lin P, Christiansen L, et al. Association of mild acetabular dysplasia with an increased risk of incident hip osteoarthritis in elderly white women: the study of osteoporotic fractures. Arthritis Rheum 2000;43:400–4.
7. Lane NE, Nevitt MC, Cooper C, et al. Acetabular dysplasia and osteoarthritis of the hip in elderly white women. Ann Rheum Dis 1997;56:627–30.
8. Ganz R, Parvizi J, Beck M, et al. Femoroacetabular impingement: a cause for osteoarthritis of the hip. Clin Orthop Relat Res 2003;112–20.
9. Eijer H, Myers SR, Ganz R. Anterior femoroacetabular impingement after femoral neck fractures. J Orthop Trauma 2001;15:475–81.
10. Myers SR, Eijer H, Ganz R. Anterior femoroacetabular impingement after periacetabular osteotomy. Clin Orthop Relat Res 1999;93–9.
11. Klaue K, Durnin CW, Ganz R. The acetabular rim syndrome. A clinical presentation of dysplasia of the hip. J Bone Joint Surg Br 1991;73:423–9.
12. Leunig M, Casillas MM, Hamlet M, et al. Slipped capital femoral epiphysis: early mechanical damage to the acetabular cartilage by a prominent femoral metaphysis. Acta Orthop Scand 2000;71:370–5.
13. Siebenrock KA, Schoeniger R, Ganz R. Anterior femoro-acetabular impingement due to acetabular retroversion. Treatment with periacetabular osteotomy. J Bone Joint Surg Am 2003;85:278–86.
14. Reynolds D, Lucas J, Klaue K. Retroversion of the acetabulum. A cause of hip pain. J Bone Joint Surg Br 1999;81:281–8.

15. Martin HD, Kelly BT, Leunig M, et al. The pattern and technique in the clinical evaluation of the adult hip: the common physical examination tests of hip specialists. Arthroscopy 2010;26:161–72.

16. Ganz R, Klaue K, Vinh TS, et al. A new periacetabular osteotomy for the treatment of hip dysplasias. Technique and preliminary results. Clin Orthop Relat Res 1988;26–36.

17. Wiberg G. Studies on dysplastic acetabula and congenital subluxation of the hip joint. With special reference to the complication of osteo-arthritis. Acta Chirurgiae Scandanavica 1939;83:5–135.

18. Murphy SB, Ganz R, Müller ME. The prognosis in untreated dysplasia of the hip. A study of radiographic factors that predict the outcome. J Bone Joint Surg Am 1995;77:985–9.

19. Bellabarba C, Sheinkop MB, Kuo KN. Idiopathic hip instability. An unrecognized cause of coxa saltans in the adult. Clin Orthop Relat Res 1998;261–71.

20. Shu B, Safran MR. Hip instability: anatomic and clinical considerations of traumatic and atraumatic instability. Clin Sports Med 2011;30:349–67.

21. Smith MV, Sekiya JK. Hip instability. Sports Med Arthrosc 2010;18:108–12.

22. Philippon M, Schenker M, Briggs K, et al. Femoroacetabular impingement in 45 professional athletes: associated pathologies and return to sport following arthroscopic decompression. Knee Surg Sports Traumatol Arthrosc 2007;15:908–14.

23. Philippon MJ, Weiss DR, Kuppersmith DA, et al. Arthroscopic labral repair and treatment of femoroacetabular impingement in professional hockey players. Am J Sports Med 2010;38:99–104.

24. Schilders E, Dimitrakopoulou A, Bismil Q, et al. Arthroscopic treatment of labral tears in femoroacetabular impingement a comparative study of refixation and resection with a minimum two-year follow-up. J Bone Joint Surg Br 2011;93:1027–32.

25. Larson CM, Giveans MR. Arthroscopic debridement versus refixation of the acetabular labrum associated with femoroacetabular impingement. Arthroscopy 2009;25:369–76.

26. Larson CM, Giveans MR, Stone RM. Arthroscopic debridement versus refixation of the acetabular labrum associated with femoroacetabular impingement: mean 3.5-year follow-up. Am J Sports Med 2012;40:1015–21.

27. Philippon MJ, Briggs KK, Hay CJ, et al. Arthroscopic labral reconstruction in the hip using iliotibial band autograft: technique and early outcomes. Arthroscopy 2010;26:750–6.

28. Sierra RJ, Trousdale RT. Labral reconstruction using the ligamentum teres capitis: report of a new technique. Clin Orthop Relat Res 2009;467:753–9.

29. Walker J, Pagnotto M, Trousdale R, et al. Preliminary pain and function after labral reconstruction during femoroacetabular impingement surgery. Clin Orthop Relat Res 2012;470(12):3414–20.

30. Philippon MJ. The role of arthroscopic thermal capsulorrhaphy in the hip. Clin Sports Med 2001;20:817–29.

31. Domb BG, Giordano BD, Philippon MJ. Arthroscopic capsulotomy, capsular repair, and capsular plication of the hip: relation to atraumatic instability. Arthroscopy 2012. [Epub ahead of print].

32. Wenger DR, Ditkoff TJ, Herring JA, et al. Protrusio acetabuli in Marfan's syndrome. Clin Orthop Relat Res 1980;134–8.

33. Clohisy JC, Carlisle JC, Beaule PE, et al. A systematic approach to the plain radiographic evaluation of the young adult hip. J Bone Joint Surg Am 2008;90(Suppl 4): 47–66.

34. Li PL, Ganz R. Morphologic features of congenital acetabular dysplasia: one in six is retroverted. Clin Orthop Relat Res 2003;245–53.

35. Dora C, Zurbach J, Hersche O, et al. Pathomorphologic characteristics of post-traumatic acetabular dysplasia. J Orthop Trauma 2000;14:483–9.

36. Sankar WN, Schoenecker JG, Mayfield ME, et al. Acetabular retroversion in Down syndrome. J Pediatr Orthop 2012;32:277–81.

37. Sankar WN, Brighton BK, Kim Y-J, et al. Acetabular morphology in slipped capital femoral epiphysis. J Pediatr Orthop 2011;31:254–8.

38. Dora C, Bühler M, Stover MD, et al. Morphologic characteristics of acetabular dysplasia in proximal femoral focal deficiency. J Pediatr Orthop B 2004;13:81–7.

39. Goodman DA, Feighan JE, Smith AD, et al. Subclinical slipped capital femoral epiphysis. Relationship to osteoarthrosis of the hip. J Bone Joint Surg Am 1997;79:1489–97.

40. Nötzli HP, Wyss TF, Stoecklin CH, et al. The contour of the femoral head-neck junction as a predictor for the risk of anterior impingement. J Bone Joint Surg Br 2002;84:556–60.

41. Ito K, Minka MA 2nd, Leunig M, et al. Femoroacetabular impingement and the cam-effect. A MRI-based quantitative anatomical study of the femoral head-neck offset. J Bone Joint Surg Br 2001;83:171–6.

42. Siebenrock KA, Wahab KH, Werlen S, et al. Abnormal extension of the femoral head epiphysis as a cause of cam impingement. Clin Orthop Relat Res 2004;54–60.

43. Gosvig KK, Jacobsen S, Sonne-Holm S, et al. Prevalence of malformations of the hip joint and their relationship to sex, groin pain, and risk of osteoarthritis: a population-based survey. J Bone Joint Surg Am 2010;92:1162–9.

44. Jung KA, Restrepo C, Hellman M, et al. The prevalence of cam-type femoroacetabular deformity in asymptomatic adults. J Bone Joint Surg Br 2011;93:1303–7.

45. Murphy SB, Millis MB. Periacetabular osteotomy without abductor dissection using direct anterior exposure. Clin Orthop Relat Res 1999;92–8.

46. Murphy SB, Millis MB, Hall JE. Surgical correction of acetabular dysplasia in the adult. A Boston experience. Clin Orthop Relat Res 1999;38–44.

47. Trumble SJ, Mayo KA, Mast JW. The periacetabular osteotomy. Minimum 2 year followup in more than 100 hips. Clin Orthop Relat Res 1999;54–63.

48. Peters CL, Erickson JA, Hines JL. Early results of the Bernese periacetabular osteotomy: the learning curve at an academic medical center. J Bone Joint Surg Am 2006;88:1920–6.

49. Burstein D, Velyvis J, Scott KT, et al. Protocol issues for delayed Gd(DTPA)(2-)-enhanced MRI (dGEMRIC) for clinical evaluation of articular cartilage. Magn Reson Med 2001;45:36–41.

50. Jessel RH, Zurakowski D, Zilkens C, et al. Radiographic and patient factors associated with pre-radiographic osteoarthritis in hip dysplasia. J Bone Joint Surg Am 2009;91:1120–9.

51. Trousdale RT, Ekkernkamp A, Ganz R, et al. Periacetabular and intertrochanteric osteotomy for the treatment of osteoarthrosis in dysplastic hips. J Bone Joint Surg Am 1995;77:73–85.

52. Cunningham T, Jessel R, Zurakowski D, et al. Delayed gadolinium-enhanced magnetic resonance imaging of cartilage to predict early failure of Bernese periacetabular osteotomy for hip dysplasia. J Bone Joint Surg Am 2006;88:1540–8.

53. Gautier E, Ganz K, Krügel N, et al. Anatomy of the medial femoral circumflex artery and its surgical implications. J Bone Joint Surg Br 2000;82:679–83.

54. Shore BJ, Millis MB, Kim Y-J. Vascular safe zones for surgical dislocation in children with healed Legg-Calvé-Perthes disease. J Bone Joint Surg Am 2012;94: 721–7.
55. Ganz R, Gill TJ, Gautier E, et al. Surgical dislocation of the adult hip a technique with full access to the femoral head and acetabulum without the risk of avascular necrosis. J Bone Joint Surg Br 2001;83:1119–24.
56. Shore BJ, Novais EN, Millis MB, et al. Low early failure rates using a surgical dislocation approach in healed Legg-Calvé-Perthes disease. Clin Orthop Relat Res 2012;470:2441–9.
57. Beck M, Leunig M, Parvizi J, et al. Anterior femoroacetabular impingement: part II. Midterm results of surgical treatment. Clin Orthop Relat Res 2004;418:67–73.
58. Murphy S, Tannast M, Kim Y-J, et al. Debridement of the adult hip for femoroacetabular impingement: indications and preliminary clinical results. Clin Orthop Relat Res 2004;178–81.
59. Beaulé PE, Le Duff MJ, Zaragoza E. Quality of life following femoral head-neck osteochondroplasty for femoroacetabular impingement. J Bone Joint Surg Am 2007;89:773–9.
60. Ferguson SJ, Bryant JT, Ganz R, et al. An in vitro investigation of the acetabular labral seal in hip joint mechanics. J Biomech 2003;36:171–8.
61. Ferguson SJ, Bryant JT, Ganz R, et al. The influence of the acetabular labrum on hip joint cartilage consolidation: a poroelastic finite element model. J Biomech 2000;33:953–60.
62. Ferguson SJ, Bryant JT, Ganz R, et al. The acetabular labrum seal: a poroelastic finite element model. Clin Biomech (Bristol, Avon) 2000;15:463–8.
63. Wenger DE, Kendell KR, Miner MR, et al. Acetabular labral tears rarely occur in the absence of bony abnormalities. Clin Orthop Relat Res 2004;145–50.
64. Telleria JJ, Lindsey DP, Giori NJ, et al. An anatomic arthroscopic description of the hip capsular ligaments for the hip arthroscopist. Arthroscopy 2011;27: 628–36.
65. Simpson JM, Field RE, Villar RN. Arthroscopic reconstruction of the ligamentum teres. Arthroscopy 2011;27:436–41.
66. Amenabar T, O'Donnell J. Arthroscopic ligamentum teres reconstruction using semitendinosus tendon: surgical technique and an unusual outcome. Arthroscopy Techniques 2012, in press.
67. Philippon MJ, Pennock A, Gaskill TR. Arthroscopic reconstruction of the ligamentum teres: technique and early outcomes. J Bone Joint Surg Br 2012;94:1494–8.

Surgery for Osteoarthritis of the Knee

John C. Richmond, MD

KEYWORDS

- Knee • Osteoarthritis • Surgery • Arthroscopy • Osteotomy • Arthroplasty

KEY POINTS

- The indications for arthroscopy have narrowed.
- Orthopedic surgeons continue to explore surgical options less invasive than total knee replacement for isolated unicompartmental arthritis of the knee joint, including arthroscopic meniscectomy, grafting of symptomatic areas of bone marrow lesions, unloading osteotomy, and unicompartmental knee replacement.
- Current total knee arthroplasty designs can be expected to survive 20 years or more in the older, less active population. New materials may extend that survivorship.

When more conservative modalities of management for knee osteoarthritis (OA) are no longer or not effective, then surgery is usually indicated. Currently available surgical techniques for the treatment of OA of the knee range from arthroscopy to total joint arthroplasty. These techniques include procedures regarded as less invasive than total joint arthroplasty, including osteotomies and joint-preserving unicompartmental replacements. Total joint arthroplasty of either the hip or the knee has been demonstrated to be one of the most cost-effective medical interventions available (**Fig. 1**). A recent study from Europe has confirmed again that total knee arthroplasty is a more cost-effective medical intervention than coronary artery bypass surgery.[1] Total joint arthroplasty is one of the most studied treatments in OA because of the very high volume of joint replacements performed (more than 600,000 total knee replacements are performed each year in the United States, and the number is increasing annually).[2] This high volume and the significant expense of the procedure have resulted in many well-performed studies investigating the long-term survivorship and effectiveness of this intervention in treating OA of the knee. Although total knee replacement remains an excellent procedure in the older population (>70 years of age), there are significant issues concerning the long-term durability of total knee arthroplasty in the younger

The author has nothing to disclose.
Department of Orthopedic Surgery, New England Baptist Hospital, 125 Parker Hill Avenue, Boston, MA 02120, USA
E-mail address: jrichmon@nebh.org

Rheum Dis Clin N Am 39 (2013) 203–211
http://dx.doi.org/10.1016/j.rdc.2012.10.008   rheumatic.theclinics.com
0889-857X/13/$ – see front matter © 2013 Elsevier Inc. All rights reserved.

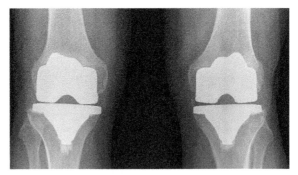

Fig. 1. Bilateral total knee arthroplasties, an extremely cost-effective treatment for end-stage osteoarthritis of the knee, noted for high durability and excellent long-term survival.

population (<55 years of age). One long-term study of more than 10,000 total knees demonstrated the failure of total knee replacement at 10 years was approximately 3 times higher in the population under the age of 55 years than in the population over the age of 70 years (15% vs 6%).[3] With this significantly higher risk of failure, multiple other alternative treatments often are recommended in this younger age group. This article reviews the alternative surgical treatments to total knee arthroplasty, including arthroscopy, a new grafting procedure for subchondral edema, osteotomy, and unicompartmental arthroplasty.

ARTHROSCOPY

Arthroscopic treatment in OA can range from lavage only to more complicated procedures that include removal of frayed articular cartilage (chondroplasty or debridement), removal of unstable meniscal tears and loose bodies, and synovectomy for hypertrophic synovium. For the first 25 years of arthroscopic surgery in the United States, debridement and/or lavage of the osteoarthritic knee was an accepted treatment, with little challenge as to its efficacy. In 2002, however, Moseley and colleagues[4] published a controlled trial of arthroscopic debridement/lavage versus sham surgery for OA of the knee in *The New England Journal of Medicine*. This study, albeit imperfect, demonstrated that placebo surgery was as effective as lavage or debridement for the osteoarthritic knee. Following that article, 2 additional randomized controlled trials failed to demonstrate the benefit of arthroscopic lavage with meniscal and/or chondral debridement in OA over conservative care.[5,6] Any beneficial effect demonstrated by either of these treatments for painful OA of the knee without mechanical symptoms is likely related to the cyclic nature of the symptoms in OA or to the placebo effect.[7]

There are, however, times when arthroscopic treatment of the osteoarthritic joint can be of benefit, particularly in that patient who has relatively mild to moderate OA and a mechanically significant meniscal tear or loose body causing locking, buckling, or catching.[8,9] In these cases, the surgery is not performed for the OA but rather to treat the mechanical derangement. More severe OA does less well than mild or moderate OA when treated arthroscopically. When preoperative weight-bearing views demonstrate bone on bone in an involved compartment, arthroscopy has a limited role. Arthroscopic removal of impinging osteophytes that block full extension and removal of significant areas of synovitis that are causing recurrent effusions have been beneficial in published case series.[10]

Over the past decade, bone marrow lesions (**Fig. 2**) have been recognized a significant pain generator in the osteoarthritic knee.[11,12] Sharkey and colleagues[13] have
developed a minimally invasive technique used in conjunction with arthroscopy to
treat these bone marrow lesions. Using fluoroscopic guidance and a spatial frame
to position a small cannula into the lesion, liquid calcium phosphate bone substitute
is injected. This liquid calcium phosphate bone substitute rapidly hardens at body
temperature and its osteoconductive properties promote healing of the lesion.
Although it is very early in its evaluation, the results are promising, but further
follow-up is needed.

In summary, for OA of the knee, the author recommends arthroscopic surgery be
considered only in patients who have mild to moderate OA as demonstrated radiographically on the Kellgren-Lawrence scale and symptoms suggestive of mechanical
derangement. Secondary indications for arthroscopy in more advanced OA (Kellgren-
Lawrence stage 3) are the presence of anterior osteophytes in the intercondylar notch
that block extension or significant synovitis, leading to recurrent effusions. In these
cases, resection of the osteophytes to regain extension and major synovectomy to
reduce the recurrent effusions has proven beneficial and may delay more invasive
surgery. Finally, those patients with OA of the knee and significant bone marrow
lesions may benefit from minimally invasive grafting of the lesions with a calcium phosphate bone substitute.

OSTEOTOMY

Unicompartmental OA can exist in any of the 3 compartments (medial, lateral, or patellofemoral) of the joint. It is most common in the varus knee, involving the medial
compartment. The data as to efficacy and long-term outcomes following osteotomy
are much better established for the medial compartment than for the lateral or patellofemoral compartments. Osteotomy to unload an overloaded compartment was first
described in the 1960s for the medial compartment and in the 1970s for the patellofemoral compartment. Osteotomy for the treatment of lateral compartment tibiofemoral
OA has been much less widely studied.

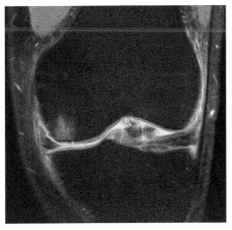

Fig. 2. Fat-suppressed coronal magnetic resonance image demonstrating bone marrow
lesion (high signal) in the medial femoral condyle of a patient with mild OA of the knee.

THE VARUS KNEE WITH MEDIAL COMPARTMENT ARTHROSIS

Osteotomy typically has been considered for a younger and more active population than joint replacement arthroplasty, where their high level of activity may result in premature failure of the prosthesis.[3] It is recommended specifically for this group so that these patients can continue with high-impact, strenuous work or recreational activities. There is consensus that high-impact activities are deleterious after joint replacement arthroplasty and may lead to precocious failure of the implant through wear of the polyethylene and potential loosening of the prosthesis. It has been recommended that nothing more strenuous than cycling, low-impact aerobics, cross-country or light downhill skiing, or doubles tennis be performed following joint replacement arthroplasty.[14] Patients desirous of maintaining a more strenuous and active lifestyle, independent of age, can be considered for osteotomy when they have isolated unicompartmental disease. The Cochrane Review of valgus high tibial osteotomies concluded that these procedures improve function and reduce pain.[15] The reviewers concluded there was insufficient evidence to support osteotomy over unicompartmental arthroplasty. As noted previously, however, osteotomy should be preferred in the more vigorously active younger person desirous of strenuous work or athletic endeavors.

Identification of candidates for osteotomy requires long leg alignment views to determine the axis of weight-bearing of the extremity as well as weight-bearing films of the knees performed both in the anterior-posterior direction with the knee in full extension and in the posterior-anterior direction with the knee flexed ("Rosenberg views").[16] When the weight-bearing axis falls in the medial compartment, valgus high tibial osteotomy is an appropriate procedure. The goal of the procedure is to unload the damaged compartment and transfer weight-bearing to the well-maintained lateral compartment. The combination of this mechanical overload of the noninvolved compartment and the destructive processes involved in OA ultimately leads to progression of the OA to involve the remainder of the joint, eventually necessitating total joint arthroplasty in the future.

There are multiple techniques for valgus-producing high tibial osteotomies as well as many different ways to fix these postoperatively. None has proved superior to the others. There are few direct comparative studies in the literature, and few meaningful differences have been demonstrated.[17,18] A closing wedge osteotomy, in which a wedge of bone is removed laterally from the tibia, with internal fixation using hardware, has the longest track record. There is detailed information about the durability of this osteotomy and the ease of revision to total joint arthroplasty when the osteotomy ultimately fails because of the progression of the arthritis. Available data within the literature indicate there is at least a 50% 10-year rate of success for osteotomy before revision to total knee replacement.[19] Newer techniques for performing and for fixing the osteotomy have proven more durable, with Pinczewski's group from Australia reporting a nearly 80% 10-year survival, with more than 50% holding up for 15 years.[20] Revisions of osteotomies performed with modern techniques of fixation to total knee arthroplasty when the OA progresses have results comparable with those of primary total knee arthroplasties.[21]

PATELLOFEMORAL OSTEOARTHRITIS

Isolated OA of the patellofemoral joint is not a common problem. Recognition of this condition is based on patellofemoral symptoms, with significant damage to the articular surface noted on plain radiographs, magnetic resonance imaging scanning, or arthroscopy, with preservation of the tibiofemoral articulation. In the past, treatment of this condition has included patellectomy. Patellectomy has fallen out of favor because of the potential loss of quadriceps strength and the need for a functioning patella to have optimal results with later total knee arthroplasty. Elevation of the tibial tubercle to decrease joint reactive forces across the patellofemoral joint was performed first in the 1960s and 1970s.[22] It has become a reliable alternative treatment when reasonable articular surface remains and the areas of most severe cartilage breakdown or exposed bone can be unloaded appropriately.[23] Because there is a spectrum from chondromalacia patella and patellar instability to patellofemoral arthrosis, there are no meaningful data in the literature to define accurately the indications or predictors for long-term success of procedures designed to unload the osteoarthritic patellofemoral joint by elevation of the tibial tubercle.

THE VALGUS KNEE WITH LATERAL COMPARTMENT OSTEOARTHRITIS

Significantly less information is available in the literature for treating the valgus knee with lateral compartment collapse via an osteotomy, in part because this condition is less common than the varus knee with medial degeneration. Also, patients who have lateral degeneration tend to be women, older, and more sedentary than patients who have varus medial compartment OA. Because of the alignment of the knee and the relationship of the weight-bearing surface of the tibia to the floor, any realignment osteotomy for lateral compartment arthrosis usually needs be performed on the distal femur. This procedure is more complicated, and fewer surgeons consider it a treatment technique. From the few series in the literature, the rates of success and durability of the procedure seem to be similar to those of proximal tibial osteotomy for varus malalignment and medial compartment arthrosis.[24] As in tibial osteotomies, there is no scientific evidence to support 1 technique over another.

UNICOMPARTMENTAL ARTHROPLASTY

Unicompartmental arthroplasty has been performed for many years. Current designs are considered superior to designs manufactured in the 1980s.[25,26] Success with these implants is definitely surgeon-specific, and many arthroplasty surgeons prefer the reliability of total joint arthroplasty over unicompartmental replacement. Many series, however, have noted that patient satisfaction is higher with unicompartmental arthroplasty than with total knee arthroplasty (**Fig. 3**). It is theorized that this satisfaction is related to the preservation of 2 otherwise normal compartments within the joint. The problems with unicompartmental arthroplasty are related to the progression of the OA in the remaining 2 compartments. This progression leads to a significantly higher rate of revision over a 10- to 15-year timeframe than seen with total joint arthroplasty.[26] These data indicate the reason for failure is progression of the arthritis in the contralateral tibiofemoral compartment, not problems with the implant itself. The rates of success for the revision of these unicompartmental replacements to total knee arthroplasty seem to be similar to the rates of success for primary total knee arthroplasty. Interestingly, unicompartmental arthroplasty is touted as being best suited for the younger patient, in whom the preservation of normal tissues, with minimal bone resection, is a potential benefit when revision becomes necessary. It also is promoted for older patients who have isolated disease, whose OA is not likely to progress to a degree that will affect the outcome of surgery before their demise.[27,28] For the younger, more active patient who has abnormal alignment, osteotomy seems to be a better choice than uincompartmental replacement. For the older, more sedentary patient, unicompartmental arthroplasty is supported by the literature as a more reliable operation.[29,30] A recent literature review highlighted this and reinforced that

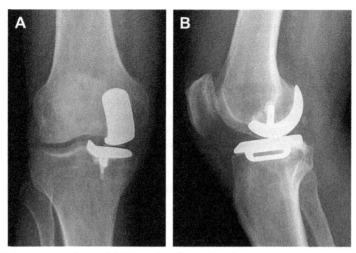

Fig. 3. (*A*) Anteroposterior and (*B*) lateral radiographs of a unicompartmental arthroplasty. These devices have the advantage of sparing normal parts of a joint with isolated compartmental degeneration, but they do not hold up as long as total joint replacements.

these procedures are indicated for different populations: high tibial osteotomies for younger, more active people, unicompartmental arthroplasty for older and more sedentary people.[31] Advancing technology has led to robot-assisted and custom-manufactured unicompartmental arthroplasty. To date, there is no evidence that these designs are better than the currently available designs, although they do hold promise to reduce technical issues with implantation and improve the fit of the prosthesis.

PATELLOFEMORAL REPLACEMENTS

Patellofemoral replacement has had a dubious long-term track record going back to the 1970s and 1980s. At that time, the implants were primitive, and the instrumentation to implant them was unreliable at best.[32] Current modifications of the implants and instrumentation have made the procedure more technically reproducible, and presently there are several midterm studies demonstrating survivorship in the range of 85% at 10 years.[33,34] Revision of a patellofemoral replacement to total knee arthroplasty does not seem to compromise the results.[35] As with the unicompartmental devices for tibiofemoral articulation, new custom-made implants have been designed. These implants show promising early results, but to date patellofemoral replacement has little if any evidence base to support their use. Isolated patellofemoral replacement, like a unicompartmental arthroplasty, probably is best performed by the surgeons most experienced in the technique.

EMERGING TECHNOLOGY FOR TOTAL KNEE REPLACEMENT

As noted in the introduction to this article, total knee arthroplasty is a very cost-effective, durable procedure for the treatment of OA of the knee joint. A recent review has indicated that the results are better, and the complications fewer, when the procedure is performed in specialty hospitals rather than general hospitals.[36] This difference probably is related to the volume both in the operating room and on the floors, with the development of clinical pathways to improve clinical outcomes. Because the designs in total knee arthroplasty that were introduced in the 1980s have been in use for 20+ years, survival past 20 years can be expected in the older (>65 years) patient who is not morbidly obese.[37]

During the past 10 years, many new technologies have been introduced into the realm of total joint arthroplasty, and a review of the most publicized and potentially important changes is warranted. These changes include minimally invasive total knee arthroplasty and computer-assisted or navigated total knee replacement. Unfortunately, these technologies have become marketing tools for surgeons, hospitals, and orthopedic implant manufacturers. In general, the length of the incision used for total knee replacement has become shorter. Many surgeons believe that total knee replacement through these mini-incisions is very demanding technically. Computer navigation can assist with joint replacement arthroplasty through these small incisions because bony anatomic landmarks can be identified precisely without extensile exposure. It allows the surgeon to obtain excellent alignment of the prosthesis (with higher reproducibility than traditional alignment guides). Computer navigation involves a significant learning curve as well as prolonged operative time and expense. The benefit of improved alignment may extrapolate to long-term durability of the prosthesis, although this benefit is yet to be demonstrated.[38,39] Although a number of surgeons have embraced the technology, many high-volume arthroplasty surgeons think that the additional operative time, increased expense, and limited improvements in alignment do not warrant its adoption.

Several orthopedic implant manufacturers have introduced total knee prostheses that are marketed as gender specific. There are anatomic differences between men and women, which previously had not been accounted for in the manufacturing of the implant. The gender-specific knee replacement for women has been promoted as being better because it reflects the anatomic variations between men and women recognized when the prosthesis was designed. To date, there is no evidence to support an advantage of these gender-specific devices for women; in fact, when the literature for traditional total knee arthroplasty is reviewed in detail for outcomes based on sex, the risk of failure is not greater in women than in men.[40]

An additional recent change in total knee arthroplasty has been the introduction of highly cross-linked polyethylene. This material has been shown to be a significant advancement for hip replacement, by dramatically decreasing the wear rate of polyethylene liners. This material has been introduced as the liner for the tibial tray in some total knee arthroplasty designs, but the results need to be assessed carefully, because it has reduced fracture toughness and produces smaller wear particles, both of which may be theoretical problems with knee replacement.[41]

SUMMARY

The surgical treatment of OA of the knee continues to evolve. The indications for arthroscopy have narrowed. Orthopedic surgeons continue to explore less invasive surgical options than total knee replacement for isolated unicompartmental arthritis of the knee joint. As in all therapeutic interventions, the practice of evidence-based medicine will drive surgeons to use only those surgical techniques that have been proven safe and efficacious by long-term prospective outcome studies.

REFERENCES

1. Räsänen P, Paavolainen P, Sintonen H, et al. Effectiveness of hip or knee replacement surgery in terms of quality-adjusted life years and costs. Acta Orthop 2007; 78(1):108–15.

2. Murphy L, Schwartz TA, Helmick CG, et al. Lifetime risk of symptomatic knee osteoarthritis. Arthritis Rheum 2008;59(9):1207–13.
3. Rand JA, Trousdale RT, Ilstrup DM, et al. Factors affecting the durability of primary total knee prostheses. J Bone Joint Surg Am 2003;85:259–65.
4. Moseley JB, O'Malley K, Petersen NJ, et al. A controlled trial of arthroscopic surgery for osteoarthritis of the knee. N Engl J Med 2002;347:81–8.
5. Herrlin S, Hållander M, Wange P, et al. Arthroscopic or conservative treatment of degenerative medial meniscal tears: a prospective randomised trial. Knee Surg Sports Traumatol Arthrosc 2007;15(4):393–401.
6. Kirkley A, Birmingham TB, Litchfield RB, et al. A randomized trial of arthroscopic surgery for osteoarthritis of the knee. N Engl J Med 2008;359:1097–107.
7. Siparsky P, Ryzewicz M, Peterson B, et al. Arthroscopic treatment of osteoarthritis of the knee: are there any evidence-based indications? Clin Orthop Relat Res 2007;455:107–12.
8. Dearing J, Nutton RW. Evidence based factors influencing outcome of arthroscopy in osteoarthritis of the knee. Knee 2008;14(3):159–63.
9. Aaron RK, Skolnick AH, Reinert SE, et al. Arthroscopic debridement for osteoarthritis of the knee. J Bone Joint Surg Am 2006;88:936–43.
10. Steadman JR, Ramappa AJ, Maxwell RB, et al. An arthroscopic treatment regimen for osteoarthritis of the knee. Arthroscopy 2007;23(9):948–55.
11. Felson DT, Chaisson CE, Hill CL, et al. The association of bone marrow lesions with pain in knee osteoarthritis. Ann Intern Med 2001;134(7):541–9.
12. Felson DT, Niu J, Guermazi A, et al. Correlation of the development of knee pain with enlarging bone marrow lesions on magnetic resonance imaging. Arthritis Rheum 2007;56(9):2986–92.
13. Sharkey PF, Cohen SB, Leinberry CF, et al. Subchondral bone marrow lesions associated with knee osteoarthritis. Am J Orthop 2012;41(9):413–7.
14. Healy WL, Iorio R, Lemos MJ. Athletic activity after joint replacement. Am J Sports Med 2001;29(3):377–88.
15. Brouwer RW, Raaij van TM, Bierma-Zeinstra SMA, et al. Osteotomy for treating knee osteoarthritis. Cochrane Database Syst Rev 2005;(1):CD004019.
16. Rosenberg TD, Paulos LE, Parker RD, et al. The forty-five-degree posteroanterior flexion weight-bearing radiograph of the knee. J Bone Joint Surg Am 1988;70(10):1479–83.
17. Brouwer RW, Bierma-Zeinstra SM, van Koeveringe AJ, et al. Patellar height and the inclination of the tibial plateau after high tibial osteotomy: the open versus the closed-wedge technique. J Bone Joint Surg Br 2005;87:1227–32.
18. Brouwer RW, Bierma-Zeinstra SM, van Raaij TM, et al. Osteotomy for medial compartment arthritis of the knee using a closing wedge or an opening wedge controlled by a Puddu plate: a one-year randomised, controlled study. J Bone Joint Surg Br 2006;88:1454–9.
19. Billings A, Scott DF, Camargo MP, et al. High tibial osteotomy with a calibrated osteotomy guide, rigid internal fixation, and early motion. Long-term follow-up. J Bone Joint Surg Am 2000;82:70–9.
20. Hui C, Salmon LJ, Kok A, et al. Long-term survival of high tibial osteotomy for medial compartment osteoarthritis of the knee. Am J Sports Med 2011;39:64–70.
21. Meding JB, Keating EM, Ritter MA, et al. Total knee arthroplasty after high tibial osteotomy: a comparison study in patients who had bilateral total knee replacement. J Bone Joint Surg Am 2000;82:1252.
22. Maquet P. Advancement of the tibial tuberosity. Clin Orthop Relat Res 1976;115: 225–30.

23. Farr J, Schepsis A, Cole B, et al. Anteromedialization: review and technique. J Knee Surg 2007;20(2):120–8.
24. Backstein D, Morag G, Hanna S, et al. Long-term follow-up of distal femoral varus osteotomy of the knee. J Arthroplasty 2007;22(4 Suppl 1):2–6.
25. Emerson RH Jr, Higgins LL. Unicompartmental knee arthroplasty with the Oxford prosthesis in patients with medial compartment arthritis. J Bone Joint Surg Am 2008;90(1):118–22.
26. Borus T, Thornhill T. Unicompartmental knee arthroplasty. J Am Acad Orthop Surg 2008;16(1):9–18.
27. Soohoo NF, Sharifi H, Kominski G, et al. Cost-effectiveness analysis of unicompartmental knee arthroplasty as an alternative to total knee arthroplasty for unicompartmental osteoarthritis. J Bone Joint Surg Am 2006;88(9):1975–82.
28. Slover J, Espehaug B, Havelin LI, et al. Cost-effectiveness of unicompartmental and total knee arthroplasty in elderly low-demand patients. A Markov decision analysis. J Bone Joint Surg Am 2006;88(11):2348–55.
29. Naal FD, Fischer M, Preuss A, et al. Return to sports and recreational activity after unicompartmental knee arthroplasty. Am J Sports Med 2007;35:1688–95.
30. Stukenborg-Colsman C, Wirth CJ, Lazovic D, et al. High tibial osteotomy versus unicompartmental joint replacement in unicompartmental knee joint osteoarthritis: 7–10-year follow-up prospective randomised study. Knee 2001;8(3):187–94.
31. Dettoni F, Bonasia DE, Castoldi F, et al. High tibial osteotomy versus unicompartmental knee arthroplasty for medial arthrosis of the knee: a review of the literature. Iowa Orthop J 2010;30:131–40.
32. Grelsamer RP, Stein DA. Current concepts review: patellofemoral arthritis. J Bone Joint Surg Am 2006;88:1849–60.
33. van Jonbergen HP, Werkman DM, Barnaart LF, et al. Long-term outcomes of patellofemoral arthroplasty. J Arthroplasty 2010;25(7):1066–71.
34. Walker T, Perkinson B, Mihalko WM. Instructional course lecture: patellofemoral arthroplasty: the other unicompartmental knee replacement. J Bone Joint Surg Am 2012;94(18):1712–20.
35. van Jonbergen HP, Werkman DM, van Kampen A. Conversion of patellofemoral arthroplasty to total knee arthropasty: a matched case control study of 13 patients. Acta Orthop 2009;80(1):62–6.
36. Cram P, Vaughan-Sarrazin MS, Wolf B, et al. A comparison of total hip and knee replacement in specialty and general hospitals. J Bone Joint Surg Am 2007; 89(8):1675–84.
37. Bae DK, Song SJ, Park MJ, et al. Twenty-year survival analysis in total knee arthroplasty by a single surgeon. J Arthroplasty 2012;27(7):1297–304.
38. Bauwens K, Matthes G, Wich M, et al. Navigated total knee replacement. A meta-analysis. J Bone Joint Surg Am 2007;89:261–9.
39. Fu Y, Wang M, Liu Y, et al. Alignment outcomes in navigated total knee arthroplasty: a meta-analysis. Knee Surg Sports Traumatol Arthrosc 2012;20(6): 1075–82.
40. Rankin EA, Bostrom M, Hozack W, et al. Gender-specific knee replacements: a technology overview. J Am Acad Orthop Surg 2008;16:63–7.
41. Lachiewicz PF, Geyer MR. The use of highly cross-linked polyethylene in total knee arthroplasty. J Am Acad Orthop Surg 2011;19(3):143–51.

Targeting Care

Tailoring Nonsurgical Management According to Clinical Presentation

Jillian Eyles, BAppSc(Physiotherapy)[a],*,
Barbara R. Lucas, BAppSc(Physiotherapy), MEd, MPH[a],
David J. Hunter, MBBS, MSc, PhD, FRACP[b,c]

KEYWORDS

- Osteoarthritis • Clinical predictors • Treatment response

KEY POINTS

- Numerous studies have explored patient characteristics, including body mass index, psychological factors, muscle strength, tibiofemoral alignment, radiographic changes, and signs of inflammation, as potential predictors of response to nonsurgical interventions for the management of osteoarthritis (OA) of the hip and knee.
- Often the sample sizes used by these studies have been inadequate in yielding sufficient numbers of responders to the interventions to allow for analysis of the potential predictors identified.
- Several well-designed studies have been adequately powered to provide some evidence for clinical characteristics that do or do not predict response to nonsurgical interventions for participants with hip and knee OA.

INTRODUCTION

The activity limitation attributed to osteoarthritis (OA) places it within the world's top 10 most disabling conditions.[1] Globally, OA affects approximately 18.0% of women and 9.6% of men older than 60 years.[2] In 2003 the annual costs to the United States economy of OA and other rheumatic conditions was an estimated $128 billion.[3] These enormous costs are projected to rise steeply with the steadily increasing prevalence of rheumatic conditions.[3]

This prevalent, expensive, disabling disease is incurable, so it follows that current treatments focus on symptomatic relief. Commonly reported treatment goals for this

Disclosures: None.
[a] Department of Physiotherapy, Royal North Shore Hospital, Pacific Highway, St Leonards, New South Wales 2065, Australia; [b] Department of Rheumatology, Royal North Shore Hospital, Pacific Highway, St Leonards, New South Wales 2065, Australia; [c] Sydney Medical School-Northern, Kolling Building Level 7, Royal North Shore Hospital, Reserve Road, St Leonards, New South Wales 2065, Australia
* Corresponding author.
E-mail address: jeyles@nsccahs.health.nsw.gov.au

group include reductions in joint pain, stiffness, activity limitation, participation restriction, and improvements in quality of life and well-being. To assist clinicians in achieving these goals with their patients, numerous international evidence-based guidelines for management of hip and knee OA have become available.[4-10] There is uniformity in most of the recommendations made by the guidelines,[11] and agreement that conservative management of hip and knee OA should combine both nonpharmacologic and pharmacologic treatment modalities.[4-10]

The recommendations made in the guidelines for the management of hip and knee OA are broad. The evidence-based, expert consensus guidelines from the Osteoarthritis Research Society International (OARSI) (2008) include no fewer than 20 recommendations for the nonsurgical management of hip and knee OA[4]; however, the treatments are not arranged systematically to indicate the order of priority in which they should be undertaken. With so many recommended management options tabled, it would be advantageous to know which treatments are most likely to be effective for the individual with hip or knee OA according to clinical presentation.

This review examines the evidence available for the identification of clinical characteristics that predict patient response to nonsurgical treatments for hip and knee OA. The summation of this evidence may assist clinicians to target treatments most likely to benefit patients according to clinical presentation, and identify areas for further research.

BODY MASS INDEX

Obesity is a known risk factor for the development of arthritis[12] and is a strong predictor for long-term progression of the disease.[13] There is evidence that obesity is a risk factor for knee OA, but the relationship between obesity and the risk of developing hip OA is less clear.[14,15] International guidelines nonetheless recommend weight reduction in individuals with hip and knee OA who are overweight or obese.[8,9,11,16] There is strong evidence that weight loss is an effective treatment for knee OA, yet little evidence exists regarding weight loss as an effective treatment for obese patients with hip OA.

It seems reasonable that body mass index (BMI) may be a clinical characteristic that predicts response to weight-loss interventions but, surprisingly, evidence exists that it does not. A post hoc analysis of a randomized controlled trial (RCT) involving 111 overweight veterans with knee OA investigated 9 clinical characteristics as possible predictors of weight change between baseline, 16 weeks, and 32 weeks. The minimum amount of weight loss required to define a treatment responder was not provided. Multiregression analysis revealed that BMI was not predictive of weight loss in response to the interventions for overweight veterans with knee OA.[17] The external validity of this study is limited by confining the recruitment of participants to veterans.

Two studies found that BMI was not predictive of response to a Dutch multimodal, stepped-care model of pain management for hip and knee OA. Snijders and colleagues[18] investigated the efficacy of the Dutch model in a cohort of 183 participants with hip and knee OA. The model combined pharmacologic and nonpharmacologic treatments. Two possible definitions of positive treatment response were described: (1) Outcome Measures in Rheumatoid Arthritis Clinical Trials/Osteoarthritis Research Society International (OMERACT-OARSI) Responder Criteria, and (2) patient-reported numeric rating scale (NRS) for pain of 4 or less. At 12-week reassessment, 86 patients were responders according to definition (1), and 71 fulfilled definition (2). BMI was 1 of 11 potential predictors of response included in analyses, and was not a significant predictor of response to this program[18]; however, in identifying true predictors of response the study was underpowered. A more recent study used the same Dutch model, focusing specifically on a stepped-care protocol used to progress the use of acetaminophen and nonsteroidal anti-inflammatory drugs (NSAIDs) at standardized intervals according to patient-reported pain levels.[19] The definition of treatment responder was a patient-reported NRS pain 4 or less, and 100 participants met this target. The study was underpowered in analyzing 13 patient characteristics, including BMI, as possible predictors of response. Further research is required to determine whether BMI can predict a positive treatment response in this multimodal stepped-care model of pain management.

Two well-powered studies examined the potential of BMI as a predictor of response to cyclooxygenase-2 (COX-2) inhibitors. Bingham and colleagues[20] pooled the results of 2 similar RCTs comparing the efficacy of etoricoxib and celecoxib with that of placebo. The OMERACT-OARSI Responder Criteria determined that 562 participants were responders to the COX-2 inhibitors following 12 weeks of the intervention. BMI, one of 16 variables analyzed as potential predictors of response, failed to predict a positive treatment response to the COX-2 inhibitors.[20] Similar results were found by Detora and colleagues,[21] who combined the results of 3 6-week RCTs comparing the COX-2 inhibitor rofecoxib with placebo in 1501 patients with hip and knee OA. Responder criteria were not defined. Patient data were analyzed according to subgroups representing 14 baseline characteristics including BMI. Analysis of covariance failed to identify any baseline measures associated with treatment response.[21] To date, good evidence exists that baseline BMI does not predict a response in patients with hip and knee OA treated with COX-2 inhibitors.

A single study explored BMI as a predictor of response to intra-articular corticosteroid injection (CSI) for the management of hip OA. Robinson and colleagues[22] followed 120 patients with hip OA for 12 weeks following CSI. Participants were classified as responders to the CSI at 12 weeks if a reduction in baseline Western Ontario and McMaster Universities Osteoarthritis Index (WOMAC) pain subscale of greater than 15% was achieved; 48 participants met this criterion. Logistic regression determined that BMI, one of 14 variables analyzed, was not a significant predictor of response to hip CSI[22]; however, the study was underpowered in detecting true predictors of treatment response.

Four cohort studies explored possible predictors of response to intra-articular (IA) hyaluronic acid derivatives for hip and knee OA. Short-term efficacy and tolerability of IA Hylan G-F 20 were assessed in 4253 patients with symptomatic knee OA.[23] Responder criteria were not defined, and the primary outcome was pain measured at baseline and 3 weeks on a 4-point Likert scale. At 3 weeks after IA Hylan G-F 20, 88.4% of patients assessed their pain as better or much better. Logistic regression of 7 potential predictors of short-term pain reduction determined that underweight patients were more likely than their obese counterparts to report reduced knee pain. The method of recruitment threatens the validity of this evidence; the investigators invited 840 orthopedic surgeons to report on at least 5 consecutive patients receiving Hylan G-F 20 for relief of knee OA pain, introducing significant selection bias.

Longer-term outcomes of patients with knee OA receiving IA Hylan G-F 20 were explored in 3 cohort studies.[24–26] A retrospective cohort of 155 patients with knee OA was reassessed 7 to 14 months following IA Hylan G-F 20.[24] The definition of responder was not specified. Analysis of 16 possible predictors found that BMI was not a significant predictor of patient satisfaction, although this study was underpowered in identifying the possible predictors, and the retrospective design was prone to significant recall bias. Longer-term outcomes of Hylan G-F 20 were also studied in a small cohort of 32 patients with mild to moderate knee OA 6 months following IA Hylan G-F 20.[25] Clinical response was defined using the OMERACT-OARSI "high improvement" criterion. Only 15 participants were responders, and 8 variables, including BMI, were investigated as predictors of response, leaving the study underpowered for the detection of significant predictors. BMI was not significantly correlated with patient response. A prospective cohort study examining 84 patients with knee OA for 6 months following knee IA Hylan G-F 20 found that Short-Form-36 (SF-36) health survey scores were significantly improved at 6 months after injection.[26] The responder criteria were not described. Three factors, including the subjects' percentage above ideal body weight, were analyzed for correlations with positive treatment outcomes seen in the SF-36 health survey categories Physical Function, Role-Physical, and Role-Emotional. The subjects' percentage above ideal body weight was not predictive of improvement. The high number of patients lost to follow-up (23%) affected the validity of this study. Evidence for BMI and percentage above ideal body weight as clinical characteristics predictive of longer-term response to knee IA Hylan G-F 20 was inconclusive, owing to low validity and power.

BMI was not a significant predictor of response to IA Hylan G-F 20 in people with hip OA. Migliore and colleagues[27] evaluated 250 patients with hip OA who received IA Hylan G-F 20. Treatment response was defined as a 30% or greater improvement in baseline Lequesne scores or NSAID usage at 6 months, but the number of participants classified as responders was unclear. Ten possible predictors of treatment response were analyzed; BMI was not a significant predictor of response to hip IA Hylan G-F 20.[27] The large number of dropouts (42%) affected the validity of this study.

Patients with a lower BMI may be more likely to experience a reduction in chronic knee pain following treatment with glucosamine sulfate. A prospective correlational study of 39 participants with chronic knee pain followed patients receiving 1.5 g glucosamine sulfate daily for 12 weeks.[28] Participants were not required to have been diagnosed specifically with OA, which affected the external validity of this study. The definition of treatment responder was not described, and 7 patient characteristics were examined as potential predictors of reduction of pain rated on a visual analog scale (VAS). The study was underpowered in determining the effects of 7 potential predictors.

To date, most of the evidence suggests that BMI is not a consistent predictor of response to nonsurgical treatments for people with hip and knee OA. Some evidence exists that BMI is not predictive of response to a weight-loss program in overweight veterans with knee OA.[17] There is good evidence that BMI does not predict response to COX-2 inhibitors for the management of hip and knee OA.[20,21] The evidence is weak that BMI is not predictive of treatment response to either a multimodal stepped-care pain management model,[18,19] hip CSI,[22] hip IA Hylan G-F 20,[27] or glucosamine for chronic knee pain.[28] The evidence for BMI as a predictor of response to knee IA Hylan G-F 20 is weak and conflicting.[23–26] Further research is required to determine whether BMI is a clinical characteristic that can foretell a response to nonsurgical treatments for people with hip and knee OA.

PSYCHOLOGICAL FACTORS

Complex interactions exist between psychological factors and perceived symptoms of OA. Compared with their peers, people with OA report an increased prevalence of depression and depressed mood.[29] The intensity of perceived OA pain has been demonstrated to be predictive of depression severity in this cohort.[29] Poor mental health has been associated with worse overall hip and knee OA pain, and deterioration in mental health has been found to precede short-term exacerbations of OA pain.[30] Treatment of depression in people with arthritis appears to improve depressive symptoms, reduce OA pain, and improve function and quality of life,[31] and therefore is an important consideration in the management of OA.

Many treatments prescribed for hip and knee OA management, particularly exercise, weight-loss programs, and medications; require active participation from the patient. The compliance with and efficacy of these treatments may be influenced by the individual's mental state as to how rehabilitation outcomes are affected. The prospective cohort study "Predictors for response to rehabilitation in patients with hip or knee OA"[32] featured 250 patients with hip and knee OA who participated in a 3- to 4-week multimodal rehabilitation program combining exercise therapy, hydrotherapy, relaxation strategies, distraction techniques, patient education, manual therapy, thermotherapy, and electrotherapy. Participants were assessed at baseline and 6 months following the program. Three different definitions of treatment responder were used: (1) the minimal clinically important difference (MCID) (18%) improvement shown on the WOMAC, (2) improvement on the Transition scale, and (3) MCID improvement on WOMAC and improvement on the Transition scale. The transition scale was described as a measure of the current state of health of the OA joint compared with its state 6 months earlier.[32] There were 21 personal, lifestyle, and psychological measures investigated as potential predictors of the 3 definitions of responder. Depression and anxiety were evaluated using the Hospital Anxiety and Depression Scale, and mental health was assessed using the mental component of the SF-36. The absence of depressive symptoms was determined to be a strong predictor of all 3 of the responder definitions, suggesting that depression may hinder the achievement of positive treatment outcomes of patients with hip and knee OA following a 3- to 4-week rehabilitation program. This study did not attempt to answer the question as to why patients did not achieve the same results as their nondepressed counterparts, but one may hypothesize that perhaps those patients with depression have more difficulty complying with a comprehensive rehabilitation program. This area is an interesting one for further research.[32]

The presence of depression may affect the ability of overweight people with OA to lose weight. A post hoc analysis of an RCT aimed to identify predictors of positive treatment response resulting from weight-loss interventions for 111 overweight veterans with knee OA.[17] Veterans were randomized into groups receiving 24 weeks of nutritional counseling, a home exercise program, a combination of both, or usual care. There were no differences in weight loss between intervention groups, and 9 variables were investigated as possible predictors of weight change between baseline, 16 weeks, and 32 weeks of the RCT. The amount of weight loss required to indicate successful treatment response was not indicated. Symptoms of depression were evaluated using The Center for Epidemiologic Studies Depression Scale, which measured 20 items to achieve a score out of 60. The presence of depression was indicated by a score of 16 or greater. The absence of depression was the only independent predictor of weight loss at 16 weeks and 32 weeks.[17] This study is limited by its failure to define treatment responders; however, it does suggest that depressive symptoms may limit the ability of veterans to lose weight.

Depression and anxiety did not seem to predict the treatment response of patients with knee OA to CSI. A small study of 59 patients with knee OA receiving CSI examined 10 possible predictors of a favorable response, defined as a 15% or greater reduction of pain rated on VAS, to injection of methylprednisolone acetate.[33] The Hospital Anxiety and Depression score at baseline was not found to consistently predict treatment response. Given that 59 patients were used to investigate

10 predictors of response, this study was underpowered in detecting meaningful effects of the potential predictors.

Mental health scores do not seem to predict response to a combined nonpharmacologic and pharmacologic pain-management program. Predictors for response to analgesics were explored in relation to a cohort study of 347 patients investigating treatment outcomes of a stepped model of care for hip and knee OA. The model initially offered education, lifestyle and weight-loss advice, physiotherapy, and acetaminophen, then progressed to other medications at intervals as guided by a pain NRS.[19] Treatment response was defined as achievement of pain NRS of 4 or greater, and there were 100 responders. Thirteen possible predictors of response were explored, including mental health. The SF-36 questionnaire was used to assess health-related quality of life, and the mental component summary (MCS) scores of the SF-36 were used to reflect mental health. Mental health rated by the MCS was not a significant predictor of response to the stepped model of pharmacologic pain management for patients with hip and knee OA; however, this study was underpowered regarding the analysis of 13 possible predictors.

Self-reported participant mood failed to predict treatment outcome in a small cross-over RCT of 11 patients with osteoarthritis receiving 2 different NSAIDs.[34] During 2 treatment periods of 4 weeks' duration, participants received ketoprofen and piroxicam. A 4-week washout period followed the initial drug treatment before commencement of the second drug. Participants were classified as treatment responders if they showed 30% or better improvement of 5 of the 7 variables measured at baseline, including pain, tenderness, swelling, patient and physician global assessments, acute-phase protein levels, and disability. There were 20 baseline variables explored as possible predictors of response including mood, assessed using an 18-item questionnaire. Mood was not a significant predictor of treatment outcome; however, the small sample size of this study leaves it underpowered for the detection of meaningful effects of the predictors investigated.

In summary, 2 well-designed, adequately powered studies used specific measures of depression that were predictive of response to intervention.[17,32] Both studies demonstrated the relationship between the absence of depressive symptoms and positive nonpharmacologic treatment outcomes. The treatments investigated in these studies included a comprehensive rehabilitation program and weight-loss interventions. These treatment modalities require high levels of active participation of the patients involved, which may be affected by the presence of depressive symptoms. Of interest, the 3 studies investigating drug-therapy regimes, perhaps not requiring such a high level of active participation by the subjects, consistently found different measures of psychological factors incapable of predicting treatment response.[19,33,34] Two of these studies were underpowered[33,34] and the third, which was inadequately powered, did not measure depression specifically.

MUSCLE STRENGTH

In view of the biomechanical influence and protective functions of skeletal muscles surrounding joints, muscle weakness is considered to be an important possible factor in the development and progression of OA. Evidence for the significance of muscle strength in the pathogenesis of OA remains unclear.[35,36] Higher quadriceps strength may have a protective effect against the development of symptomatic OA.[36] Whether muscle weakness precedes the onset of OA, or if it is a feature of already established disease seen on radiography, or is only related to the onset of pain and other symptoms, is an area for further research.

The evidence for the role of muscle strength in the progression of OA is varied. Limited evidence exists to support muscle strength as a predictor of progression of knee OA.[13] Nevertheless, over time people with knee OA who have greater quadriceps strength report less pain and superior functional ability compared with their weaker counterparts.[37] Quadriceps strength has been studied widely in relation to knee OA; however, muscles around the hip that stabilize the pelvis also have an effect on adduction forces around the knee, which may result in increased compression of the medial compartment[38] and influence the pathogenesis and progression of OA. Hip OA has also been associated with significantly reduced lower limb muscle strength[39]; however, limited evidence is available to explain the role of hip and thigh musculature in the development and progression of the disease. Further research is required to explain this possible relationship.

Treatments for hip and knee OA have long included specific exercises designed to strengthen muscles surrounding the joints involved. High-level evidence exists regarding the reduction of pain and dysfunction in knee OA through therapeutic exercises.[40] The evidence to date for the efficacy of exercise in hip OA is less convincing,[41] yet exercise is often prescribed. Wright and colleagues[42] published a study aiming to identify baseline characteristics of patients with hip OA likely to respond favorably to physical-therapy interventions. As part of a larger RCT, 91 patients were randomized to groups receiving manual therapy, exercise therapy, a combination of both, or usual care. The OMERACT-OARSI Responder Criteria determined treatment responders. Ten variables were analyzed as predictors of treatment response. Measures of muscle strength using a hand-held dynamometer were not predictive of treatment success. Only 22 of the 68 participants were responders, which left the study underpowered in identifying predictors of response.[42]

There has been recent interest in the nature of lower limb muscle weakness in people with knee OA. Decreased quadriceps strength in knee OA has been attributed to both loss of muscle cross-sectional area[43] and reduced ability to activate the muscles.[44] In a cohort of 111 subjects taken from a larger RCT, baseline ability to activate quadriceps was examined as 1 of 9 possible predictors of changes in strength of the muscle following a 6-week exercise program for subjects with knee OA. Primary outcome measures were quadriceps strength and quadriceps activation, measured using a burst-superimposition maximum isometric quadriceps torque test; however, a definition of treatment response was not identified. Although activation of lower quadriceps was associated with lower strength, baseline activation of quadriceps did not predict the magnitude of gain in quadriceps strength following exercise therapy.[45] These results suggest that patients with OA should benefit from strengthening exercises regardless of baseline activation of quadriceps.

Baseline muscle strength does not seem to predict the degree of symptomatic relief achieved following a weight-loss program in obese people with knee OA. The 192 participants, who were part of a larger RCT, were randomized to 2 different dietary interventions. Significant response to the interventions included the OMERACT-OARSI Responder Criteria and improvement on Knee Injury and Osteoarthritis Outcome (KOOS) scores. Although weight loss was achieved in most of the subjects, only 64% achieved the OMERACT-OARSI responder criterion. There were 23 variables investigated as possible predictors of response to the weight-loss programs, including measurements of baseline hamstrings and quadriceps strength using isometric dynamometry. Baseline muscle strength was not predictive of symptomatic relief in response to the weight-loss program.[46] The study was underpowered in detecting significant predictors from a possible 23 variables.

One study investigated muscle strength as a predictor of response to a pharmacologic agent. Jones and Doherty[33] performed a crossover RCT comparing CSI with saline (placebo) in 59 subjects with knee OA. Ten possible predictors of treatment response were analyzed. Treatment response, defined as a decrease of 15% or more in pain rated on a VAS, was not predicted by baseline quadriceps strength measured using a commercial strain gauge. This study was significantly underpowered for the analysis of 10 predictors of response.

Further research into the role of muscle strength in the pathogenesis of OA and subsequent progression of the disease may be helpful in refining recommendations for therapies aimed at OA prevention and further joint deterioration as a consequence of OA. To date, muscle strength has not been demonstrated to predict response to nonsurgical interventions for hip and knee OA.

TIBIOFEMORAL JOINT ALIGNMENT

Varus (bow-legged) or valgus (knock-kneed) tibiofemoral joint alignments are clinical characteristics observed in some people with knee OA. Joint alignment affects the distribution of load borne by the medial and lateral compartments of the articular surface of the knee. Static knee alignment is conventionally determined using full-length weight-bearing radiographs of the lower limb with knees extended. Lines are drawn from the center of the femoral head to the talus through the middle of the femoral and tibial shafts to indicate the load-bearing mechanical axis, then measurements are made of various angles subtended from where those lines intersect.[47–49] Neutral alignment is commonly defined as 0° to 2° of varus,[50] meaning that in a normal knee the mechanical axis passes medial to the knee joint, resulting in 60% to 70% of weight-bearing forces passing through the medial articular surface.[51] Varus malalignment results in higher loads borne through the medial compartment of the knee, whereas increased compressive forces through the lateral articular surface accompany valgus malalignment.

Dynamic knee alignment can be assessed using 3-dimensional gait analysis. In varus knees the measurement of knee-adduction moment during the stance phase of walking is an indirect measure of joint compressive forces sustained within the medial tibiofemoral joint compartment.[49,52,53] Static and dynamic alignment is an important consideration, given that altered distribution of forces placed through the joint surface may lead to damage of articular structures, possibly increasing the risk for development of OA or worsening existing disease.

It remains unclear as to whether knee-joint malalignment precedes incident knee OA[47,48]; however, varus alignment is considered to be a significant predictor of knee OA disease progression.[13] Knee malalignment has been demonstrated to interact with other risk factors for OA progression, increasing the likelihood of disease acceleration. Possible interactive factors include greater quadriceps strength,[54] the stage of disease observed in the individual,[55] and obesity.[48]

The evidence for the relationship between knee malalignment and reported OA symptoms remains unclear.[55,56] Nevertheless, some nonsurgical treatments in OA management guidelines aim to reduce pain and dysfunction associated with tibiofemoral malalignment. Orthotic bracing, shoe wedges, and muscle strengthening are recommended with a view to improving the biomechanics of the joint.[4,6,7,9,10] Several studies have investigated knee-joint alignment as a predictor response to nonsurgical management of OA. An RCT by Lim and colleagues[57] examined the effect of a 12-week quadriceps-strengthening program on knee-adduction moment, pain, and function in 107 subjects with knee OA. Knee alignment was assessed on radiographs, and participants were stratified according to whether they had more neutral (<5°) or more varus (≥5°) alignment. Specific responder criteria were not described. Patients in the strengthening group achieved significant improvements in strength regardless of alignment. Self-reported function, performance measures, and knee-adduction moment determined using 3-dimensional gait analysis were unchanged by the intervention in both alignment groups. Pain, assessed using the WOMAC pain subscale, was significantly improved in the strengthening group subset that was more neutrally aligned. Neutral knee-joint alignment may mediate improvements in knee OA pain following a 12-week quadriceps-strengthening program.

Immediate changes in static alignment and knee-adduction moment were not predictive of response to lateral-wedge insoles at 3 months. A cohort of 40 volunteers with knee OA were provided with laterally wedged insoles to assess the immediate effects of the insoles on knee OA pain, knee-adduction moment, and static alignment.[49] The lateral wedges immediately reduced knee-adduction moment calculated using 3-dimensional gait analysis and walking pain measured using the WOMAC pain subscale, but had no effect on static alignment as determined on full-length leg radiographs. Alignment was defined as the angle subtended by the intersection of the femoral and tibial mechanical axes. Varus malalignment was determined when the angle was less than 180°, with valgus indicated by an angle of greater than 180°. After 3 months of wearing the insoles, significant improvements in pain and function persisted. A definition of treatment responder was not specified; nevertheless, 10 predictors at baseline of outcome after 3 months were explored. Neither immediate changes in static alignment nor knee-adduction moment were predictive of decreased pain and improvement in function 3 months following the intervention.[49] The size of this cohort limited the ability of the study to identify true predictors of response to the intervention.

A larger RCT of 192 obese subjects with knee OA allocated patients to 2 different weight-loss interventions.[46] Knee-joint alignment was assessed using a "Plug-in-Gait" model with a 6-camera stereophotogrammetric system and markers on anatomic landmarks. A knee was categorized as varus when alignment was greater than 0°, and valgus if less than 0°. Baseline knee alignment was one of 23 variables examined as possible predictors; however, it failed to predict improvements in KOOS or achievement of OMERACT-OARSI Responder Criteria following weight-loss interventions.[46] In view of the fact that only 64% of patients were treatment responders according to OMERACT-OARSI criteria, the study was underpowered in detecting effects of significant predictors.

It is interesting to consider the definitions of knee malalignment used in the 3 studies discussed above. Lim and colleagues[57] used a more extreme definition of 5° or more to indicate varus malalignment. By contrast, the 2 other studies categorized subjects to knee-malalignment groups if the mechanical axis did not appear as a straight line.[46,49] This disparity may have increased the severity of malalignment observed within the participants assigned to the varus group investigated by Lim and colleagues, compared with the subjects categorized to knee-malalignment groups in the other studies. Participants with varus malalignment studied by Lim and colleagues[57] did not experience improvements in pain following strength training, whereas neutrally aligned subjects reported significant pain reduction. Perhaps the higher severity of varus malalignment was key to the determination of knee-joint alignment as a predictor of outcome after intervention in this study. Future research considering knee malalignment as a predictor of treatment response to conservative treatments should consider carefully the definition of joint alignment.

ASSESSMENT BY RADIOGRAPHY AND MAGNETIC RESONANCE IMAGING

The presence of radiographic osteophytes (OP) and joint-space narrowing are commonly used to diagnose OA. These features are combined to determine radiographic disease severity according to scoring systems such as the Kellgren-Lawrence grade (KLG).[58] Despite known limitations, radiographs are inexpensive, accessible, and easy to interpret, so are commonly used in research for the classification of subjects to determine eligibility, and for stratification of samples according to radiographic severity. Radiographic joint-space width (JSW) or minimum joint-space width (mJSW) is recommended for use in clinical trials; however, magnetic resonance imaging (MRI) is preferred particularly for the assessment of cartilage morphology.[59]

Relatively few articles analyze radiographic severity of hip and knee OA as possible predictors of response to nonsurgical, nonpharmacologic treatments. Two of the 3 articles doing so examined the ability of radiologic and MRI OA severity to predict response to weight-loss interventions. A small RCT of 30 obese female participants with knee OA compared 2 dietary weight-loss interventions.[60] Within the intervention group 90% of participants achieved a clinically significant weight reduction of greater than 10%, and 33% had a 50% improvement in symptoms of knee OA. A strict definition of treatment responder was not provided. Structural joint damage was assessed at baseline using both the KLG classification and low-field MRI (0.2 T) to assess various measures of cartilage abnormalities, bone marrow lesions, effusions, and synovitis of the medial, lateral, and patellofemoral compartments of the knee. Five baseline radiographic characteristics and clinical outcomes following the weight-loss interventions were investigated for correlations. None of the imaging variables were able to forecast symptomatic response to treatment[60]; however, this study was likely underpowered in identifying significant predictors.

A second RCT randomized 192 obese patients with knee OA into 8 weeks of 2 experimental dietary interventions.[46] Results were calculated for the entire cohort, as the method of weight loss was not relevant for this analysis. OA symptoms were evaluated at baseline and at 16 weeks using the OMERACT-OARSI Responder Criteria and changes in KOOS. High-field MRI was assessed using the Boston-Leeds Osteoarthritis of the Knee Score (BLOKS) to measure joint damage at baseline. Conventional radiography determined the baseline KLG and mJSW. MRI and radiographic measures failed to find any relationship between variables assessing structural damage to the knee and symptomatic improvements following the dietary interventions.[46] Only 64% of patients were treatment responders according to OMERACT-OARSI criteria, therefore this study may also be insufficiently powered to detect the effects of 23 potential predictors.

A third study examining the ability of radiographic features to predict response to nonsurgical, nonpharmacologic interventions was conducted by Hinman and colleagues.[49] A cohort of 40 patients with knee OA wore full-length 5° lateral-wedge insoles for 3 months. Improvements were observed in WOMAC pain and function subscales following the intervention. Tibiofemoral OA severity was assessed at baseline using the KLG scoring system. Following analysis of 10 possible predictors of outcome, greater disease severity indicated by higher KLG scores was predictive of worse pain at 3 months. This study does not define responder criteria, and the small sample size reduced the ability to identify predictors of response to lateral-wedge insoles.

Two studies examined radiographic severity using KLG as potentially predictive of response to interventions combining both nonpharmacologic and drug therapies for hip and knee OA. Both investigated cohorts of patients with hip and knee OA participating in a Dutch multimodal, stepped-care pain-management program.[18,19] During the 12-week program subjects received standardized nonpharmacologic management and pain-relieving medications, prescribed and altered at set intervals depending on self-reported pain at reassessment. The definition of positive treatment response in the initial cohort of 183 patients was fulfillment of either the OMERACT-OARSI Responder Criteria or NRS of 4 or less.[18] The later study of 347 subjects required NRS of 4 or less at 12 weeks to indicate successful response to the intervention.[19] Both studies analyzed OA severity as determined by KLG scores as possible predictors of positive treatment outcomes. The first study tested 11 possible predictors of response to intervention, and found that disease severity did not forecast improvements in overall pain and function as a result of the 12-week pain management program.[18] In the second study, 13 predictors were tested for correlation with treatment response at the 4 different steps of the treatment model. Greater OA severity was independently associated with a higher chance of pain relief achieved in response to the use of acetaminophen.[19] This correlation was discovered because unlike in the first study, the predictors of response were tested at each of the separate steps of the program. There were 59 responders to acetaminophen, so the study was underpowered for the testing of 13 predictors. Although the evidence is tenuous, this finding lends support to the recommendations made by international OA management guidelines to trial acetaminophen as a first-line pharmacologic treatment of hip and knee OA,[4–10] even in those patients with severe disease.

Evidence to the contrary was presented by Case and colleagues[61] in the results from a double-blind, placebo-controlled RCT comparing the efficacy of acetaminophen and diclofenac sodium for the management of pain in knee OA. Eighty-two patients were randomized to 3 groups receiving either one of the drugs or placebo. The primary outcome at baseline, 2 weeks, and 12 weeks was the WOMAC scale. The diclofenac sodium group alone achieved significant improvement ($\geq 20\%$) in all 3 WOMAC subscales following the intervention. The subjects were stratified according to prestudy medication, baseline pain, and disease severity indicated by KLG to identify subsets of patients who were consistent in their response to the treatments. None of the subgroups consistently demonstrated preferential response to acetaminophen or diclofenac sodium. This study suffered from a high number of dropouts (>25%). Three of the 5 subjects who withdrew from the diclofenac sodium treatment arm (n = 25) did so as a result of adverse effects. Despite the evidence presented in this study for the superior efficacy of diclofenac sodium, the relatively high risk of unwanted side effects lends further weight to the OA treatment guidelines that recommend a trial of acetaminophen before commencing NSAID therapy,[4–10] and it can be presumed that this follows regardless of radiographic severity.

Four articles investigated radiologic predictors of response to CSI for hip OA. Of these, only one reported that radiographically determined disease severity was a significant predictor of positive response to steroid injection.[62] This retrospective cohort study reviewed radiographs, radiology reports, and medical records of 361 patients who had received fluoroscopically guided IA methylprednisolone acetate 80 mg, or methylprednisolone with bupivacaine. The definition of treatment responder was a 50% decrease in pain reported on a VAS. An immediate positive response to injection was evident in 68.2% of hips and a delayed response was apparent in 71.4%. OA severity was measured at baseline using KLG classification, and the grades were split into groups for analysis. Multivariate regression determined that radiographic severity of OA was an independent predictor of treatment response. Patients with advanced disease were much more likely to experience both immediate and delayed onset of pain relief. The investigators suggested that people with advanced hip OA are likely to achieve a better response to CSI than those with mild or moderate disease.[62] Although a sizable number of participants was recruited, these inferences should be considered cautiously in view of the inherent risk of bias associated with the retrospective cohort design of this study.

By contrast, Robinson and colleagues,[22] using a similar fluoroscopically guided injection of methylprednisolone and bupivacaine into the hip joint of 120 people with hip OA, concluded that radiographically determined OA severity was not predictive of response to intervention. This cohort study assessed symptomatic response to 40-mg and 80-mg doses of the steroid. A decrease in the WOMAC pain by greater than 15% was considered to indicate positive treatment response, and 75 patients were classified as responders at 6 weeks. The investigators concluded that the higher dose (80 mg) of methylprednisolone was more effective and lasted longer. Twelve possible predictors of treatment response included KLG scoring. Forward logistic regression found that KLG was incapable of predicting reduced pain in response to hip CSI.[22] This study was underpowered in detecting predictors of response among 12 variables.

Similar conclusions were made regarding a small prospective cohort of 27 patients with hip OA assessed at baseline and 2, 12, and 26 weeks following hip IA lignocaine and methylprednisolone.[63] The main outcome measure was pain measured on VAS. The degree of radiologic severity according to KLG classification and mJSW had no significant bearing on the reported pain relief following steroid injection to the hip; however, the small sample size decreased the power to detect significant predictors. The fourth RCT compared ultrasound-guided CSI with IA hyaluronic acid, saline (control), and standard care (no injection) in 77 subjects with hip OA.[64] Response to treatment was delineated by the OMERACT-OARSI Responder Criteria, and there were 14 responders to steroid injection. CSI was significantly more effective than the 3 other treatments. Univariate regression analysis determined that of 5 predictors analyzed, radiographic severity using Croft grading and mJSW were not predictive of treatment response to CSI; however, the study was underpowered in analyzing 5 predictors.[64] Further research is required to explore the value of radiographic and MRI clinical characteristics indicating disease severity as potential predictors of response to hip CSI.

Three cohort studies attempted to identify radiographic characteristics of patients with hip and knee OA that were predictive of treatment response to IA Hylan G-F 20.[24,25,27] Migliore and colleagues[27] followed 250 patients who received ultrasound-guided IA Hylan G-F 20 into OA hips. Treatment response was defined as improvement of greater than 30% or more in Lequesne index or NSAID use. Significant improvements were reported for all outcome measures at 3, 6, 9, and 12 months when compared with baseline. Multiregression analysis of 8 baseline variables determined that KLG was unable to predict treatment response.[27] A high number of dropouts limited the validity of this study. The second study followed a small cohort of 32 patients with mild to moderate knee OA for 6 months following IA Hylan G-F 20.[25] The OMERACT-OARSI "High Improvement" responder criteria for OA were used to define responders to treatment. Fifteen participants met the responder criteria. Eight predictors of treatment response were explored, including mJSW, which was not predictive of positive response to Hylan G-F 20 injection.[25] The study was underpowered and limited by the exclusion of patients with severe OA. Conrozier and colleagues[24] studied a cohort of 155 patients across the spectrum of mild through severe knee OA. Knee joint-space loss in a single compartment seen on radiographs and meniscal calcinosis noted on MRI scans were predictive of a good outcome after IA Hylan GF-20. The definition of treatment responder was not adequately described in this retrospective cohort, so it is difficult to define the improvement actually predicted by these measures.[24] Nevertheless, weak evidence exists that knee joint-space loss in a single compartment and meniscal calcinosis may predict response to IA Hylan G-F 20, and this warrants further research.

Bennett and colleagues[28] investigated the symptomatic response of 39 subjects with chronic knee pain treated with 1.5 g oral glucosamine sulfate for 12 weeks. Primary outcome measures at baseline and 3 months included pain VAS rated on movement, VAS for restriction in function, and patient-rated global change score. These outcomes were all found to be significantly improved at 12 weeks, but the responder criteria were not specified. Seven possible predictors of reduced pain and improved functional ability were analyzed using regression modeling. The investigators concluded that lower levels of osteophytes in the patellofemoral joint, BMI, and functional self-efficacy were predictors of successful glucosamine treatment. The presence of osteophytes within the medial and lateral compartments of the tibiofemoral joint was not correlated with response to the intervention.[28] The study was underpowered for the identification of true predictors of response, and the participants did not require formal diagnosis of OA, so these results must be viewed accordingly.

Overall, there was weak evidence that radiographic measures of OA severity may have predictive value in the identification of potential responders to lateral-wedge insoles,[49] CSI,[62] and glucosamine sulfate. MRI assessment was predictive of response in a single study concerned with Hylan G-F 20 injections in the knee.[24] A greater number of studies exist that were unable to predict response to treatment based on radiographic disease severity or MRI. There is good evidence that KLG scores are not predictive of response to hip CSI.[22] Further research is required to clarify the roles performed by radiography and MRI regarding clinical characteristics that predict response to the nonsurgical treatment of hip and knee OA.

INFLAMMATION

Abnormal progressive remodeling of joint tissues occurs in response to local inflammatory processes arising within osteoarthritic joints.[65] Physical examination may reveal clinical signs such as presence of joint swelling, effusion, and heat. With recent improvements in imaging techniques, synovial hypertrophy has become a surrogate marker of local inflammation within a joint.

Signs of inflammation were examined as potential predictors of response to weight-loss interventions for participants with knee OA. The clinical cohort described by Gudbergsen and colleagues[46] participated in a 4-month dietary intervention. Responders were required to fulfill the OMERACT-OARSI Responder Criteria. Joint-damage severity was assessed on MRI using the BLOKS, which included scoring for synovitis and effusion. Although synovitis and effusion were not predictive of OMERACT-OARSI response, there was some evidence that the effusion score correlated with changes in the KOOS activities of daily living score from baseline to 4 months. Responder criteria for the KOOS score were not provided. There were 23 variables assessed as potential predictors of response; 123 patients were responders, therefore this study was insufficiently powered for this many predictors. The presence of inflammatory markers such as effusion and synovitis requires further investigation as predictors of symptomatic response to weight-loss interventions for overweight patients with OA.

Systemic pharmacologic agents such as NSAIDs and COX-2 inhibitors are prescribed for their analgesic properties and also to reduce inflammatory activity in affected joints. Two studies found that the presence of swelling was not predictive of response to these drug therapies. The data of 3 6-week RCTs comparing rofecoxib with placebo were combined to analyze the consistency of response of patients with hip or knee OA classified into subgroups determined by 14 demographic and disease factors.[21] Three outcome measures were analyzed in relation to the subgroups: pain walking on a flat surface (WOMAC), patient global assessment of response to therapy, and global assessment of disease status. The definition of treatment responder was not provided. Overall, the subgroups did not show consistent interactive effects with all 3 outcome measures. The absence of knee swelling in participants with knee OA significantly correlated with improved scores on the patient global assessment of response to therapy, but not the 2 remaining outcome measures.[21] Another study investigated swelling among numerous possible predictors of response of patients with OA and rheumatoid arthritis to ketoprofen and piroxicam.[34] The trial was very small with only 11 participants with OA, so was underpowered in determining significant predictors of response.[34] Further investigation into signs of inflammation as possible predictors of response to NSAIDs and COX-2 inhibitors would be helpful to the clinician attempting to tailor pharmacologic management according to clinical presentation.

IA corticosteroids aim to directly reduce inflammatory processes occurring within joint tissues. An RCT by Chao and colleagues[66] examined inflammatory characteristics assessed on ultrasonography as predictors of response to IA corticosteroid injection for knee OA. Participants were categorized as inflammatory if synovial hypertrophy (synovitis) with or without effusion was detected on gray-scale ultrasound examination of the affected knee(s) at baseline. Within the intervention group, 16 patients presented with synovitis on ultrasonography and 18 did not. At 4 weeks there were no significant differences between the inflammatory and noninflammatory subgroups. Significantly lower WOMAC pain scores of the noninflammatory subgroup at 12 weeks suggested that those without inflammatory characteristics experienced prolonged beneficial effects from corticosteroids. The presence of effusion had no influence on response to corticosteroid injection.[66]

The presence of hip-joint synovitis on ultrasound assessment of patients with hip OA was predictive of treatment response to CSI. An RCT compared standard care (no injection), injection of normal saline (placebo), nonanimal stabilized hyaluronic acid, and methylprednisolone acetate.[64] Of the participants receiving CSI, 14 participants were classified as responders according to the OMERACT-OARSI criteria. The investigators concluded that synovitis was predictive of response at 4 and 8 weeks following injection; however, this study was underpowered in establishing clear associations between the 5 variables analyzed as possible predictors. By contrast, Robinson and colleagues[22] found that evidence of hip synovitis and effusion on ultrasonography were not predictive of clinical response to IA methylprednisolone injection. The cohort study defined response to intervention as greater than 15% reduction in baseline WOMAC pain score at 6 and 12 weeks following injection. This study was also underpowered in identifying predictors of response. Further research using greater numbers of subjects is required to explore ultrasound-determined inflammatory characteristics as predictors of response to CSI of osteoarthritic hips.

Inflammatory characteristics identified on physical examination of patients with knee OA failed to predict response to CSI. The presence of local inflammation indicated by knee-joint fluid, local heat, synovial thickening, and stiffness were explored as possible predictors of response to IA methylprednisolone in an RCT of 59 participants with symptomatic knee OA.[33] No predictors of response were identified, perhaps as a result of this study being underpowered. Pendleton and colleagues[67] examined similar clinical signs of inflammation, namely presence of heat, effusion, and synovial thickening, in addition to the presence of effusion and synovitis on knee ultrasonography, as predictors of improvements in baseline WOMAC pain scale 1 and 6 weeks following CSI. The presence of heat was associated with a 29% greater reduction in night pain; otherwise, clinical and ultrasonographic inflammatory signs were not predictive of response. The study was underpowered and did not publish any measures of data variability. Adequately powered, well-designed research is necessary to determine whether clinical and ultrasonographic signs of inflammation are predictive of outcomes following CSI for knee OA.

Moderate effusion was associated with a good outcome following IA injection with Hylan G-F 20 in patients with symptomatic OA. Conrozier and colleagues[24] followed a cohort of 155 patients who received 3 IA Hylan G-F 20 injections and were evaluated 7 to 14 months later. Treatment outcomes included patient satisfaction, safety, and changes in pain and function, which were assessed on 4-point Likert scales. This study was limited by the lack of validated outcome measures and the retrospective study design.

Only one study investigated signs of inflammation as predictive of outcome to nonsurgical, nonpharmacologic intervention. There is weak evidence that that synovitis and effusion seen on MRI are unable to predict response to weight loss in patients with OA.[46] Numerous studies were concerned with signs of inflammation as predictors of outcomes to pharmacologic agents, but few were sufficiently powered. Some evidence exists that knee-joint swelling may predict good outcomes from rofecoxib[21] and that patients without synovitis observed on ultrasonography experience prolonged pain relief following CSI injection in comparison with patients with knee OA presenting with synovitis.[66] The evidence for synovitis on ultrasonography as a predictor of response for outcomes following hip CSI is conflicting.[22,64] There is little evidence to support the use of clinical inflammatory signs as predictors of response to CSI for knee OA.[33,67] Further research is required to determine whether signs of inflammation are useful predictors of response to conservative therapies for people with hip and knee OA.

OTHER CLINICAL CHARACTERISTICS THAT MAY PREDICT RESPONSE TO INTERVENTION

For the purposes of this review, the authors have selected patient characteristics deemed worthy of examination as potential predictors of response to interventions for those with hip and knee OA. There is a wider range of presenting features than those covered here, analyzed as potential predictors of response and further discussed in the literature. Among the articles identified through literature searches for the predictors chosen, age and gender were commonly analyzed as potential predictors of response to intervention, but appeared to hold little predictive capacity overall. Four well-powered studies investigating predictors of response to COX-2 inhibitors,[20,21] a rehabilitation program,[32] and exercise therapy[45] provided moderate to good evidence that age was not a powerful predictor of response to these interventions. Further investigation of age as a predictor of response to alternative interventions for patients with hip and knee OA is justified.

One adequately powered study determined female gender to be a characteristic predictive of treatment success following participation in a rehabilitation program.[32] By contrast, 3 well-powered studies found that gender was not predictive of treatment success for COX-2 inhibitors and exercise therapy.[20,21,45] Additional research into gender as a predictor of treatment response to different nonsurgical modalities is required.

WOMAC subscales of pain and function are often used as primary outcome measures in OA research. Of the studies extracted from literature searches performed

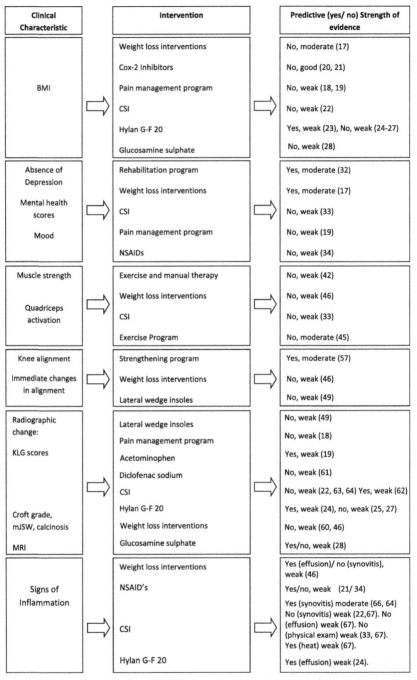

Clinical Characteristic	Intervention	Predictive (yes/ no) Strength of evidence
BMI	Weight loss interventions	No, moderate (17)
	Cox-2 Inhibitors	No, good (20, 21)
	Pain management program	No, weak (18, 19)
	CSI	No, weak (22)
	Hylan G-F 20	Yes, weak (23), No, weak (24-27)
	Glucosamine sulphate	No, weak (28)
Absence of Depression / Mental health scores / Mood	Rehabilitation program	Yes, moderate (32)
	Weight loss interventions	Yes, moderate (17)
	CSI	No, weak (33)
	Pain management program	No, weak (19)
	NSAIDs	No, weak (34)
Muscle strength / Quadriceps activation	Exercise and manual therapy	No, weak (42)
	Weight loss interventions	No, weak (46)
	CSI	No, weak (33)
	Exercise Program	No, moderate (45)
Knee alignment / Immediate changes in alignment	Strengthening program	Yes, moderate (57)
	Weight loss interventions	No, weak (46)
	Lateral wedge insoles	No, weak (49)
Radiographic change: / KLG scores / Croft grade, mJSW, calcinosis / MRI	Lateral wedge insoles	No, weak (49)
	Pain management program	No, weak (18)
	Acetominophen	Yes, weak (19)
	Diclofenac sodium	No, weak (61)
	CSI	No, weak (22, 63, 64) Yes, weak (62)
	Hylan G-F 20	Yes, weak (24), no, weak (25, 27)
	Weight loss interventions	No, weak (60, 46)
	Glucosamine sulphate	Yes/no, weak (28)
Signs of Inflammation	Weight loss interventions	Yes (effusion)/ no (synovitis), weak (46)
	NSAID's	Yes/no, weak (21/ 34)
	CSI	Yes (synovitis) moderate (66, 64) No (synovitis) weak (22,67). No (effusion) weak (67). No (physical exam) weak (33, 67). Yes (heat) weak (67).
	Hylan G-F 20	Yes (effusion) weak (24).

Fig. 1. Summary of evidence available for particular features of clinical presentation shown by people with hip and knee osteoarthritis. BMI, body mass index; CSI, intra-articular corticosteroid injection; KLG, Kellgren-Lawrence Grade; mJSW, minimum joint space width; MRI, magnetic resonance imaging; NSAIDs, nonsteroidal anti-inflammatory drugs.

around the chosen predictors, 2 well-designed studies examined WOMAC pain and function scores as predictors of response to COX-2 inhibitors. One found that that baseline WOMAC pain was not predictive of response to etoricoxib and celecoxib. Lower levels of function on the WOMAC decreased the odds of response to the drugs, but the difference in WOMAC function scores between responders and nonresponders was not clinically significant.[20] The second study concluded that baseline WOMAC function was not predictive of response to rofecoxib.[21] Although baseline WOMAC pain and function scores were not predictive of response to COX-2 inhibitors, these measures may prove to be interesting predictors of response to different nonsurgical interventions in other research.

SUMMARY

This review identified and summarized the evidence available for particular features of clinical presentation shown by individuals with hip and knee OA that were predictive of response to nonsurgical interventions. The studies are summarized in **Fig. 1**. Good evidence exists that BMI is not predictive of response to COX-2 inhibitors for hip and knee OA,[20] and there is moderate evidence that BMI does not predict weight reduction following weight-loss interventions for overweight people with knee OA.[17] There is some evidence to suggest that the absence of depressive symptoms predicts successful outcomes from both weight-loss interventions in overweight people with knee OA[17] and a 3- to 4-week rehabilitation program for participants with hip and knee OA.[32] Moderate evidence was cited that activation of quadriceps muscle was not predictive of improvements in quadriceps strength attained by participants with knee OA during a strengthening program.[45] Patients with medial knee OA who were neutrally aligned were more likely than their more varus-aligned counterparts to achieve significant pain relief following a quadriceps-strengthening program.[57] Evidence was lacking for any radiographic or MRI changes that were significant predictors of response to nonsurgical interventions; however, patients with knee OA presenting without inflammatory characteristics on ultrasonography (synovitis) were more likely to experience prolonged benefit from CSI than were inflammatory patients.[66]

The practice of analyzing patient characteristics as potential predictors of response to interventions is becoming increasingly popular. Researchers attempting to identify predictors of clinical response to nonsurgical treatments for hip and knee OA require the use of larger sample sizes, or restriction of the number of variables analyzed such that 10 to 15 responders are studied per possible predictor.[68] Identification of further characteristics capable of predicting response to intervention would indeed provide clinicians with additional tools to tailor the nonsurgical care of patients with hip and knee OA according to their clinical presentation.

REFERENCES

1. World Health Organization. Chronic diseases and health promotion: chronic rheumatic conditions. Available at: http://www.who.int/chp/topics/rheumatic/en/. Accessed September 17, 2012.
2. Murray C, Lopez A. The global burden of disease. A comprehensive assessment of mortality and disability from diseases, injuries, and risk factors in 1990 and projected to 2020. Cambridge (MA): Harvard School of Public Health on behalf of the World Health Organization and The World Bank; 1996.
3. Centers for Disease Control and Prevention (CDC). National and state medical expenditures and lost earnings attributable to arthritis and other rheumatic conditions—United States. MMWR Morb Mortal Wkly Rep 2007;56:4–7.

4. Zhang W, Moskowitz R, Nuki G, et al. OARSI recommendations for the management of hip and knee osteoarthritis, Part II: OARSI evidence-based, expert consensus guidelines. Osteoarthritis Cartilage 2008;16(12):137–62.

5. Zhang W, Doherty M, Arden NK, et al. EULAR evidence based recommendations for the management of hip osteoarthritis: report of a task force of the EULAR Standing Committee for International Clinical Studies Including Therapeutics (ESCISIT). Ann Rheum Dis 2005;64:669–81.

6. Pendleton A, Arden N, Dougados M, et al. EULAR recommendations for the management of knee osteoarthritis: report of a task force of the Standing Committee for International Clinical Studies Including Therapeutic Trials (ESCISIT). Ann Rheum Dis 2000;59:936–44.

7. Royal Australian College of General Practitioners. Guideline for the non-surgical management of hip and knee osteoarthritis. South Melbourne (Australia): Royal Australian College of General Practitioners; 2009.

8. Zhang W, Nuki G, Moskowitz RW, et al. OARSI recommendations for the management of hip and knee osteoarthritis: part III: changes in evidence following systematic cumulative update of research published through January 2009. Osteoarthritis Cartilage 2010;18(4):476–99.

9. NICE and Royal College of Physicians Guidelines on Osteoarthritis. Osteoarthritis—national clinical guideline for care and management in adults. United Kingdom 2008. Available at: http://guidance.nice.org.uk/CG59. Accessed September 18, 2012.

10. Hochberg MC, Altman RD, April KT, et al. American College of Rheumatology 2012 recommendations for the use of nonpharmacologic and pharmacologic therapies in osteoarthritis of the hand, hip, and knee. Arthritis Care Res (Hoboken) 2012;64(4):465–74.

11. Misso M, Pitt V, Jones K, et al. Quality and consistency of clinical practice guidelines for diagnosis and management of osteoarthritis of the hip and knee: a descriptive overview of published guidelines. Med J Aust 2008; 189(7):394–9.

12. Janssen I, Mark AE. Separate and combined influence of body mass index and waist circumference on arthritis and knee osteoarthritis. Int J Obes 2006;30(8): 1223–8.

13. Chapple CM, Nicholson H, Baxter GD, et al. Patient characteristics that predict progression of knee osteoarthritis: a systematic review of prognostic studies. Arthritis Care Res (Hoboken) 2011;63(8):1115–25.

14. Heliövaara M, Mäkelä M, Impivaara O, et al. Association of overweight, trauma and workload with coxarthrosis: a health survey of 7,217 persons. Acta Orthop Scand 1993;64(5):513–8.

15. Karlson E, Mandl L, Aweh G, et al. Total hip replacement due to osteoarthritis the importance of age, obesity, and other modifiable risk factors. Am J Med 2003; 114(2):93–8.

16. Brand C, Hunter DJ, Hinman RS, et al. Improving are for people with OA of the hip and knee: how has national policy for OA been translated into service models in Australia. Int J Rheum Dis 2011;14:181–90.

17. Wolf S, Foley S, Budiman-Mak E, et al. Predictors of weight loss in overweight veterans with knee osteoarthritis who participated in a clinical trial. J Rehabil Res Dev 2010;47(3):171–81.

18. Snijders GF, den Broeder AA, van Riel PL, et al. Evidence-based tailored conservative treatment of knee and hip osteoarthritis: between knowing and doing. Scand J Rheumatol 2011;40(3):225–31.

19. Snijders GF. Treatment outcomes of a Numeric Rating Scale (NRS)-guided pharmacological pain management strategy in symptomatic knee and hip osteoarthritis in daily clinical practice. Clin Exp Rheumatol 2012;30(2):164–70.
20. Bingham CO 3rd, Smugar SS, Wang H, et al. Predictors of response to cyclooxygenase-2 inhibitors in osteoarthritis: pooled results from two identical trials comparing etoricoxib, celecoxib, and placebo. Pain Med 2011;12(3):352–61.
21. Detora L, Krupta D, Bolognese J, et al. Rofecoxib shows consistent efficacy in OA clinical trials, regardless of specific patient demographic and disease factors. J Rheumatol 2001;28(11):2494–503.
22. Robinson P, Keenan AM, Conaghan PG. Clinical effectiveness and dose response of image-guided intra-articular corticosteroid injection for hip osteoarthritis. Rheumatology 2007;46(2):285–91.
23. Kemper F, Gebhardt U, Meng T, et al. Tolerability and short-term effectiveness of Hylan G-F 20 in 4253 patients with osteoarthritis of the knee in clinical practice. Curr Med Res Opin 2005;21(8):1261–9.
24. Conrozier T, Mathieu P, Schott A, et al. Factors predicting long-term efficacy of Hylan GF-20 viscosupplementation in knee osteoarthritis. Joint Bone Spine 2003;70:128–33.
25. Anandacoomarasamy A, Bagga H, Ding C, et al. Predictors of clinical response to intraarticular Hylan injections—a prospective study using synovial fluid measures, clinical outcomes and magnetic resonance imaging. J Rheumatol 2008;35(4):685–90.
26. Goorman S, Watanabe T, Miller E, et al. Functional outcome in knee osteoarthritis after treatment with Hylan G-F 20: a prospective study. Arch Phys Med Rehabil 2000;81:479–83.
27. Migliore A, Tormenta S, Massafra U, et al. Intra-articular administration of Hylan G-F 20 in patients with symptomatic hip osteoarthritis: tolerability and effectiveness in a large cohort study in clinical practice. Curr Med Res Opin 2008; 24(5):1309–16.
28. Bennett AN, Crossley KM, Brukner PD, et al. Predictors of symptomatic response to glucosamine in knee osteoarthritis: an exploratory study. Br J Sports Med 2007;41(7):415–9.
29. Roseman T, Backenstrass M, Rosemann A, et al. Predictors of depression in a sample of 1021 primary care patients with osteoarthritis. Arthritis Rheum 2007;57(3):415–22.
30. Wise BL, Niu J, Zhang Y, et al. Psychological factors and their relation to osteoarthritis pain. Osteoarthritis Cartilage 2010;18:883–7.
31. Lin EH, Katon W, Von Korff M, et al. Effect of improving depression care on pain and functional outcomes among older adults with arthritis: a randomized controlled trial. JAMA 2003;290(18):2428–9.
32. Weigl M, Angst F, Aeschlimann A, et al. Predictors for response to rehabilitation in patients with hip or knee osteoarthritis: a comparison of logistic regression models with three different definitions of responder. Osteoarthritis Cartilage 2006;14(7):641–51.
33. Jones A, Doherty M. Intra-articular corticosteroids are effective in osteoarthritis but there are no clinical predictors of response. Ann Rheum Dis 1996;55:829–32.
34. Walker J, Sheather-Reid R, Carmody J, et al. Nonsteroidal antiinflammatory drugs in rheumatoid arthritis and osteoarthritis. Arthritis Rheum 1997;40(11):1944–54.
35. Palmieri-Smith RM, Thomas AC, Karvonen-Gutierrez C, et al. Isometric quadriceps strength in women with mild, moderate, and severe knee osteoarthritis. Am J Phys Med Rehabil 2010;89(7):541–8.

36. Segal NA, Torner JC, Felson D, et al. Effect of thigh strength on incident radiographic and symptomatic knee osteoarthritis in a longitudinal cohort. Arthritis Rheum 2009;61(9):1210–7.

37. Amin S, Baker K, Niu J, et al. Quadriceps strength and the risk of cartilage loss and symptom progression in knee osteoarthritis. Arthritis Rheum 2009;60(1): 189–98.

38. Roos EM, Herzog W, Block JA, et al. Muscle weakness, afferent sensory dysfunction and exercise in knee osteoarthritis. Nat Rev Rheumatol 2012;7(1):57–63.

39. Suetta C, Aagaard P, Magnusson S, et al. Muscle size, neuromuscular activation, and rapid force characteristics in elderly men and women: effects of unilateral long-term disuse due to hip osteoarthritis. J Appl Physiol 2007;102:942–8.

40. Fransen M, McConnell S. Land-based exercise for osteoarthritis of the knee: a metaanalysis of randomized controlled trials. J Rheumatol 2009;36(6):1109–17.

41. Fransen M, McConnell S, Hernandez-Molina G, et al. Does land-based exercise reduce pain and disability associated with hip osteoarthritis? A meta-analysis of randomized controlled trials. Osteoarthritis Cartilage 2010;18(5):613–20.

42. Wright A, Cook C, Flynn T, et al. Predictors of response to physical therapy intervention in patients with primary hip osteoarthritis. Phys Ther 2011;91(4):510–24.

43. Sattler M, Dannhauer T, Hudelmaier M, et al. Side differences of thigh muscle cross-sectional areas and maximal isometric muscle force in bilateral knees with the same radiographic disease stage, but unilateral frequent pain—data from the osteoarthritis initiative. Osteoarthritis Cartilage 2012;20(6):532–40.

44. Pietrosimone BG, Hertel J, Ingersoll CD, et al. Voluntary quadriceps activation deficits in patients with tibiofemoral osteoarthritis: a meta-analysis. PM R 2011; 3(2):153–62 [quiz: 62].

45. Scopaz KA, Piva SR, Gil AB, et al. Effect of baseline quadriceps activation on changes in quadriceps strength after exercise therapy in subjects with knee osteoarthritis. Arthritis Rheum 2009;61(7):951–7.

46. Gudbergsen H, Boesen M, Lohmander LS, et al. Weight loss is effective for symptomatic relief in obese subjects with knee osteoarthritis independently of joint damage severity assessed by high-field MRI and radiography. Osteoarthritis Cartilage 2012;20(6):495–502.

47. Hunter DJ, Niu J, Felson DT, et al. Knee alignment does not predict incident osteoarthritis: the Framingham osteoarthritis study. Arthritis Rheum 2007;56(4): 1212–8.

48. Brouwer G, vanTol A, Bergink A, et al. Association between valgus and varus alignment and the development and progression of radiographic osteoarthritis of the knee. Arthritis Rheum 2007;56(4):1204–11.

49. Hinman RS, Payne C, Metcalf BR, et al. Lateral wedges in knee osteoarthritis: what are their immediate clinical and biomechanical effects and can these predict a three-month clinical outcome? Arthritis Rheum 2008;59(3):408–15.

50. Cooke T, Sled E, Scudamore R. Frontal plane knee alignment: a call for standardised measurement. J Rheumatol 2007;34:1796–801.

51. Andriacchi T. Dynamics of knee malalignment. Orthop Clin North Am 1994;25: 395–403.

52. Bennell KL, Hunt MA, Wrigley TV, et al. Hip strengthening reduces symptoms but not knee load in people with medial knee osteoarthritis and varus malalignment: a randomised controlled trial. Osteoarthritis Cartilage 2010;18(5):621–8.

53. Foroughi N, Smith RM, Lange AK, et al. Progressive resistance training and dynamic alignment in osteoarthritis: a single-blind randomised controlled trial. Clin Biomech (Bristol, Avon) 2011;26(1):71–7.

54. Sharma L, Dunlop D, Cahue S, et al. Quadriceps strength and osteoarthritis progression in malaligned and lax knees. Ann Intern Med 2003;138:613–9.

55. Sharma L, Song J, Felson D, et al. The role of knee alignment in disease progression and functional decline in knee osteoarthritis. JAMA 2001;286:792.

56. Lim BW, Hinman RS, Wrigley TV, et al. Varus malalignment and its association with impairments and functional limitations in medial knee osteoarthritis. Arthritis Rheum 2008;59(7):935–42.

57. Lim BW, Hinman RS, Wrigley TV, et al. Does knee malalignment mediate the effects of quadriceps strengthening on knee adduction moment, pain and function in medial knee osteoarthritis? A randomized controlled trial. Arthritis Rheum 2008;59(7):943–51.

58. Guermazi A, Burstein D, Conaghan P, et al. Imaging in osteoarthritis. Rheum Dis Clin North Am 2008;34(3):645–87.

59. Conaghan PG, Hunter DJ, Maillefert JF, et al. Summary and recommendations of the OARSI FDA osteoarthritis Assessment of Structural Change Working Group. Osteoarthritis Cartilage 2011;19(5):606–10.

60. Gudbergsen H, Boesen M, Christensen R, et al. Radiographs and low field MRI (0.2T) as predictors of efficacy in a weight loss trial in obese women with knee osteoarthritis. BMC Musculoskelet Disord 2011;12:56.

61. Case JP, Baliunas AJ, Block JA. Lack of efficacy of acetaminophen in treating symptomatic knee osteoarthritis: a randomized, double-blind, placebo-controlled comparison trial with diclofenac sodium. Arch Intern Med 2003;163(2):169–78.

62. Deshmukh AJ, Panagopoulos G, Alizadeh A, et al. Intra-articular hip injection: does pain relief correlate with radiographic severity of osteoarthritis? Skeletal Radiol 2011;40(11):1449–54.

63. Plant M, Borg A, Dziedzic K, et al. Radiographic patterns and response to corticosteroid hip injection. Ann Rheum Dis 1997;56:476–80.

64. Atchia I, Kane D, Reed M, et al. Efficacy of a single ultrasound-guided injection for the treatment of hip osteoarthritis. Ann Rheum Dis 2011;70:110–6.

65. Loeser RF, Goldring SR, Scanzello CR, et al. Osteoarthritis: a disease of the joint as an organ. Arthritis Rheum 2012;64(6):1697–707.

66. Chao J, Wu C, Sun B, et al. Inflammatory characteristics on ultrasound predict poorer longterm response to intraarticular corticosteroid injections in knee osteoarthritis. J Rheumatol 2010;37(3):650–5.

67. Pendleton A, Millar A, O'Kane D, et al. Can sonography be used to predict the response to intra-articular corticosteroid injection in primary osteoarthritis of the knee? Scand J Rheumatol 2008;37(5):395–7.

68. Babyak M. What you see may not be what you get: a brief, non-technical introduction to overfitting in regression-type models. Psychosom Med 2004;66:411–21.

Index

Note: Page numbers of article titles are in **boldface** type.

Rheum Dis Clin N Am 39 (2013) 235–243
http://dx.doi.org/10.1016/S0889-857X(12)00139-1
0889-857X/13/$ – see front matter © 2013 Elsevier Inc. All rights reserved.

rheumatic.theclinics.com

Moving?

Make sure your subscription moves with you!

To notify us of your new address, find your **Clinics Account Number** (located on your mailing label above your name), and contact customer service at:

Email: journalscustomerservice-usa@elsevier.com

800-654-2452 (subscribers in the U.S. & Canada)
314-447-8871 (subscribers outside of the U.S. & Canada)

Fax number: 314-447-8029

Elsevier Health Sciences Division
Subscription Customer Service
3251 Riverport Lane
Maryland Heights, MO 63043

*To ensure uninterrupted delivery of your subscription, please notify us at least 4 weeks in advance of move.

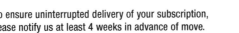

ELSEVIER

Printed and bound by CPI Group (UK) Ltd, Croydon, CR0 4YY

03/10/2024

01040442-0007